AF339298

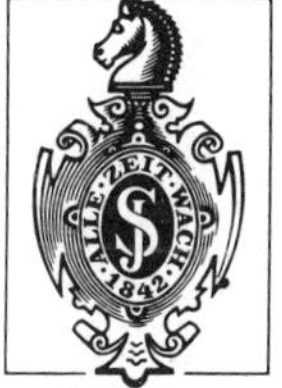
ALLE·ZEIT·WACH
1842

D. Bergqvist

Postoperative Thromboembolism

Frequency, Etiology, Prophylaxis

With 7 Figures and 48 Tables

Springer-Verlag
Berlin Heidelberg New York 1983

David Bergqvist
Associate Professor
University of Lund
Department of Surgery
Malmö General Hospital
S-21401 Malmö

ISBN 3-540-12062-9 Springer-Verlag Berlin Heidelberg New York
ISBN 0-387-12062-9 Springer-Verlag New York Heidelberg Berlin

Library of Congress Cataloging in Publication Data
Bergqvist, David, 1941 — Postoperative thromboembolism. Rev. and translation of: Postoperativ tromboembolism. 1981.
Bibliography: p. Includes index. 1. Surgery--Complications and sequelae. 2. Thromboembolism. I. Title.
RD98.4.B4713 1983   617'.01   82-19402
ISBN 0-387-12062-9

Printed in the United States of America

Composition: Schreibsatz-Service Weihrauch, Würzburg

Contents

VI

Foreword

Our knowledge of postoperative thromboembolic complications has increased enormously over the past 2 decades, particularly where diagnosis and prophylaxis are concerned. The ^{125}I-fibrinogen method of diagnosing thrombosis has completely changed our concept of the frequency, occurrence, and natural course of thrombosis, and it has formed the basis of most thromboprophylactic studies.

Concurrently with the development of this diagnostic method, two methods for the prophylaxis of thrombosis have come into vogue, namely low-dose heparin and dextran. Both these methods were tested in very extensive studies during the seventies, and their value has been unequivocally proved, for reducing both the frequency of thrombosis with and without symptoms, and the frequency of fatal pulmonary embolism.

Thromboprophylaxis is not particularly common in surgery; however, and its general use is far from uncontested. It has been argued that not only does it complicate surgical activities and make them more expensive, but it also involves an unacceptable number of other complications.

Our new knowledge of the thromboembolism problem has not made it easier for surgeons. The literature has become increasingly difficult to survey, and partly contradictory. The risk of thrombosis in connection with surgery is a real one, however, and now more notably so than before. There are two main reasons for this, one being the fact that the number of elective, extensive surgical operations in elderly patients, e.g., hip joint surgery, has increased markedly. This type of surgery is not performed because of a vital indication, but in order to improve the patient's quality of life. Thrombosis complicating this type of surgery is particularly difficult to accept, but the frequency of thrombosis in connection with hip joint surgery is in fact higher than in connection with most other surgical operations. This is mainly due to the high age of the patients and the extent of the operation. The other reason why the thromboembolism problem is more pronounced today is that other postoperative complications, fatal as well as nonfatal, have decreased during the past decades. Thromboembolism is thus on the way to becoming the predominant general postoperative complication.

Dr. David Bergqvist has been working both clinically and experimentally on the problems involved in thrombosis and hemostasis for many years. He is thus extremely well qualified to make a critical survey of this complex problem. His book is full of literature references and facts, making it a valuable reference work. Summaries of the various problems also make the book easy to read. I see this book as being primarily and aid to surgeons in forming their own opinion on the complex question of diagnosis and prophylaxis of postoperative complications in the form of thromboembolism.

Sven-Erik Bergentz
Professor of Surgery
University of Lund
Sweden

Preface

The purpose of this work is to present an up-to-date review of our knowledge of the problems in connection with postoperative thromboembolism, and particularly to analyze the prophylactic possibilities available today. I hope that this book will be useful to the various groups of personnel interested in these problems. This edition is a revision of the Swedish one published in 1981).

In some tables, on the frequency of thrombosis and embolism in different situations, I have given mean values. I am well aware of the fact that from a scientific point of view this is not a proper procedure, since the different studies may vary considerably. Still, I think that such a procedure is justified in a review of this kind, as it gives an immediate impression of the magnitude to be expected, especially in tables where the number of data is considerable.

Several people have contributed valuable information to this manuscript, and to them I am greatly indebted: Dr. L.-O. Andersson, Prof. S.-E. Bergentz, Dr. Agneta Bergqvist, Dr. Harriet Hedin, Dr. Ulla Hedner, Prof. Inga Marie Nilsson, Dr. W. Richter, Dr. E. Svensjö, and Prof. B. Zederfeldt. Errors which may remain are of course my sole responsibility. I am deeply grateful extensive editorial work for the carried out by Mrs. Gunilla Lundborg and also for the secretarial work of Mrs. Birgit Alm, which has been invaluable.

The English translation was skilfully performed by Mrs. Stina Lundberg, and Kathryn J. and Carlos Esquived, M.D., are gratefully acknowledged for the final revision of the English text.

Malmö, April, 1982   David Bergqvist

Introduction

In the acute phase of the disease a thrombus in the deep venous system can embolize to the lungs, with a possible fatal outcome, or, in rare cases, give rise to venous gangrene, which is also a life-threatening complication. Otherwise, the acute symptoms of thrombosis are of little clinical importance, and can sometimes be altogether absent. In the long run, however, it may induce post-thrombotic venous insufficiency with long-lasting suffering for the patient and large costs for the community. These complications mean that some kind of prophylaxis is justified for groups of patients at high risk of thrombosis, and intensive research is in progress in an attempt to find the ideal anti-thrombotic agent.

This review gives the background of the problems involved in thromboembolism in connection with surgery and trauma. It also analyzes the different thromboprophylactic alternatives available today.

Definitions

A thrombus can be defined as a semisolid mass which is formed by the components of the blood during circulation in or ex vivo, i.e., under dynamic conditions. A clot, on the other hand, is formed by the same components in noncirculating blood in vivo, in vitro, or post mortem, i.e., under static conditions.

The clot is morphologically homogeneous, whereas the thrombus consists of a platelet head and a fibrin tail. The relationship between the head and tail depends, for instance, on the blood flow when the thrombus is formed. The morphological difference between an arterial and a venous thrombus is well known, and the higher the flow rate the higher the proportion of platelets in the head.

Thrombosis is the disease resulting from thrombus formation.

History

Thrombosis has been known as a disease since about 2000 B.C., but the expression thrombosis was coined by Claudius Galenos (130–200 A.D.).

Pulmonary embolism was described for the first time by Wiseman (1676) and Malpighy (1886), the latter in *De Polypo Cordis Dissertatio*, but the relationship between thrombosis and embolism was not clarified until the 1840s by Rudolf Virchow. Egeberg in Oslo in 1845 considered such a relation as very probable when he found fatal pulmonary embolism and intrapelvic thrombi in a female dying postpartum. The modern concept of the pathogenesis and pathophysiology of thrombosis is based on Virchow's works, summarized in his famous triad (Fig. 1). Similar ideas had, however, been reported as early as 1794 by John Hunter in *A Treatise on the Blood, Inflammation and Gunshot Wounds* (Douglas 1978).

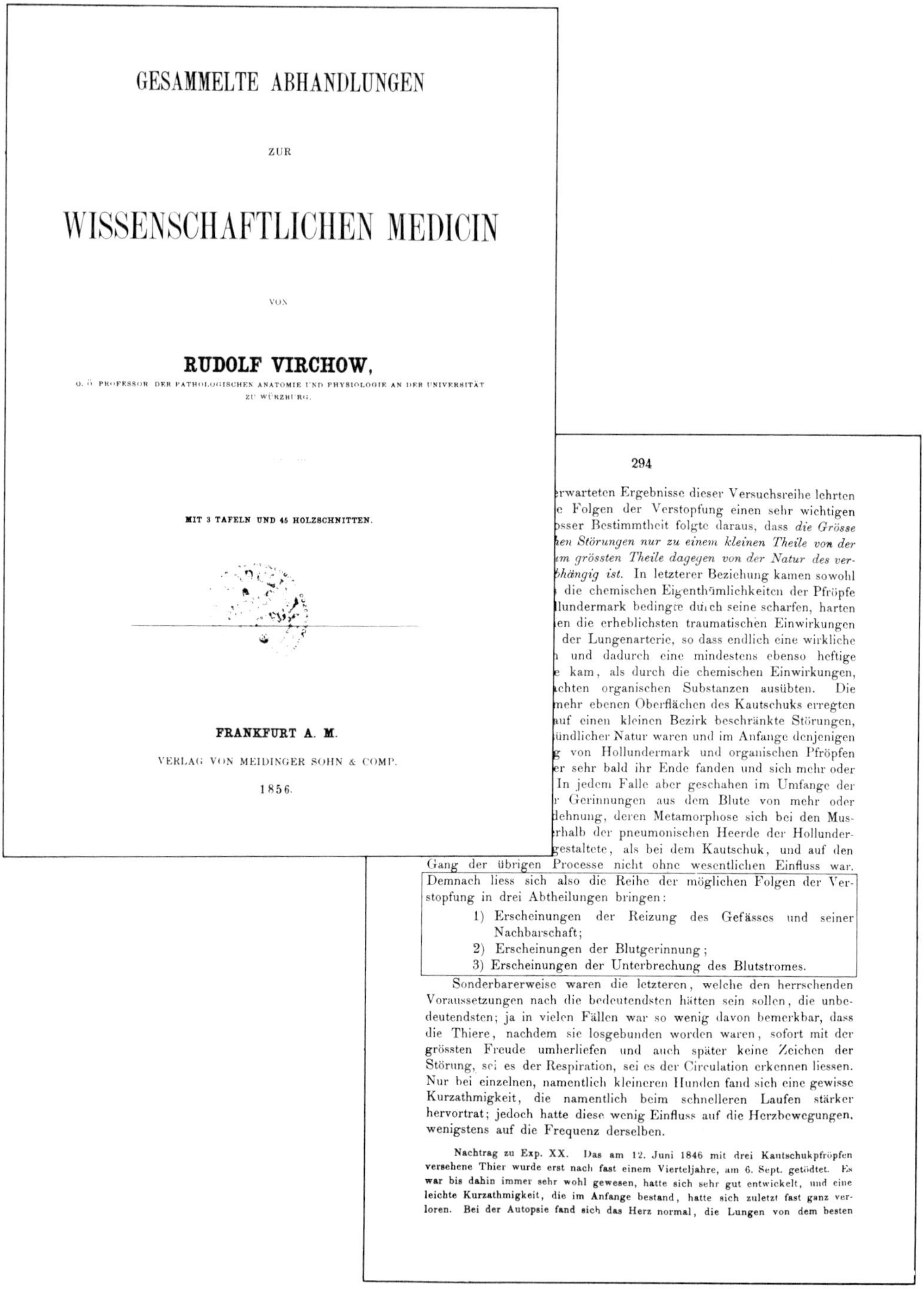

GESAMMELTE ABHANDLUNGEN

ZUR

WISSENSCHAFTLICHEN MEDICIN

VON

RUDOLF VIRCHOW,

O. Ö. PROFESSOR DER PATHOLOGISCHEN ANATOMIE UND PHYSIOLOGIE AN DER UNIVERSITÄT
ZU WÜRZBURG.

MIT 3 TAFELN UND 45 HOLZSCHNITTEN.

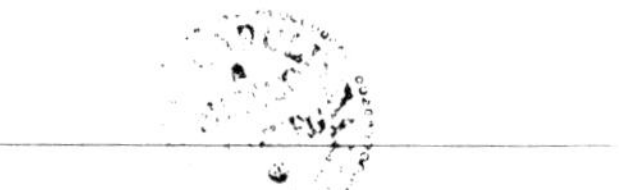

FRANKFURT A. M.

VERLAG VON MEIDINGER SOHN & COMP.

1856.

294

…rwarteten Ergebnisse dieser Versuchsreihe lehrten …e Folgen der Verstopfung einen sehr wichtigen …sser Bestimmtheit folgte daraus, dass *die Grösse …en Störungen nur zu einem kleinen Theile von der …m grössten Theile dagegen von der Natur des ver-…hängig ist.* In letzterer Beziehung kamen sowohl … die chemischen Eigenthümlichkeiten der Pfröpfe …lundermark bedingte durch seine scharfen, harten …en die erheblichsten traumatischen Einwirkungen … der Lungenarterie, so dass endlich eine wirkliche …n und dadurch eine mindestens ebenso heftige …e kam, als durch die chemischen Einwirkungen, …chten organischen Substanzen ausübten. Die …mehr ebenen Oberflächen des Kautschuks erregten …auf einen kleinen Bezirk beschränkte Störungen, …ündlicher Natur waren und im Anfange denjenigen …g von Hollundermark und organischen Pfröpfen …er sehr bald ihr Ende fanden und sich mehr oder … In jedem Falle aber geschahen im Umfange der …r Gerinnungen aus dem Blute von mehr oder …dehnung, deren Metamorphose sich bei den Mus-…rhalb der pneumonischen Heerde der Hollunder-…gestaltete, als bei dem Kautschuk, und auf den
Gang der übrigen Processe nicht ohne wesentlichen Einfluss war.

Demnach liess sich also die Reihe der möglichen Folgen der Verstopfung in drei Abtheilungen bringen:

> 1) Erscheinungen der Reizung des Gefässes und seiner Nachbarschaft;
> 2) Erscheinungen der Blutgerinnung;
> 3) Erscheinungen der Unterbrechung des Blutstromes.

Sonderbarerweise waren die letzteren, welche den herrschenden Voraussetzungen nach die bedeutendsten hätten sein sollen, die unbe-deutendsten; ja in vielen Fällen war so wenig davon bemerkbar, dass die Thiere, nachdem sie losgebunden worden waren, sofort mit der grössten Freude umherliefen und auch später keine Zeichen der Störung, sei es der Respiration, sei es der Circulation erkennen liessen. Nur bei einzelnen, namentlich kleineren Hunden fand sich eine gewisse Kurzathmigkeit, die namentlich beim schnelleren Laufen stärker hervortrat; jedoch hatte diese wenig Einfluss auf die Herzbewegungen. wenigstens auf die Frequenz derselben.

Nachtrag zu Exp. XX. Das am 12. Juni 1846 mit drei Kautschukpfröpfen versehene Thier wurde erst nach fast einem Vierteljahre, am 6. Sept. getödtet. Es war bis dahin immer sehr wohl gewesen, hatte sich sehr gut entwickelt, und eine leichte Kurzathmigkeit, die im Anfange bestand, hatte sich zuletzt fast ganz ver-loren. Bei der Autopsie fand sich das Herz normal, die Lungen von dem besten

Fig. 1. "Virchow's triad", from the original work of 1856

Although much has happened in thrombosis research during the past 100 years, the investigation of its pathophysiology is still focused on changes in the vessel walls, on the properties of the blood, and on blood flow conditions.

During the latter part of the nineteenth century, the hemostatic phenomenon in microcirculation was described (Zahn 1872), and the first studies were carried out to establish a relationship between hemostasis and thrombosis, i.e., the role of the platelets (Bizzozero 1882). This relationship is still of interest today when postoperative thromboprophylaxis is discussed, since there are few methods which alter the development of thrombosis without concurrently affecting the hemostatic mechanism to some extent.

Thrombosis as a postoperative complication was reported for the first time in 1894 by von Strauch. Pulmonary embolism as an important postoperative cause of death began to attract attention around the turn of the century. As early as 1864 Azam reported a case of fatal pulmonary embolism following a fracture of the tibia, where the subsequent autopsy showed extensive thrombosis in the fractured leg, a finding that was a complete surprise to the clinicians. A survey among different surgeons in the United States made it clear that patients who underwent operations in the lower part of the abdomen and/or gynecologic surgery were at high risk for the development of postoperative thrombosis (Cordier 1905). The same study also noted that abdominal hysterectomy was more dangerous in this respect than vaginal hysterectomy, a well-known fact today. Lister made an analysis of *status presens* in 1927, pointing out that increasing age is an important risk factor for the development of post-traumatic pulmonary embolism. At about the same time Gustaf Petrén in Lund, Sweden, made an analysis of causes of postoperative mortality and concluded: "The often unexpected and unforseeable occurrence of deaths from pulmonary embolism, their increased number and our, in the main, helplessness in the face of them, both prophylactically and therapeutically, make pulmonary embolism the greatest crux of present-day practical surgery."

Studies then appeared showing that operations on different organ systems gave rise to different frequencies of postoperative thromboembolic complications (Schönbauer 1928). Also, after relatively simple procedures such as operations for inguinal hernias fatal pulmonary embolism was a real danger (Bergquist 1938).

A great deal of interest in thrombosis and particularly prevention of venous thrombosis has existed in Sweden for a long time. Lennander (1899) stressed the importance of generous administration of fluids in order to maintain an adequate circulation. On

Table 1. Rate of thrombosis in different vascular sections in 24 autopsies
In total 42 extremities exhibited thrombosis (Frykholm 1939)

Site	Number of legs
Calf muscle veins	39
Calf muscle veins and main crural veins	25
Main crural veins (isolated thrombosis)	2
Veins of the abductor canal	16
Veins of the pelvis	5

the basis of autopsy studies, Frykholm (1939) was able to show that thrombosis in the veins of the calf muscles is a common phenomenon (Table 1), and that the thrombotic process progresses in a centripetal direction. This, to some degree, verified the findings published a few years previously by Rössle in Germany (1937).

On the basis of his observations, Frykholm suggested that the rational method for thromboprophylaxis ought to be mechanical:

— "If a rational mechanical prophylaxis is to be carried through, *the head of the bed should be raised*, and it should be raised high enough for the patient to slide downwards and make him actively push his feet against the footboard in order to stay up. He should be kept in a position in which a spontaneous thrombosis hardly ever occurs, namely the vertical position."

This kind of prophylaxis almost equals early mobilization, the importance of which has been known since about 1940 (Ochsner and DeBakey 1940, Backer-Gröndahl 1944, Johansson and Holmdahl 1945, Dahl-Iversen 1945, Westerborn 1946, Lindvall 1946, Borgström 1950, Gibbs 1957). In fact, it had already been pointed out at the turn of the century that early mobilization had a thromboprophylactic effect (Ries 1899, Richardson 1904, Kümmel 1908, Björkenheim 1909).

New sensitive diagnostic methods have, nonetheless, proven that early mobilization is not sufficient protection and that postoperative thromboembolic complications are still a problem. Therefore trials with different drugs have become the focus of interest.

Heparin is a naturally occurring product in the body. It was first isolated from liver or hepar (McLean 1916); hence its name (Howell and Holt 1918). The chemical structure was established by Jorpes (1935, 1946), and further clinical development was carried out by two other well-known Swedes: Clarence Crafoord and Gunnar Bauer.

Crafoord (1936) used prophylactic heparin in high doses postoperatively, whereas De Takats (1950) suggested that low doses of heparin could be used in order to prevent venous thromboembolism. These thoughts were later developed further by Sharnoff and co-workers, who in an uncontrolled study (Sharnoff et al. 1960, Sharnoff 1966) were able to demonstrate a decrease in the frequency of fatal pulmonary embolism.

Swedish scientists were also involved with the development of oral anticoagulants, i.e., dicumarol and antiprothrombin (AP). Thus, Lehmann produced and clinically tried the active substance contained in spoiled sweet clover, which had long been known to induce bleeding in animals (Lehmann 1942b, 1976). The clinical development was conducted simultaneously in the United States and Sweden, but the exchange of necessary scientific information was prevented by the Second World War.

By coincidence, in November 1942 the Mayo group presented its experience with the treatment of 17 cases, while in the same month, at the Swedish Medical Society's national conference, Lehmann discussed his results from treating 17 cases. Bruzelius (1945) published his large thrombosis material from Lund, Sweden, where AP had been used. He reported the results of prophylactic AP treatment on 1448 patients who had undergone surgery. The frequency of fatal postoperative pulmonary embolism was 0.16% for AP prophylaxis compared with 0.49% in a historical reference. The effect was verified by Borgström (1950), who investigated untreated and AP-treated patients assigned to either group by their referral number. It was later shown by Storm (1958) that the prophylactic effect could be further improved if the patients were given anti-coagulant therapy preoperatively.

Dextran is a Swedish product developed by Grönwall and Ingelman (1944). Dextran was introduced in 1947 as a plasma volume expander, and was later shown to improve the peripheral flow as well as to have an antithrombotic effect. The antithrombotic effect was demonstrated experimentally by Borgström et al. (1959), and for the first time in patients with a clinical diagnosis of thrombosis by Koekenberg (1961). The development of low molecular weight dextran with favorable rheologic properties has primarily been achieved by Gelin and his group in Gothenburg (Gelin 1962).

In 1954 DeBakey carried out a rather pessimistic review on prophylaxis and held the view that much of the confusion on the subject of thromboembolism derived from the difficulty of establishing the diagnosis and that consequently there was no firm basis for evaluating prophylactic methods.

With the knowledge that clinical diagnosis of thrombosis is very difficult (see e.g., Phillips 1963, Haeger 1965, Flanc et al. 1968) and with the discovery of various objective diagnostic methods, thromboprophylaxis has entered a new phase of very rapid development. It is primarily after the establishment of the ^{125}I-fibrinogen test as a suitable objective screening method that more extensive studies on the frequency and prevention of thrombosis have been possible. This diagnostic method has also yielded important knowledge of the natural history of postoperative thrombosis, e.g., the early postoperative or even intraoperative onset, the high frequency, and the marked involvement of the veins in the calf. In spite of numerous studies showing the difficulty and unreliability of clinical diagnosis, a surprising number of clinicians still rely on this method (Negus 1978, Bergqvist 1980b, Kettunen 1981).

During the 1940s the thromboprophylactic effect of AP was quite extensively studied in Lund (Sweden). Clinical diagnosis was still performed but the use of controlled studies at different times was abandoned in favor of controlled studies performed at the same time, where the patient number decided the group assignment of the patients (Strömbeck 1948, Borgström 1950).

Modern prophylaxis research was introduced in 1959, when Sevitt and Gallagher published a study on the effect of oral anticoagulants on thromboembolic complications following surgery for hip fracture. The study was designed as a randomized prospective investigation using objective diagnosis, namely emboli verified by autopsy. Such a design is an absolute must when it comes to continued studies of the prophylaxis against postoperative thromboembolism. In this book priority is given to controlled studies using objective methods for establishing the diagnosis of thromboembolism.

Frequency of Thromboembolic Complications

Thrombosis may occur in any part of the venous system, and in a number of different situations. This review will primarily be limited to postoperative and post-traumatic deep venous thrombosis of the lower extremities.

Postoperative thrombosis forms an important part of thrombosis as a whole. In a survey of consecutive thrombus-positive phlebographies, Nylander et al. (1977) found that 24% of the thrombi were postoperative and 8% post-traumatic, i.e., about one-third of the entire material. This agrees surprisingly well with the figues compiled by Gjöres (1956) from interviews with patients who at some time had developed thrombosis. This is in contrast to arm vein thrombosis where operation is rarely the only cause (Sundqvist et al. 1981).

When assessing the need for thromboprophylaxis, not only venous thrombosis but also pulmonary embolism should be considered. As an introduction, a short review of the different methods available for diagnosing these conditions is presented.

Diagnosis of Deep Vein Thrombosis

The frequency of detected post-traumatic and postoperative thrombosis varies according to the diagnostic method, time of diagnosis, patient population, and type of surgery.

The clinical diagnosis of deep venous thrombosis has proved to be very unreliable. In addition, there seems to be no correlation between the acute complication of pulmonary embolism and the presence of local symptoms of thrombosis. For clinicians, the so-called silent fatal pulmonary embolism is a fact.

Table 2. Pathophysiologic properties of venous thrombosis used for diagnosis

Property	Diagnostic method
Filling of the vascular lumen	
Morphology	Phlebography, nuclear venography
Reduced venous reservoir	Plethysmography
Reduced venous emptying	Plethysmography, ultrasound
Fibrin formation from fibrinogen	^{125}I-fibrinogen test
Thrombolysis	^{99}Tc^{m}-plasmin test
Increased temperature	
Inflammation	Thermography
Increased resting blood flow in the skin	Thermography, plethysmography
Collateral venous flow	Phlebography, thermography

The unreliability of clinical diagnosis has naturally resulted in the search for more objective methods to establish or rule out thrombosis. There are a number of objective diagnostic methods today. These methods are based on different pathophysiologic properties of thrombus formation; therefore, their sensitivities may vary in different conditions and in different regions of the extremity involved (Table 2). Basic knowledge of these conditions is necessary for the accurate interpretation of the results. A schematic summary of the diagnostic principles is presented in Figure 2.

The methods most often used for the documentation of postoperative thrombosis are phlebography and the ^{125}I-fibrinogen test. When postoperative thrombosis is of concern, the diagnostic method employed must be capable of following large numbers of patients during the period of highest risk, i.e., from the time of surgery until 1–2 weeks postoperatively. This fact explains why the comparatively simple ^{125}I-fibrinogen test has come into vogue so rapidly.

Phlebography is the oldest diagnostic procedure. It is well established and may still be considered a good reference method. The great advantage of phlebography is that it gives an anatomic and morphologic diagnosis, thereby giving an idea of the prognosis, since the risk of pulmonary embolism is greater the more proximal the thrombus. Also, the risk of post-thrombotic venous insufficiency appears to be greater if the valve mechanism of the popliteal vein is involved.

Otherwise, very little is known about the possibility of predicting the development of complications by studying the radiologic findings. The method is, however trying for the investigator as well as the patient, and it is laborious for extensive screening investigations. For optimal information, bilateral preoperative and post-

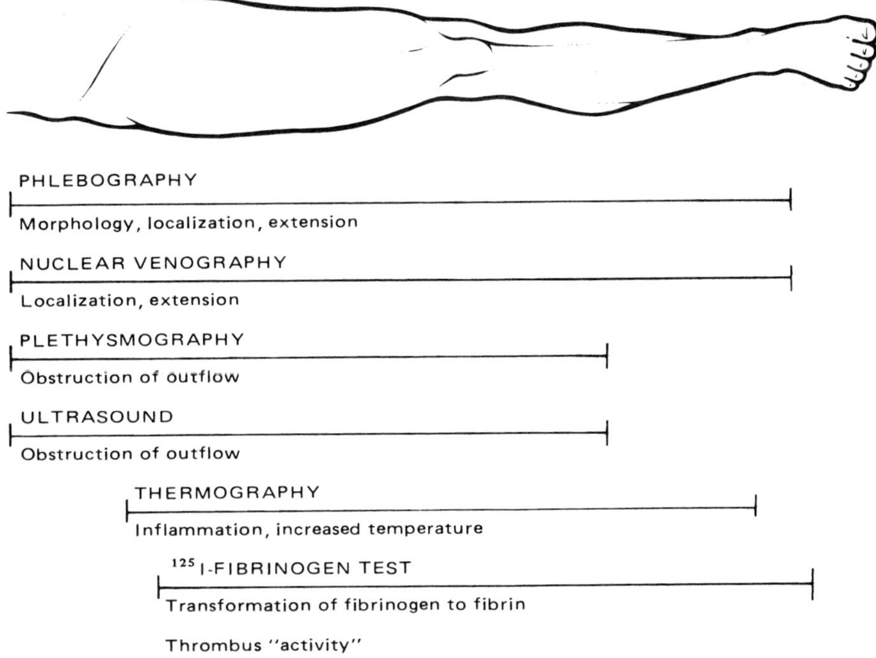

Fig. 2. Principles of some thrombodiagnostic methods and their anatomic limitations

operative phlebography should be performed on at least one occasion. Furthermore, altough obvious, it should be pointed out that phlebography is not an absolute method. A difference in interpretation between up to 10% of radiologists may occur (McLachlan et al. 1979). Certain venous segments are difficult to visualize, and even if they are not completely filled with contrast medium it does not necessarily indicate the presence of a thrombus. The greatest difficulties are encountered when visualization of the deep femoral vein is required (Culver et al. 1970, Schmitt 1977). There are also quite a few artifacts, making the interpretation difficult and giving rise to diagnostic problems (Lea Thomas and Carty 1975).

Some investigators have also claimed that phlebography has been the cause of thrombosis in serveral cases (Cranley 1975, Albrechtsson and Olsson 1976). A frequency as high as 50% has been reported. However, this is probably due to differences in technique, since other investigators have not been able to find the same high rate of complications (WJ William 1973, Berge et el. 1978, 1981, Kristiansen et al. 1981). Obviously, the patient population may influence the results.

The ^{125}I-fibrinogen test is a very sensitive method which can detect thrombi as small as 1 cm in size (Becker 1972b). The introduction of the ^{125}I-fibrinogen test has provided important information about the natural history of postoperative thrombosis, for instance, that the frequency is much higher than previously known, that the great majority are localized in the calf, that the onset of most thrombi occurs in very close connection with the surgical operation, and that postoperative thrombi, although giving no symptoms, can still give rise to pulmonary embolism.

The method has been of great epidemiologic value and has been useful in the analysis of risk factors in the etiology of postoperative thrombosis. A good correlation with phlebography has been demonstrated (Flanc et al. 1968, Negus et al. 1968, Kakkar et al. 1969b, Browse 1972, Jung et al. 1975, Hirsh and Gallus 1975, Kakkar 1977). One of the drawbacks of the fibrinogen test is the fact that pelvic thrombi cannot be detected because of the high background activity (the high flow in the pelvic blood vessels and the excretion of free ^{125}I in the urine). Another important limitation is that the fibrinogen test becomes positive with fibrin formation, a hematoma for example. Consequently, the ^{125}I-fibrinogen test should not be used in patients with recent surgery of the lower extremities. The use of the test in surgery of the hip is discussed in more detail on p. 20.

Other conditions associated with a positive test are: superficial thrombophlebitis, healing wound, fractures, ulcerations, cellulitis, arthritis, and extensive edema (Warlow and Ogston 1973, Jung et al. 1975, Poulose et al. 1976, Kakkar 1977). A possible way of differentiating between deep vein thrombosis and superficial thrombophlebitis is with a modification of the fibrinogen test — the ^{125}I-fibrinogen-sum-coincidence method (Jacobsson et al. 1980). By using a specific characteristic of ^{125}I-decay, the depth of thrombi can be determined with good agreement with phlebography.

Hepatitis virus cannot be isolated from fibrinogen during its preparation (Cronberg et al. 1963). There is thus a theoretic risk of transmission of hepatitis when using ^{125}I-fibrinogen. The donors of this fibrinogen are selected very carefully, and only two cases of hepatitis have been reported out of several thousands of injections given (Laiwah et al. 1970). In a study on the frequency of hepatitis in patients given ^{125}I-fibrinogen, a comparison was made with a group of matched controls. No difference between the two groups could be established (Hicks and Hazell 1973).

One of the most discussed subjects with regard to the fibrinogen test has been the clinical relevance of the thrombi detected (a positive test) (Levy et al. 1975, Douss 1976, Blaisdell 1979). The principal application of this method is, however, not to diagnose postoperative thrombosis for treatment purposes, but to use it as a scientific instrument in prospective studies, where the prevalence of thrombosis in a certain population is to be established.

It is impossible, judging from the result of a test, to foresee whether or not a particular patient will develop thromboembolic complications. On the other hand, it is known that the risk of pulmonary embolism is greater with a positive test (Warlow and Ogston 1973, Browse et al. 1974a, Ruckley 1975, 1976), and that the risk is even greater with a positive test above the knee than a positive test below the knee (Kakkar et al. 1969b).

To predict which patients will develop a post-thrombotic syndrome is even more difficult; but from the small amount of data available it appears that the risk is greater after a positive test than after a negative one (see also p. 30). If a thrombus is localized in the popliteal vein, there is a great risk of valve destruction followed by venous insufficiency (Shull et al. 1979). A positive test at knee level should therefore be heeded.

An important question is how to treat thrombi detected by the fibrinogen test. One possible way to analyze this problem would be by a controlled study to determine whether a particular treatment will reduce the frequency of fatal pulmonary embolism or not. This would require a very large patient population and is almost impractical. Knowing that most thrombi diagnosed by the fibrinogen test are small and localized in the calf, many surgeons are reluctant to treat them just after an operation, because of an increased risk of complications with the antithrombotic therapy. As a practical measure, treatment is recommended when the trombus is growing proximally and extending above the knee, preferably after verification by phlebography.

When the ^{125}I-fibrinogen test is used as a screening tool it is important to specify the diagnostic criteria applied, the time interval between surgery and injection of fibrinogen, and the length of time of the measurements made. Standardization is necessary in order to produce comparable studies (Roberts 1975, Bergqvist 1977). Other factors influencing the result of the ^{125}I-fibrinogen test are: normal postoperative increase in the fibrinogen content and extravascular accumulation of ^{125}I-fibrinogen. In addition a decrease in radioactivity by natural degradation leads to reduced sensitivity with increasing time after the trauma. This is at least of theoretic interest (Shah et al. 1980).

Other diagnostic methods which by their simplicity might be suitable for screening such as plethysmography, ultrasound, and thermography are relatively insensitive in detecting small thrombi of the legs; unfortunately, most of the postoperative thrombi fall into such a category (Milne et al. 1971, Bergqvist et al. 1973, Bergqvist 1977, Bergqvist and Hallböök 1978b, Bernstein et al. 1979).

Diagnosis of Pulmonary Embolism

The frequency of detected pulmonary embolism depends on the diagnostic method used and when the investigation is carried out. While there are reliable and sensitive methods for diagnosing venous thrombosis, our methods of diagnosing pulmonary embolism are considerably fewer, and there is no suitable and simple reference method. As in venous thrombosis, clinical diagnosis is very uncertain. The classic triad of symptoms of dyspnea, pleuritis, and hemoptysis is unusual, being present in less than one-fourth of patients having pulmonary embolism (Stein et al. 1981).

Pulmonary angiography is the most reliable method in vivo; however, it is not suitable as a postoperative screening procedure.

Diagnosis at autopsy requires that the pathologist be alert to the problem. In one study the frequencey of detection of pulmonary embolism increased from 12% on routine autopsy to 51% when the pathologists were actively seeking the diagnosis (Morrell and Dunnill 1968). Thus, frequency figures may be unreliable if small emboli are not considered. Pathologists may have differing viewpoints on the primary cause of death. Therefore the concept of fatal pulmonary embolism may also be ambiguous. It is advisable that thromboprophylactic studies include both the autopsy findings as often as possible and total mortality, since the latter may remain unchanged even with a decreased incidence of thromboembolic complications. Needless to say these thromboembolic complications ought to be investigated in detail. The follow-up time should extend over at least 1 month postoperatively since emboli may develop quite late (Andreasen and Krieger Lassen 1965). In trauma cases, the follow-up time should be even longer (Sevitt 1962).

The diagnosis is more difficult when scintigraphic methods are used. These are, however, the methods that by their relative simplicity are suitable for screening.

Perfusion scintigraphy has a high sensitivity, and a negative examination almost excludes pulmonary embolism. The specificity is low, nonetheless, and particulary chronic obstructive pulmonary disease gives rise to diagnostic difficulties (P. Johnson 1971, Quinn 1971, Lippmann and Fein 1981). Normal ventilation in an area with a perfusion defect suggests embolism as the cause. In this situation the ventilation scintigram has been valuable (McNeil et al. 1974, O. Williams et al. 1974, McNeil 1976, Knight and Metrewelli 1977, Neumann et al. 1980, Cheely et al. 1981), even though the combination of perfusion and ventilation scintigraphy has been seriously questioned by other authors (Robin 1977).

A less accurate diagnostic procedure is the combination of perfusion scintigraphy and roentgenogram of the chest, preferably both pre- and postoperatively. A segmental perfusion defect, when a chest X-ray gives no other explanation, is in all probability caused by pulmonary embolism (Talbot and Griffiths 1974). Nevertheless, some apparently healthy patients have preoperative segmental perfusion defects, and a preoperative examination is therefore valuable (Bergqvist et al. 1980a).

The interpretation of the scintigram may be difficult since the assessment frequently varies with the investigator. Furthermore, the same investigator may give different interpretations of the same scintigram on different occasions, and may also be influenced by the clinical picture (Herlev Hospital Study Group 1979). Therefore the physician interpreting the scintigrams of prophylactic studies should be unaware of the clinical history and the prophylactic method.

The use of ^{111}In-labeled platelets is a new diagnostic possibility with promising preliminary data (Moser et al. 1980).

Other examinations, such as chest X-ray, ECG, and various biochemical tests including arterial pO_2 and fibrinogen degradation products, are too unspecific and hence of little value for establishing the incidence of pulmonary embolism in prospective studies.

Incidence of Thrombosis

Preoperative Thrombosis

In most studies of postoperative venous thrombosis, the patients were, of course, evaluated during the postoperative period but with little or no assessment of their pre-operative status. A few studies with adequate preoperative examinations have already demonstrated the presence of venous changes, and in some patients even thrombosis. As early as 1941, Pettersson reported some cases of intraoperative pulmonary embolism, which means that the thrombus must have started to form preoperatively.

Becker et al. (1970) found thrombotic changes on preoperative phlebograms in five out of 56 patients who underwent transvesical prostatectomy; in four, the pictures remained unchanged postoperatively. These patients might have been considered as having postoperative thrombosis had only a postoperative examination been performed. A ^{125}I-fibrinogen test would have probably given negative results.

In a study of patients who underwent elective hip surgery with bilateral pre- and postoperative phlebograms, 13 of 40 legs showed venous abnormalities, three of which had deep venous thrombosis (Table 3; Bergqvist et al. 1976a). These three cases were negative on fibrinogen testing prior to the operation, but became positive postoperatively, developing the disease simultaneously according to phlebography.

Using the fibrinogen test, Heatley et al. (1976) examined 50 patients hospitalized more than 4 days before gastrointestinal surgery. Of these patients, 11 developed signs of preoperative thrombosis, and in ten the diagnosis was confirmed by phlebography. Eight of these had malignant disease. There is a high risk of developing thrombosis in patients with gynecologic malignancy, even without surgery. Von Hugo et al. (1981) found a frequency of 43% in women treated with radiotherapy. Nine of 107 surgical patients (8.4%) with varied diagnoses were found to have preoperative thrombosis using the fibrinogen test (Laaksonen et al. 1973).

With the same diagnostic method, thrombosis was detected in 14% of 300 medical patients with different illnesses (Prescott et al. 1978). This figure agrees relatively well with that reported by Gallus et al. (1973b). A similar frequency was seen in patients who were treated for chronic obstructive pulmonary disease (Prescott et al. 1981) or acute respiratory failure (Moser et al. 1981).

Stevens et al. (1968) performed phlebograms on patients with hip fractures. Forty-seven patients were confined to their beds for more than a week preoperatively and 15% of these exhibited preoperative thrombosis. Of 24 patients undergoing surgery

Table 3. Results from 40 preoperative phlebograms in patients with arthrosis of the hip

Diagnosis	Number of legs
Varicose veins	9
Deep venous thrombosis	3[a]
Venous ectasias	1

[a]Preoperatively negative ^{125}I-fibrinogen test. All patients with thrombosis showed progression of the disease by phlebography, and the ^{125}I-fibrinogen test became positive.

on the 3rd day, two (8%) had thrombosis. In a small study (11 patients) using [111] In-labeled platelets for diagnosis there were four patients who developed thrombosis after the hip fracture but before the operation (Fenech et al. 1981).

In studies employing the [125] I-fibrinogen examination and where measurements were not begun until the postsurgical period the incidence of "postoperative" thrombosis is falsely high, as it also includes thrombosis developed preoperatively.

Incidence Following General Surgery

With the introduction of the [125] I-fibrinogen test the high incidence of postoperative thrombosis became evident. Good studies using phlebography as a screening method in general surgery are scarce, but a few studies were carried out in the beginning of the fibrinogen test era in order to check the sensitivity of this method. A good correlation between the two methods was demonstrated (Warlow and Ogston 1973). A 30% incidence of thrombosis about 1 week postoperativley was demonstrated by phlebography (Smyrnis and Kolios 1973). Among 83 patients who had undergone abdominal surgery, the Groote Schuur Hospital Thromboembolus Study Group (1979) found 18 cases of deep venous thrombosis of the calf by phlebography, and four with isolated iliofemoral thrombosis. The rate of thrombosis naturally varies between different groups of patients and will be dealt with in more detail in the discussion of patients at risk (p. 51). In surgery of the upper abdomen for benign disorders, the incidence is very low (Hartsuck and Greenfield 1973, Bergman et al. 1975, Johansson et al. 1975).

In a small study Kakkar et al. (1971) reported a 26% incidence of thrombosis in elective surgery for inguinal hernias. This figure is surprisingly high. Otherwise, the frequency varies considerably between 13% and 59% (Table 4).

Splenectomy has been considered to be an operation which entails a high risk of thrombosis secondary to a long-standing postoperative increase in the number of platelets (Rosenthal 1925, Chesner 1946, Mills and Lucia 1949, Gelpi and Ende 1958). The risk is enhanced in persistent anemia postsplenectomy (Hirsh and Dacie 1966). In small series where objective diagnosis has been employed (Douss 1976, Butler et al. 1977, Starksen et al. 1978), the incidence of thrombosis following splenectomy was the same as that of other types of surgery in the upper abdomen. Splenectomy because of Hodgkin's disease shows no excess of deep vein thrombosis whereas splenectomy because of non-Hodgkin lymphoma shows high incidence (Dawson et al. 1981).

The incidence of thrombosis following abdominoperineal resection of the rectum — a relative large operation including dissection of the pelvis — is about 30% (Hartsuck and Greenfield 1973, Åberg et al. 1974).

Malignancy seems to increase the risk of proximal thrombosis postoperatively (Bergqvist and Hallböök 1980).

The incidence of thrombosis in acute general surgery is largely unknown. Using the [125] I-fibrinogen examination, Sagar et al. (1975) found no evidence of deep venous thrombosis in a small series of fertile women undergoing appendectomies for acute appendicitis.

It is both desirable and necessary that the patients suffering from acute surgical disorders be carefully studied to determine the incidence of thromboembolic complications as well as their need for prophylaxis. There are many reasons for assuming

Table 4. The frequency of thrombosis in different general surgery materials
Diagnosis of thrombosis by the ^{125}I-fibrinogen test

Author	Number of patients	Number of thrombosis	Incidence of thrombosis (%)	Comments
Bergqvist and Hallböök (1980)	14	51	27	Abdominal surgery, past 50 yrs
Butler et al. (1977)	6	34	18	Splenectomy
Carter and Eban (1974)	17	97	18	Past 45 yrs
Clagett et al. (1975)	10	49	20	
Douss (1976)	91	326	28	Past 40 yrs
Encke et al. (1976)	13	34	38	Abdominal surgery
Fey et al. (1975)	43	73	59	One-third past 55 yrs
Forsberg and Törngren (1977)	46	153	31	"Major surgery"
Gallus et al. (1976)	61	392	16	Past 40 yrs
Groote Schuur Hosp. (1979)	27	99	27	Abdominal surgery, past 40 yrs
Hutter et al. (1976)	36	100	36	Past 40 yrs, some urologic operations
Int. Multicentre Trial (1975)	164	667	25	"Major surgery", past 40 yrs
Joffe (1975a)	66	130	51	85% past 40 yrs
Kakkar et al. (1970)	62	203	31	Past 40 yrs
Kakkar et al. (1969b)	40	132	30	Past 40 yrs
Koppenhagen et al. (1977)	15	50	30	All ages
Korvald et al. (1974)	6	46	13	Abdominal surgery
Lambie et al. (1970b)	49	111	44	Past 40 yrs
Multiunit Contr. Trial (1974)	47	128	37	"Major surgery", past 40 yrs
Mühe et al. (1975)	33	75	44	Past 30 yrs
Nicolaides et al. (1972b)	29	122	24	"Major surgery", past 40 yrs
Plante et al. (1979)	14	66	21	Abdominal surgery
Renney et al. (1976)	24	75	32	Past 40 yrs
Rosengarten et al. (1970)	8	25	32	Past 40 yrs
Ruckley (1976)	47	128	37	Past 40 yrs
Schaub et al. (1975)	34	95	36	Elective surgery
Strand et al. (1975)	10	50	20	Abdominal surgery, past 30 yrs
Wu et al. (1977)	6	44	14	Abdominal surgery, past 40 yrs
In total	1018	3555		
Mean frequency			*29%*	

that the risk of thrombosis is high in these patient: infection, dehydration, pre-operative confinement to bed, bleeding, blood transfusions, shock, etc.

Incidence Following Urologic Surgery

Most investigations in this area have been performed in patients who underwent surgery of the prostate. The incidence of postoperative thrombosis is higher following transvesical adenoma enucleation than following either transurethral resection or most interventions in general surgery (Table 5). The reason for this difference is not clear. The mean incidence, as measured by the ^{125}I-fibrinogen test, is about 40% after transvesical surgery and about 10% after transurethral surgery.

In the few studies performed on a mixed urologic population, the incidence varied between 25% and 59% (Sebeseri et al. 1975, Kutnowski et al 1977, Coe et al. 1978, Bergqvist and Hallböök 1980). These patients should therefore be considered a high-risk group (Collins et al. 1976).

The administration of an antifibrinolytic drug (ϵ-aminocaproic or tranexamic acid) following prostatic surgery is, in most clinics, a standard method of reducing postoperative bleeding (McNichol et al. 1961, Andersson 1964, 1965). It was of obvious value to determine whether this medication (Leandoer et al. 1968) and a few clinical case reports (Naeye 1962, Gralnick and Greipp 1971) suggested this complication. In three prospective controlled studies using objective diagnosis, no increased incidence of thrombosis could be demonstrated (Becker and Borgström 1968, Gordon-Smith et al. 1972b, Hedlund 1975). In a large double-blind study of 515 prostat-

Table 5. Incidence of thrombosis following prostatic surgery
Becker and Borgström, and Becker et al. used phlebography, and Crawford et al. phleborheography for the diagnosis. In the other studies the ^{125}I-fibrinogen test was used

Authors	Transvesical surgery		Transurethral surgery	
	Number of patients	Incidence of thrombosis (%)	Number of patients	Incidence of thrombosis (%)
Becker and Borgström (1968)	12	50		
Becker et al. (1970)	187	21		
Browse et al. (1974b)	42	50	48	29
Crawford et al. (1978)			150	4.6
Gordon-Smith et al. (1972b)	62	29		
Gruber (1975)	95	36		
Hedlund (1975)	40	45	101	10
Kakkar (1977)	85	27		
Mayo et al. (1971)	41	51	20	10
Nicolaides et al. (1972b)	25	28		
Nicolaides et al. (1972c)	21	48	29	7
Rosenberg et al. (1975)	33	33		
Schaub et al. (1975)	21	29		
Sinclair et al. (1976)	19	68	21	33
von Hospenthal et al. (1977)			47	4
Mean, based on the [125]*I-fibrinogen test*		*38%*		*11%*

ectomies, the mortality was the same in the control as in the treated group. This was also the case with the rate of fatal pulmonary embolism (Vinnicombe and Shuttleworth 1966).

Incidence Following Gynecologic Surgery

Studies of thombosis following gynecologic surgery are quite rare. The incidence of thrombosis is lower than in general surgery in spite of the fact that these operations are performed in the lower part of the abdomen and in the pelvis.

Table 6 shows the incidence of thrombosis in untreated patients, using the ^{125}I-fibrinogen test. The mean incidence is 19%. Walsh et al. (1974) analyzed different subgroups among their 262 patients. In vaginal hysterectomy the incidence was 7%, in abdominal hysterectomy 12%, and in operations for malignancy 35%.

Bernstein et al. (1980) have also demonstrated the increased risk of malignancy involved in hysterectomy. A similar difference in incidence was found by Friend and Kakkar (1972) among patients who underwent abdominal or vaginal surgery. Thus, the trend is the same as in transvesical and transurethral prostatic surgery (see above). The rate of thrombosis is not influenced when either a Pfannenstiel or a midline incision is made for hysterectomy (Walsh et al. 1974). The risk of postoperative thrombosis is considerably increased in surgery for uterine prolapse, secondary to the accompanying estrogen therapy for vaginal atrophy (Åstedt et al. 1980).

Table 6. Incidence of thrombosis in gynecologic surgery
Diagnosis of thrombosis employing the ^{125}I-fibrinogen test

Author	Number of patients	Number of patients with thrombosis	Incidence of thrombosis (%)	Type of surgery
Adolf et al. (1978)	75	22	29	Mixed, 51% abdominal hysterectomy
Ballard et al. (1973)	55	16	29	"Major gynocologic surgery"
Bonnar and Walsh (1972)	140	15	11	Hysterectomy
Endl and Auinger (1977)	43	16	37	
Friend and Kakkar (1972)	92	17	18	"Major pelvic surgery"
Ruckley (1976)	29	4	14	Unspecified gynocologic surgery
Taberner et al. (1978)	48	11	23	30 hysterectomy, 18 operations of pelvic floor
Walsh et al. (1974)	262	37	14	"Major gynocologic surgery"
Total	*701*	*122*		
Mean frequency			*19%*	

Patients who have had a cesarean section constitute a special group when post-operative thromboembolism is considered. Although these patients are young, pregnancy and the puerperium per se carry an increased risk of thrombosis. Further-more, an operation in the lower part of the abdomen is performed.

The risk of venous thrombosis during pregnancy is 5-6 times greater than for non-pregnant women in the same age group (Seigel 1972). Pregnancy is associated with an increased coagulation and a reduced fibrionlysis (Bonnar 1979, Howie 1979, Redman 1979, Moseley and Kerstein 1980). Teleologically, this is an adequate response to the increased risk of a hemorrhage which results from placental separation. Moreover, the venous hemodynamics change during pregnancy. Because of the uterine pressure, venous return decreases and peripheral venous pressure increases.

Proximal thrombi are relatively more common during pregnancy. Due to the anatomy, left-sided thrombosis is more common than right-sided (Cegelski et al. 1964, A Bergqvist et al. 1982, 1983, Bergqvist and Hedner 1983). This also seems to be the case with iliofemoral thrombosis in patients taking contraceptive pills (Brunner 1977, A Bergqvist et al. 1982). Thrombi in women taking oral contraceptives also appear to be more often localized proximally than thrombi in other categories of patients (Haeger and Nylander 1971).

The incidence of thrombosis following cesarean section has been difficult to study mainly for diagnostic reasons. In some studies using clinical diagnosis, incidences of 2% – 5 % have been found (Hiilesmaa 1960, Husni et al. 1967, Segal et al. 1975). In an early study where the indications for cesarean section were somewhat different and the postoperative mobilization slow, the frequencies of thrombosis and pulmonary embolism were very high (33% and 26% respectively; Nettelblad 1931). Bilateral phlebography can hardly be carried out in a large group of women who have just undergone surgery. The ^{125}I-fibrinogen test cannot be used in pregnant and lactating women, as free ^{125}I will be transmitted to the fetus and the milk. In a small number of non-breast-feeding vomen an ^{125}I-fibrinogen test was performed following cesarean section, and no thrombi were detected (Friend and Kakkar 1972, Jackson 1972). In an unselected group of 1969 women undergoing cesarean section, A Bergqvist and collaborators (1979) performed occlusion plethysmography preoperatively and 1 week postoperatively and diagnosed the presence of thrombi in three patients (1.8%).

Incidence Following Orthopedic Surgery

It has long been known that patients with fractures have a high frequency of throm-bosis. Bauer (1944) were able to show phlebographically the increased frequency in patients with leg fractures and how the frequency varied with the location of the fracture.

Most orthopedic operations carry a high risk of thrombosis. Patients undergoing hip operations have been thoroughly investigated. Moreover, hip joint surgery is a relatively standard operation. It is important to differ between elective hip surgery, with different forms of arthrophsty, and operations due to fracture. In the latter, patients already have a trauma before arrival at the hospital. Therefore, there is a possibility that the thrombosis-inducing process is activated before any prophylaxis can be given.

These two groups of patients also exhibit a significant difference in the incidence of thrombosis, with a considerable higher incidence in the fracture group (Bergqvist et al. 1979). Both groups can be considered high risk, however.

Patients undergoing hip joint surgery exhibit two types of thrombosis. Firstly, there is the usual postoperative thrombosis of the leg commonly encountered with all types of surgery. In a few cases the thrombus grows in a proximal direction. Secondly, there is a proximal type of thrombosis which could possibly emanate from damage of the venous wall associated with the surgical trauma. This assumption is supported by intraoperative phlebographic studies, showing a clear mechanical influence on the femoral vein during certain phases of the operation (Stamatakis et al. 1977b). In this study the thrombotic process was isolated in the iliofemoral segment in as many as 25% of the cases. The rate of calf thrombosis is identical in the operated leg to the healthy one, whereas the veins of the thigh are significatly more often involved in the operated leg (Culver et al. 1970, Nillius and Nylander 1979).

Culver et al. (1970) studied 100 patients with hip fractures by phlebography, 20 of them bilaterally. In 40 of the fractured legs, there were a total of 63 thrombi, 23 of these located above the knee. Only three of the 20 unfractured legs revealed thrombosis of the thigh (in total 13 thrombi). In a prophylactic study, the same investigators observed a similar thrombus distribution in the control group, in which bilateral phlebograms were obtained from all patients (Hamilton et al. 1970).

Table 7 shows the incidence of thrombosis found after hip fracture surgery, employing phlebography as the diagnostic method. As noted, the incidence of thrombosis is also high in the healthy leg. The time of phlebography varies between 5 days

Table 7. Incidence of thrombosis in patients who underwent surgery for hip fracture without prophylaxis
Phlebographic diagnosis

Author	Time of phlebography	Number of patients	Number of patients with thrombosis		
			Total	Fractured leg	Healthy leg
Ahlberg et al. (1968)	2−10 months	45	16	16	−
Borgström et al. (1965)	3−4 weeks	23	13	13	−
Culver et al. (1970)	Within 4 weeks	100	40	40	−
Freeark et al. (1967)	On average 12.3 days postoperatively	70	29	29	−
Hamilton et al. (1970)	5−12 days	38	18	18	10
Johnson et al. (1968)	Within 3 months	25	13	13	−
Myhre and Holen (1969)	21 days	55	20	20	−
Smyrnis et al. (1973)	6−10 days	58	35	26	15
Stevens et al. (1968)	9−21 days	71	?	21	13
Total		*485*		*196*	
Mean incidence			*44%*	*40%*	*23%*

and 10 months postoperatively, but the incidence of thrombosis exhibits no correlation with time.

In the autopsy material of Sevitt and Gallagher (1959), 29 out of 35 patients were found to have deep venous thrombosis following fracture of the hip (83%).

A similar incidence of thrombosis demonstrated by phlebography is found in elective hip surgery (Table 8). In this condition proximal thrombi are also more common in the operated leg (Table 9; Bergqvist et al. 1976a).

The use of the ^{125}I-fibrinogen test as a method of diagnosis following hip surgery has been the object of much discussion, primarily due to the fact that the test becomes positive in the presence of hematoma. Some authors also state that the sensitivity is too low after hip surgery (Sautter et al. 1979). Thus, it is impossible to make a differential diagnosis between a proximal thrombus of the thigh and the activity of the fracture and the surgical hematoma.

Table 8. Incidence of thrombosis in patients who underwent elective surgery of the hip without prophylaxis
Phlebographic diagnosis

Author	Time of phlebography	Number of patients	Number of patients with thrombosis		
			Total	Operated leg	Healthy leg
Bergqvist et al. (1976a)	21 days	20	12	10	6
Evarts and Feil (1971)	10 days	56	30	30	–
Loudon et al. (1978)	6–10 days	85	?	45	28
Soreff et al. (1975)	12–14 days	14	5	5	–
Stamatakis et al. (1977b)	?	160	81	81	–
Total		*335*		*173*	
Mean incidence			*52%*	*52%*	*32%*

Table 9. Thrombus localization following elective hip surgery. (After Bergqvist et al. 1976a)
Phlebography about 21 days postoperatively. The number of patients was 20 (40 examined legs). Twelve patients had thrombosis: six in the operated leg, two in the healthy leg, and four bilaterally (16 legs in total). In nine legs, there were multiple sites of thrombosis. No isolated proximal thrombosis was observed in any of the legs

Localization	Operated leg	Healthy leg
Superficial veins	2	1
Fibular veins	9	5
Posterior tibial veins	3	1
Anterior tibial veins	–	–
Soleal veins	3	3
Popliteal vein	2	0
Superficial femoral vein	3	0
Total	*22*	*10*

Table 10. Diagnostic comparison of phlebography (phleb) and the ^{125}I-fibrinogen uptake test (FUT) in hip surgery
Phlebography is used as the reference method. The table shows the sensitivity and specificity of the ^{125}I-fibrinogen test in relation to phlebography

Author	Number of legs	Phleb + FUT +	Phleb − FUT −	Phleb + FUT −	Phleb − FUT +	Sensi-tivity (%)	Speci-ficity (%)	Corre-lation (%)
Bergqvist et al. (1973)[a]	57	14	32	4	7	77.8	82.1	80.7
Bergqvist et al. (1976)[b]	40	10	22	6	2	62.5	91.7	80.0
Bockslaff et al. (1974)[b]	73	48	20	4	1	92.3	83.3	93.2
Field et al. (1972)[a]	63	29	25	2	7	93.5	78.1	85.7
Harris et al. (1975)[b]	88	26	34	25	3	51.0	91.9	68.2
Loudon et al. (1978)[b]	170	68	65	5	32	93.2	67.0	78.2
Myrvold et al. (1973)[a]	82	25	50	3	4	89.3	92.6	91.5
Suomalainen (1980)[b]	97	19	60	7	11	73.0	85.0	81.4
Total	*670*	*239*	*303*	*56*	*67*	*81.0*	*82.1*	*81.6*
Elective surgery	*448*	*171*	*201*	*47*	*49*	*78.4*	*80.4*	*83.0*
Fracture surgery	*202*	*68*	*107*	*9*	*18*	*88.3*	*85.6*	*86.6*
Hirsh et al. (1974) (hip surgery, unspecified)	158	87	52	5	14	94.6	78.8	88.0
Le Moine and Moser (1980) (hip surgery, unspecified)	42	9	31	0	2	100	93.9	95.2

[a]Fracture surgery.
[b]Elective surgery.

The usefulness of the ^{125}I-fibrinogen examination depends, of course, on the number of isolated proximal thrombi of the thigh. As previously mentioned Stamatakis et al. (1977b) found such thrombi in 25%, while in 134 patients who underwent elective hip surgery Nillius and Nylander (1979) encountered only eight (6%), one of which was located in the nonoperated leg. Modig et al. (1981) made a careful phlebographic analysis of 15 untreated hip arthroplasty patients. In 11 patients there were 15 legs with thrombosis, two of which had isolated femoral thrombi (13%).

The studies performed concerning the diagnostic correlation between phlebography and the ^{125}I-fibrinogen test in hip surgery are presented in Table 10. The correlation appears to be somewhat lower in elective hip surgery than in fracture-hip surgery. This finding is possibly related to the fact that the femoral vein is more displaced and injured in the former operation (Stamatakis et al. 1977b). With the

Table 11. Incidence of thrombosis in hip surgery assessed by the ^{125}I-fibrinogen test

Author	Number of patients	Number of patients with thrombosis	Incidence of thrombosis (%)	Patients with bilateral thrombosis Number	%
Hip fracture surgery					
Barrie et al. (1974)	25	12	48	10	45
Bergqvist et al. (1979)	22	19	91	10	45
Checketts and Bradley (1974)	26	13	50	8	31
Field et al. (1972)	50	27	54	14	28
Gallus et al. (1973b)	21	10	48		
Morris and Mitchell (1977b)	76	23	30	20	26
Morris and Mitchell (1976b)	80	50	63	23	29
Rogers et al. (1978)	16	12	75		
Total	*316*	*166*			
Mean incidence			*53%*		
Elective hip surgery					
Bergqvist et al. (1979)	71	45	63	26	37
Bockslaff et al. (1974)	73	52	71		
Dechavanne (1975)	20	8	40		
Douss (1976)	53	33	62	14	26
Hampson et al. (1972)	52	28	54		
Harris et al. (1977)	51	22	43		
Hume et al. (1973)	19	8	42		
Loudon et al. (1978)	85	65	76		
Mannucci et al. (1976)	65	36	55	12	18
Morris et al. (1974)	32	16	50		
Rogers et al. (1978)	37	19	51		
Sagar et al. (1976a)	32	22	69		
Schöndorf (1978)	15	9	60	3	20
Venous Thromb. Clin. Study Group (1975)	30	11	37		
Total	*636*	*376*			
Mean incidence			*59%*		

exception of the study by Harris et al. (1975), both sensitivity and specificity are acceptable; therefore the ^{125}I-fibrinogen test also ought to be a useful diagnostic screening method in hip surgery. It would, of course, be ideal to combine it with some method capable of diagnosing proximal thrombosis, e.g., phlebography, ultrasound, or plethysmography.

Hull et al. (1979b) recently performed a large study (1015 Patients) to investigate the benefit of adding impedance plethysmography to the ^{125}I-fibrinogen test in post-operative screening for thrombi. Three hundred and eighty-five of the patients had undergone hip surgery, and the incidence of thrombosis increased 6% when impedance plethysmography was employed. However, the study did not show the number of isolated proximal thrombi present in legs otherwise free of thrombosis.

In an autopsy study on 31 who underwent ^{125}I-fibrinogen examinations before death, the test proved to be of little value in the operated leg but, on the other hand, there were no thrombi in the proximal region without the presence of thrombi in the calf (Morris and Mitchell 1977a). The fact that the thrombotic process may begin in serveral places at the same time was reported by Sevitt in 1962.

The ^{125}I-fibrinogen test can thus be used as a screening method for establishing the incidence of thrombosis, while other methods are required for localization of the disease.

Table 11 presents the incidence of thrombosis in hip fracture and elective hip surgery using the ^{125}I-fibrinogen test for diagnosis in patients receiving no anti-thrombotic prophylaxis. The figures show a good correlation in the incidence of thrombosis with phlebography (Tables 7, 8). Therefore, hip surgery patients form a high-risk group for postoperative thrombosis, and in several patients a thrombus is also present in the non-operated leg. In elective hip surgery the thrombosis risk is greater if the operation is performed via a lateral approach than via a posterior approach (Gallus and Darby 1981, Sikorski et al. 1981).

As for other orthopedic operations, documentation is not as comprehensive as in hip surgery. This is partly due to the fact that the ^{125}I-fibrinogen test cannot be used in the presence of hematomas. Some studies deal with thrombosis associated with fractures of the tibia. Injuries and compressions of the veins occur at the fracture level (Nylander and Semb 1972, Preter et al. 1972, Spieler et al. 1972). In 40% − 50% of the cases a thrombus, possible to diagnose by phlebography, develops (Hjelmstedt 1968, Spieler et al. 1972, Olbert et al. 1977). A similar incidence has been demon-strated following elective knee surgery (Cohen et al. 1973, McKenna et al. 1976).

In a series of 40 patients who underwent operation in a bloodless field Kroese and Stiris (1976) detected seven cases of thrombosis (17%) at phlebography 2 − 8 days postoperatively. The patients were young (median age 40 years; 19–71), and the orthopedic operation was considered small.

The occurrence of thromboembolism after amputation of the leg because of arterial insufficiency has not been studied in detail. Harper et al. (1973) reported an incidence of thrombosis of 67%, while Barnes and Slaymaker (1976) detected no thrombi by ultrasound.

A retrospective analysis of 1229 patients in the Nordic countries who underwent an operation for scoliosis was carried out by Udén (1979). Eight cases of thrombosis were detected. They were young people who underwent a very extensive operation with prolonged immobilization. In all cases the thrombosis was proximal and involved the left lower extremity. One patient died of pulmonary embolism. In a prospective study 54 children who underwent halofemoral traction because of scoliosis, phlebograms were performed. Two of them developed thrombosis − 3.7% (Leslie et al. 1981). The phlebograms were taken 2 days before a fusion operation and after an average traction of 28 days.

After an acute injury of the spinal cord, the incidence of thrombosis appears to be very high judging from a small series thoroughly investigated by Brach et al. (1977). These patients are young, with a high rate of proximal thrombi. Most thrombi also seem to occur following various surgical procedures (laminectomy and different fusion operations). The high incidence (about 70%) has been confirmed by Rossi et al. (1980). Patients undergoing spinal surgery had an incidence of about 20% (Valladares and Hankinson 1980).

Incidence in Other Types of Surgery

The incidence of thrombosis in other types of operations has been studied only sporadically. Joffe (1975a) found thrombi in 2 of 31 patients following eye operations, and in four out of seven cases of kidney transplantation.

The renal transplant study is very small, but a few observations might be of interest. The onset of all thrombi occurred after more than a week, and all were located proximally. The late onset can possibly be ascribed to heparin treatment during postoperative dialysis. Moreover, elimination of heparin is slower in uremia (Teien and Bjørnson 1976).

In a retrospective study 11% of the patients developed clinically significant thromboembolic complications after renal transplantation − all occurring after more than 3 weeks and significantly more often in diabetic patients (Arnadottir et al. 1982).

Thrombosis occurred following thoracotomy for various reasons in 32 out of 63 (51%) untreated patients (Jackman et al. 1978).

In the studies mentioned above, the ^{125}I-fibrinogen test was used.

In reconstructive vascular surgery of the abdominal aorta and distal vessels, relatively few studies on the incidence of thrombosis have been performed. Theoretically, there are several reasons for expecting a high incidence of thrombosis: dissection of the pelvic, femoral, and popliteal veins, dissection for harvesting a venous graft, postoperative edema, reluctance to move the operated leg because of pain, or damaged muscles due to previous ischemia.

Phlebograms after femoropopliteal venous bypass were carried out by Hamer (1972), who detected nine thrombi in 21 patients (43%). Most thrombi occurred in patients whose distal anastomosis extended below the knee. A considerably lower incidence, about 8% diagnosed by phlebography, was found by Husni (1967), Porter et al. (1972), and Myhre et al. (1974) after femoropopliteal venous bypass. The relatively low incidence may partly be due to the fact that these patients often received some type of antithrombotic treatment for the clamped arterial segments, e.g., intraoperative administration of heparin or dextran. In a small series of several types of vascular reconstruction, mainly carotid artery revascularization, the incidence of positive ^{125}I-fibrinogen scans was 11% (Spebar et al. 1981).

In aortoiliac surgery, the incidence is higher using the [125]-fibrinogen test: 21% (Angelides et al. 1977), 27% (Hartsuck and Greenfield 1973), and 32% (Belch et al. 1979). Comparable figures have been observed in abdominal surgery of similar complexity. In an American study, the incidence following surgery of the abdominal aorta was considerably lower (3%; Satiani et al. 1980).

Angelides et al. (1977) found that the incidence was significantly higher in surgery of aortic aneurysms than in surgery of aortoiliac occlusive disease (33% and 12% respectively). This is difficult to explain. In the former there is a more serious ischemia of the lower extremities secondary to cross-clamping of the aorta which leads to a series of metabolic changes (Mansberger et al. 1966, Lim et al. 1969, J Andersson et al. 1979, Neglén 1980). These changes may induce pulmonary microembolism (Mulcare et al. 1976, Bowald 1979). Moreover, the frequency of thromboembolic complication is higher after operation because of aortic aneurysm rupture than after elective aneurysm operation (Abbott 1980).

Postoperative thrombosis following surgery for varicose veins has been reported as rare (Dodd and Cockett 1976, Lofgren 1976, McNamara et al. 1977, May 1979), but no systematic investigations with objective diagnosis of thrombosis have been published. In May's (1979) study of 30 000 patients only one case of fatal pulmonary embolism was found.

In a few cases thromboembolic complications have occurred following sclerotherapy of varicose veins (Gjöres 1956, Dodd and Cockett 1976, Sigg 1977, Hobbs 1978).

Patients undergoing neurosurgical operations constitute an interesting group, since the operations frequently last a long time, and every prophylactic measure must be entirely free of bleeding complications intraoperatively as well as postoperatively. During the past few years some studies have appeared showing that neurosurgery entails a similar incidence of thrombosis as general surgery. Table 12 is a compilation of these studies.

Table 12. Incidence of thrombosis in neurosurgery. Diagnosis using the ^{125}I-fibrinogen test; Skillman et al. also used phlebography

Author	Number of patients	Incidence of thrombosis (%)
Cerrato et al. (1978)	50	34
Joffe (1975b)	23	43
Skillman et al. (1978)	48	25
Turpie (1976)	63	19
Turpie et al. (1979)	96	21
Valladares and Hankinson (1980)	71	32
Total	*351*	
Mean incidence		*29%*

Incidence of Pulmonary Embolism

In most autopsy studies the incidence of pulmonary embolism is high, but, of course, these patients died due to the severity of the disease. In a report on pulmonary embolism from departments of internal medicine the fatal pulmonary embolism is often a part of a disease which has a poor prognosis in itself and the patient a short expected survival (Kraemmer-Nielsen et al. 1981). Two studies give some evidence that the frequency of autopsy proven emboli in surgical patients is decreasing, but whether or not this can be attributed to an increased use of prophylactic method remains unclear (Dismuke 1981, Ruckley 1981).

Coon and Coller (1959) analyzed 4391 autopsies from a 10-year period 1945 – 1954; 606 emboli were observed (13.8%). Age was a decisive factor, but there are indications that the primary cause was an increasing incidence of heart disease and malignancy with age. This was also the case in postoperative thromboembolism. Schwartz et al. (1976) analyzed 1350 autopsies in adults during 1 year in Vienna. They found that the frequency of pulmonary embolism was 23.5% and that in 7.8% the embolism was the immediate cause of death.

A systematic survey of 1 year autopsy material carried out by Morrell and Dunnill (1968) in Oxford, showing embolism in no less than 52%, the incidence increasing with age. They believed that 37 patients would have survived had embolism not occurred. In 56 cases (43%) pulmonary embolism was the immediate cause of death. Of the 94 patients who died postoperatively, 33% had pulmonary embolism. In these patients the incidence of fresh pulmonary embolism was also higher than in the group as a whole. Evans (1971) made an attempt to analyze the prognosis in patients dying from pulmonary embolism. He found that they should have recovered from the underlying disease but they were killed by a large embolus.

In two comprehensive Swedish autopsy studies an incidence of pulmonary embolism of at least 20% was demonstrated (Kaij 1959, Diener 1975). In Malmö, where the autopsy rate was very high and of great epidemiologic value, a study on thromboembolism was carried out during the late 1950s (Kaij 1959). Of the patients in the surgical clinic 0.19% died as a result of pulmonary embolism; the corresponding figure from the orthopedic clinic was 0.27%. The incidence of fatal pulmonary embolism among the patients who died was 9.2% and 11.5% respectively. These figures are of the same magnitude as in several other autopsy investigations in the literature (Becker 1965, Vollmar and Rüdiger 1972, Macintyre and Ruckley 1974, Feigl and Schwarz 1977).

Macroscopic pulmonary embolism was detected by Havig (1977) in 55% of 508 autopsies chosen at random at the Ulleval Hospital in Oslo. Microscopic embolism was present in a further 72 cases, making the total incidence in this investigation as high as 69%. Pulmonary embolism was thought to be the immediate cause of death in 33%; in another 19% it probably contributed to the fatal outcome. In two-thirds of the cases the source of the embolus was localized to the iliofemoral veins but in one-third to the calf or sole. Seven of 31 postoperative deaths (23%) were due to pulmonary embolism.

Thus, in an unselected autopsy group, the incidence of pulmonary embolism is high. More interesting from a surgical point of view is the incidence after surgery. As pulmonary embolism is difficult to diagnose, and as pulmonary embolism in many cases is probably asymptomatic, the fatal cases have become the center of attention in the discussion of prophylaxis of thromboembolism. Table 13 shows the incidence of fatal pulmonary embolism in a few large studies with untreated reference groups. The study of Sagar et al. (1975) differs from the others by its higher total mortality rate and the higher incidence of pulmonary embolism. The data of Atiks and Broghamers (1979) collected in the early 1960s (as opposed to the other publications, which appeared in the 1970s) have asomewhat lower incidence of fatal pulmonary embolism; in this review, however, there was no lower age limit for selecting the patients. A survey of a number of publications reporting fatal postoperative pulmonary embolism was performed by Schlosser (1977). The material comprises about 4.7 million operations from the year 1900 until the mid 1960s. The incidence of fatal pulmonary embolism is surprisingly constant, between 0.2% and 1.2%, which corresponds well with the figures from later materials presented in Table 13. In an 8-year analysis of fatal pulmonary embolism from the university of Vienna the frequency was 0.33% in 22 286 (Kohn et al. 1974). There were no emboli in patients younger than 30 years of age and only 4% of the emboli were seeen in patients of less than 50 years of age. In a poll in 1979, where data from ten clinics were used, the incidence was very similar (Bell and Zuidema 1979).

The geriatric investigation of Palmberg and Hirsjärvi (1977) shows the highest incidence of fatal pulmonary embolism in acute abdominal surgery for peritonitis and ileus (9.1%).

Embolectomized patients form a special group, and because of their general weakness and high age a very high mortality varies between different reports from approximately 15% to 40% and the incidence of fatal pulmonary embolism from 2.7% to 6.2% (MacGowan and Mooneeram 1973, Eriksson and Holmberg 1977, Szczepansky 1979, Lorentzen et al. 1980).

In a study on 2015 transurethral resections of the prostate, 51 patients died (2.5%), ten in pulmonary embolism (0.5%) (Holtgrewe and Valk 1962). According to certain authors, pulmonary embolism is the most common cause of death after prostatectomy (Antila et al. 1966).

Also after renal transplantation fatal pulmonary embolism is a real danger appearing relatively late in the course (Hill et al. 1967, Simmons et al. 1972, Gurland et al. 1973).

Of 231 patients who had undergone coronary reconstruction four died of massive pulmonary embolism (1.7%; Rao et al. 1975). All these were treated with unspecified elastic stockings (see p. 67). After coronary bypass surgery there is another source of emboli from the thrombus covering the suture line in the right atrium, especially when combined with arrhythmia (Formolo and Shors 1981).

A special situation in young patients is induced abortion. Of 104 deaths related to abortion and registered during a 4-year period in Atlanta, Georgia, United States, eight were secondary to pulmonary embolism confirmed at autopsy (Kimball et al. 1978). In a large review of pulmonary embolism, the incidence has been estimated to be one to two cases per 10 000 abortions (Tietze and Lewit 1972, Hodgson and Portmann 1974, Kimball et al. 1978). The incidence of fatal pulmonary embolism is, however, less – 0.28 per 10 000 is a rate given by Greiss (1978).

The incidence of fatal pulmonary embolism is estimated to be ten times higher following cesarean section than following vaginal delivery, and during the period

Table 13. Incidence of postoperative fatal pulmonary embolism in some large series of patients

Author	Patient category	Age group	Number of patients	Total mortality		Fatal pulmonary embolism	
				Number	%	Number	%
Atik and Broghamer (1979)	General surgery, orthopedic	All	1455	142	9.8	7	0.48
Int. Multicentre (Trial 1975)	General surgery, urologic,	>40	2076	100	4.8	16	0.77
Kiil et al. (1978)	Abdomen, thorax	>40	653	?		7	1.1
Kline et al. (1975)	Abdominal surgery	>40	435	35	8	7	1.6
Palmberg and Hirsjärvi (1977)	All types of surgery	>60	4535	?		34	0.75
Sagar et al. (1975)	Abdomen, thorax	>50	236	38	16	8	3.4
Total			*9390*			79	
Mean incidence							0.8

1970–1972 it was 1.6 per 10 000 in England and Wales (Bonnar 1979). The incidence of thromboembolic complications is nevertheless low in this particular postoperative situation.

In hip surgery, particularly surgery for fracture, the incidence of embolism is considerably higher. Table 14 is a compilation of studies where the incidence of fatal pulmonary embolism in untreated patients is presented. Otherwise, only sporadic reports on fatal pulmonary embolism in orthopedic disorders have appeared.

The incidence following amputation of the femur is the same as following hip fracture surgery (Harper et al. 1973, J Williams et al. 1978). Fractures of the tibia also entail some risk of fatal pulmonary embolism (Solonen 1963: 2 out of 36 patients; Hjelmstedt 1968: 1 out of 76; Willén et al. 1982: 2 out of 66 patients). Of great importance is the fact that fatal pulmonary embolism can occur a long time after an orthopedic trauma, sometimes 2 month later (Vance 1934, Sevitt 1962). A well-defined follow-up time is therefore important in studies dealing with post-traumatic thromboembolism.

The risk of thromboembolism in trauma secondary to fractures, in particular hip and tibial fractures, is well known. There is a number of studies on the incidence,

Table 14. Incidence of fatal pulmonary embolism in hip surgery
The patients did not receive any form of prophylaxis against thromboembolism. The diagnosis is based on autopsy findings

Author	Number of patients	Number of cases of fatal pulmonary embolism
Hip fracture surgery		
Ahlberg et al. (1968)	45	2
Barrie et al. (1974)	25	3
Borgström et al. (1965)	29	2
Dolk and Westerborn (1977)	282	7
Edwards et al. (1975)	31	4
Eskeland et al. (1966)	100	7
Galasko et al. (1976)	50	2
Hansen et al. (1976)	50	2
Morris and Mitchell (1976b)	80	6
Moskowitz et al. (1978)	23	1
Myhre and Holen (1969)	55	2
Sevitt and Gallagher (1959)	150	15
Zekert et al. (1974)	120	8
Total	*1040*	*61*
Mean incidence		*5.9%*
Elective hip surgery		
Bergqvist et al. (1979)	71	2
D'Ambrosia et al. (1975)	99	1
Morris et al. (1974)	32	1
Sagar et al. (1976a)	32	1
Schöndorf (1978)	15	1
Total	*249*	*6*
Mean incidence		*2.4%*

Table 15. Incidence of fatal pulmonary embolism following trauma

Author	Type of trauma	Number of patients	Fatal pulmonary embolism	
			Number	Incidence (%)
Aldrete et al. (1979)	Liver rupture	108	1	0.9
Alho and Rokkanen (1973)	"Severe blunt injury"	258	5	1.9
Bergqvist et al. (1980c)	Penetrating abdominal injuries	70	1	1.4
Bergqvist et al. (1982)	Abdominal trauma in the elderly	177	2	1.1
Frey et al. (1973)	Liver rupture	139	2	1.4
Fry et al. (1980)	Spleen rupture	220	2	0.9
Graham et al. (1979)	Pancreatico- duodenal injury	68	1	1.5
Hedblom (1925)	Diaphragm rupture	378	2	0.5
Relihan and Litwin (1973)	"Flail chest"	85	1	1.2
Steele and Lim (1975)	Spleen rupture	247	4	1.6
Stone and Fabian (1979)	Duodenal injury	321	2	0.6

employing objective diagnostic methods. In contrast, there are almost no studies of thromboembolism after other types of trauma. The incidence of deep venous thrombosis in this group of patients has not been investigated at all.

In some studies on trauma, the cause of death has been carefully reported, thus making it possible to estimate the risk of fatal pulmonary embolism. The incidence varies between 0.5% and 2% (Table 15). Thus, the incidence of fatal pulmonary macroembolism appears to be the same as in nontraumatic operations of the corresponding organ system. The so-called microembolism, on the other hand, is found regularly in the lungs of patients who have died more than 24 h after a traffic accident (Lindquist et al. 1972). However, the pathogenesis of the microembolism syndrome or disseminated intravascular coagulation is different from that in macroembolism.

When scintigraphic diagnosis is used, the number of detected pulmonary emboli increases markedly, most of them being asymptomatic. As is the case with the ^{125}I-fibrinogen test, the clinical significance of such emboli or perfusion defects can be discussed. Table 16 shows that the incidence varies considerably between different reports. Since there is no comparison for screening between scintigraphy and pulmonary angiography, the diagnostic criterion is somewhat uncertain. However, it appears that figures from 10% to 20% are obtained if ventilation and perfusion scintigraphy are combined (Browse et al. 1974a), if chronic obstructive pulmonary disease is excluded (Allgood et al. 1970, Abernathy and Hartsuck 1974), or if only wedge-like segmental perfusion defects without a chest X-ray correlation are chosen (Butterman et al. 1977, Bergqvist et al. 1979, Groote Schuur Hosp. 1979).

In a limited study after amputation of the leg, angiography of the pulmonary artery was used as screening method (J. Williams et al. 1975). Embolism was found in

Table 16. Incidence of postoperative pulmonary embolism assessed by pulmonary scintigraphy

Author	Patient category	Number of patients	Time of scintigraphy (postoperative day)	Perfusion scintigraphy + chest X-ray	Perfusion + ventilation scintigraphy	Perfusion defects of embolus type	
						Number	%
Abernathy and Hartsuck (1974)	General surgery	26	Approx. 7	+		5	19
Allgood et al. (1970)	General surgery, urologic	64	4.3 and 7.9	+		9	14
Bergqvist et al. (1979)	Elective hip surgery	71	7	+		14	20
Browse et al. (1974a)	General surgery	40	7		+	7	18
Butterman et al. (1977)	General surgery	175	3–5	+		41	23
	Urologic	100	3–5	+		10	10
	Gynecologic	75	3–5	+		9	12
Groote Schuur Hospital (1979)	Abdominal surgery	88	7	+		5	6
Hartsuck and Greenfield (1973)	Abdominal and pelvic surgery	196		+		114	58
Johansson et al. (1975)	Abdominal surgery	49		+		13	27
Lahnborg et al. (1974)	Abdominal surgery	54	3–4	+		24	45
Murphy et al. (1972)	Urologic	59		+		8	14
Salzman and Axilrod (1971)	Urologic	51	8	+		4	8

8 out of 70 patients. Two other patients later died of embolism, giving an incidence of 14%.

In thrombosis of the leg diagnosed by phlebograms and including distal involvement, the rate of perfusion defects on scintigraphy is high (Kistner et al. 1972, Lopez-Majano et al. 1978). This is also true for thrombi detected by the ^{125}I-fibrinogen test (Warlow and Ogston 1973). In Havig's autopsy material (1977), one-third of the pulmonary emboli arose from the veins of the calf. Browse and Lea Thomas (1974) showed that nonfatal pulmonary emboli originate from different venous sections in proportion to the incidence of thrombosis within the respective section. This means that thrombi of the calf are not an unusual source of embolism.

There are two types of surgical operations which are specifically associated with pulmonary embolism, namely venous thrombectomy and various forms of pervention of embolism directed against the vena cava. In both cases the purpose is to prevent pulmonary embolism, in the former operation also to present the development of a post-thrombotic syndrome. Intraoperative pulmonary embolism occurs in a few cases in connection with venous thrombectomy, sometimes with a fatal outcome (DeWeese et al. 1967, Smith 1968, Barner et al. 1969, Mahorner 1969, Mavor and Galloway 1969, Kitianik and Quiros 1972). Postoperative pulmonary embolism is reported in 2% − 8% and contributes markedly to the postoperative mortality (DeWeese et al. 1967, Lansing and Davis 1968, Smith 1968, Barner et al. 1969, Mahorner 1969, Kitianik and Quiros 1972). In one study of 26 patients with iliofemoral thrombosis the risk of pulmonary embolism was equal in one group treated with conventional anticoagulation and one group treated with venous thrombectomy (Plate et al. 1981). Following total or partial interruption of the vena cava, nonfatal pulmonary embolism occurred in 3% − 12%, and was fatal in about 1% (McNamara et al. 1978, DeWeese 1979, Adelson et al. 1980).

Incidence of Post-thrombotic Venous Insufficiency

One of the problems involved in the study of the post-thrombotic syndrome following postoperative thrombosis is the late development of the syndrome. Another problem is the difficulty of establishing the direct relationship between the postoperative thrombosis and the evolution of the syndrome. In an individual patient there my also be a risk of other complications and other disorders predisposing to thrombosis.

In a large sociomedical study in Basel, chronic venous insufficiency was demonstrated in 15% of 4529 individuals, 1% being leg ulcer cases (Widmer 1978). The Swedish incidence was given as 2.1% in 1956 (Gjöres 1956). In a survery of 746 patients selected at random at St. Mary's Hospital in London, Hobbs (1974) found a post-thrombotic syndrome in 4%.

The relationship to previous thrombosis has been demonstrated by Bauer (1942) among others, who showed that the frequency of symptoms is a function of time (Table 17). On the other hand, Järvinen and Asp (1975) found in their study that pronounced post-thrombotic symptoms may develop in as short a time as 3 years. Similar findings were observed by O'Donnell et al. (1977), showing that approximately

Table 17. The rate of post-thrombotic changes as a function of time. After Bauer (1942)
Number of patients: 99

Years after thrombosis	Induration of the leg (%)	Present ulcer (%)
1	3	0
5	45	20
10	72	52
>10	91	79

half of 21 patients with isolated iliofemoral thrombosis developed venous ulcers after 2 years, and as much as 80% after 5 years.

Nevertheless, the most serious complication of the post-thrombotic syndrome — the leg ulcer — as a rule requires a very long time to develop. Gjöres (1956) found that the great majority of leg ulcers (86%) occurred 20 years after the acute thrombosis.

The rate of venous leg ulcers increased with age according to Skaraborg Health Control 1977, where randomly selected individuals aged 25–75 were studied (Hallböök 1977).

A few investigations with the specific purpose of studying the course of post-operative thrombosis exist. Recanalization verified by X-ray was found by Støren and Auensen (1971) in 85% of patients 9 months after a fracture of the hip. Two-thirds of the patients had persistent edema or skin induration. Bergvall and Hjelmstedt (1968) found that the recanalization process required much more time after a tibial fracture (more than 3–4 years). In a study, Becker et al. repeated (1970) phlebograms on average 33 weeks after prostatectomy in patients with postoperative thrombosis. He found residual thrombi in about half of the patients. No correlation with clinical findings was carried out, however.

Very little is known about the incidence of the post-thrombotic syndrome following thrombosis diagnosed by the ^{125}I-fibrinogen test. Using different diagnostic methods, the few small groups of patients examined after a relatively short time showed, however, that post-thrombotic manifestations had already developed in some of them (Browse and Clemenson 1974, Hedlund 1975, Mudge and Hughes 1978, Bergqvist and Hallböök 1979b). In a follow-up investigation of 179 patients, who had undergone postoperative screening with the fibrinogen uptake test 44–65 months previously, there was no difference between fibrinogen uptake test positive and negative legs in clinical investigation, venous emptying plethysmography, ambulatory plethysmography, ambulatory venous pressure measurement, or phlebography (Lindhagen et al. 1982a). It could be concluded that the fibrinogen uptake test did not indicate the patients who were at risk of developing the post-thrombotic syndrome.

In a follow-up investigation of 38 patients with tibial fracture 13–17 years previously, venous insufficiency could be demonstrated in eight (21%), both by clinical examination and by ultrasound and phlebography. This is a much higher incidence than what could be expected for a normal population (Willen et al. 1982). As previously mentioned, this category of patients has an incidence of thrombosis of approximately 50%. The frequency of the post-thrombotic syndrome is higher after open than after closed fractures of the shaft of the femur (Dencker 1964).

It has recently been demonstrated that thrombi destroying the popliteal valve are an important cause of the post-thrombotic syndrome (Shull et al. 1979). By a combination of phlebography and ultrasound examination of the popliteal vein, and by determination of the distal venous pressure during ambulation, Shull et al. were able to show that the function of the popliteal valve was a critical factor in the occurrence of venous insufficiency accompanied by leg ulcers, apart from the appearance and degree of recanalization of the iliofemoral venous segment. This also emphasizes the importance of preventing thrombi of the calf from extending to knee level.

In another study, the results clearly indicate that thrombosis of the calf also affects the hemodynamics as in the post-thrombotic syndrome (Lawrence and Kakkar 1980). Over a period of up to 2 years 113 patients with thrombosis, confirmed by phlebography, were followed by foot volumetry. No patient with extensive thrombosis exhibited normal volumetry after 2 years, 77% having serious changes. For our purpose, it is of interest that no less than 55% of the patients with thrombosis of the calf also had volumetric changes, 14% of which had pathologic changes of the same type as in post-thrombotic venous insufficiency. These frequencies are very similar to those found in a clinical follow-up 31–47 months after deep vein thrombosis (Bieger et al. 1976). But the development of a post-thrombotic syndrome is not related in a simple way to either the size of the original thrombus or its localization (Browse et al. 1980). In a group of patients with varicose veins and/or venous ulcers Arenander (1957) found a clear correlation between the degree of alterations of the deep veins and the frequency of ulceration, although as many as 25% of the patients with phlebographically normal deep veins also had ulcers.

Time of Onset of Thromboembolism

In a number of investigations, determination of the day of onset of postoperative thrombosis has been attempted. With clinical diagnosis of thrombosis most thrombi are detected about 1 week postoperatively (i.e., Dahl-Iversen and Ramberg 1932, Linde 1941). The ^{125}I-fibrinogen test with daily measurements has made further analysis of this problem possible. Nicolaides (1973) and Schaub et al. (1975) found that almost half of the cases of thrombosis began on the day of operation, and that only 10%–15% developed after 4 days. Several authors have demonstrated similar findings with a great number of cases developing in close connection with a surgical operation (Hedlund 1975), Lahnborg and Bergström 1975, Nicolaides and Gordon-Smith 1975, Rem et al. 1975, Buttermann et al. 1977, Endl and Auinger 1977). This means that a good prophylactic method must already function during operation.

Patients who underwent kidney transplantation (Joffe 1975a) and patients with malignant diseases (Bergqvist and Hallböök 1980) exhibited a much later onset of thrombosis. Likewise, postoperative infections appear to postpone the onset of thrombosis (Törngren et al. 1980b). As already mentioned (p. 11) it should also be kept in mind that preoperative onset in seen in a certain number of patients.

In a study on patients who underwent hip surgery, two quite distinct peaks were noted, one immediately after the operation, and one more than a week later (Bergqvist et al. 1976a). Similar observations have been made by other authors in this category of patients (Hampson et al. 1974, Sagar et al. 1976a, Cooke et al. 1977b, Sikorki et al. 1981). Moreover, in the study by Mannucci et al. (1976) there is a specific group of late thrombosis when the diagnostic period is prolonged to 12 days.

Some authors have found that low-dose heparin prophylaxis will postpone the onset of thrombosis (Hampson et al. 1974, Hedlund 1975, Sagar et al. 1976a, Kutnowski et al. 1977, Coe et al. 1978). Other investigatiors however, have not been able to confirm this, (Gallus et al. 1973b, Gallus et al. 1976, Mannucci et al. 1976, Bergqvist and Hallböök 1980).

In their comprehensive epidemiologic analysis of pulmonary embolism, Coon and Coller (1959) found that the highest incidence took place within 24 h postoperatively, and that 72% occurred within 2 weeks. This led to the conclusion that many cases of thrombosis develop already on the operating table, an assumption later supported by fibrinogen test investigations. The relationship in time between various forms of trauma and fatal pulmonary embolism was analyzed by Sevitt (1962), who showed that as many as 35% of the emboli developed more than 3 weeks after the trauma. Several other postoperative studies have previously demonstrated the well-known clinical fact that fatal pulmonary embolism may manifest itself a relatively long time after the operation (Barker et al. 1941, Crutcher and Daniel 1948, Byrne and O'Neil 1952).

For analysis of prophylactic studies on thromboembolism, these time aspects are important to remember. If the follow-up period is too short, an essential part of the thromboembolic complications may be missed. It is also important that the date for completion of an investigation be fixed, in order to obtain equally long follow-up periods for different prophylactic alternatives. It is difficult to compare different studies where diagnostic methods were used only on one occasion (e.g., phlebography and isotope venography) if the time of diagnosis is not the same.

When fatal pulmonary embolism is considered, a follow-up time of at least 30 days is desirable. The onset of thrombosis in relation to the operation calls for effective prophylactic methods perioperatively (during and after operation).

Summary

The number of detected thromboembolic complications depends principally on three factors: the diagnostic method employed, the time of diagnosis, and the patient population. For postoperative screening, phlebography and the ^{125}I-fibrinogen test are the most common methods used. Phlebography yields a morphologic-anatomic diagnosis. The fibrinogen test correlates well with phlebography and has a place in scientific prospective studies. In the individual case it is difficult to foresee whether or not a thrombus diagnosed by the fibrinogen test is of clinical importance, but the risk of pulmonary embolism as well as post-thrombotic syndrome increases when a thrombus reaches knee level.

Pulmonary scintigraphy has been used as a screening method for detection of pulmonary embolism and autopsy for detection of fatal pulmonary embolism. Perfusion scintigraphy is sensitive and relatively unspecific, but the diagnostic certainty increases in combination with ventilation scintigraphy.

In most general surgery studies the postoperative incidence of thrombosis ranges between 20% and 30%. In neurosurgery the figures are about the same. After transvesical prostate surgery the incidence is about 40%, and after transurethral surgery about 10%. Gynecologic surgery carries a slightly lower risk of thrombosis than general surgery. Patients undergoing orthopedic surgery constitute a high-risk group. It is important to differ between elective and posttraumatic surgery, as the coagulation system of patients with fractures is already activated before any prophylaxis can be given. The incidence of thrombosis is 50%–70% in hip surgery.

The incidence of pulmonary embolism detected by scintigraphy is about 20%–25%. The incidence of fatal pulmonary embolism is 0.5%–1% following general surgery operations, 1%–2% after elective hip surgery, and 5%–10% following hip-fracture surgery.

Post-thrombotic venous insufficiency following postoperative thrombosis is a problem that is difficult to analyze and difficult to study, and few relevant investigations have been published. If the valve in the popliteal vein is destroyed, a high incidence of post-thrombotic syndrome ensues.

Pathogenesis of Thrombosis

Thrombosis is a significant problem in general medicine. It may occur in all venous sections of the body and in the extremities; the superficial as well as the deep venous system may be involved. The most common sites of thrombus formation are, however, the veins of the legs and the pelvis. There are factors known to predispose to thrombosis, but sometimes the etiology is unclear, and in this case they are classified as "spontaneous" or cryptogenic. The latter group is becoming smaller with the increasing knowledge of thrombosis.

Thrombosis is multifactorial, and the development of a thrombus is a complex process, which is still largely unknown. The basic concepts were elucidated in the 1850s, however (see p. 1), and with some modifications, the patient with thrombosis can be analyzed according to Virchow's triad (Table 18).

The thrombotic process and the formation of the hemostatic plug have several characteristics in common; nevertheless, there are certain fundamental differences between hemostatic plug formation and the development of venous thrombi, particularly with respect to the type of wall injury, the triggering of the process, and the hemodynamic conditions. It is probably incorrect to compare the initial phases of these two processes. Most of today's prophylactic methods, however, are too insensitive to selectively affect the thrombotic process without simultaneously interfering with the hemostatic mechanism.

In the following pathogenetic discussions, postoperative thrombosis will be given particular attention.

Table 18. Modification of Virchow's triad

1. Changes of the vessel wall
   a) Wall injury with an endothelial defect
   b) Release of plasminogen activators
   c) Prostaglandin content (PGI_2)
   d) Concentration of factor VIII-related protein
   e) Release of glucosaminoglycans
2. Changes in the blood flow
   a) Flow rate
   b) Volume flow
   c) Turbulence in valve pockets
3. Changes of the properties of the blood
   a) Platelets
   b) Coagulation factors
   c) Inhibitors
   d) Fibrinolytic activity

Changes of the Vessel Wall

The normal vascular endothelium is a nonthrombogenic surface. The endothelial cell is no longer considered to be the passive surface in the vascular system, but a metabolically complex cell controlling vascular permeability and preventing thrombotic deposits on the vessel wall. It participates in the synthesis of a series of important substances: prostaglandin, bradykinin, angiotensin, adenonucleotides, plasminogen activators, factor VIII-related protein, and glucosaminoglycans (Mason et al. 1977).

In arterial thrombus formation and hemostatic plug formation, the underlying wall injury is relatively large, with exposure of collagen and basal membrane, both being potent stimuli of platelet aggregation and platelet release reaction (Hovig 1963, Ashford and Freiman 1967, Holmsen et al. 1969). Whether there is such a wall injury in venous thrombosis is, however, doubtful. Most experimental thrombosis models presume a serious endothelial injury, with denudation of the cells and exposure of underlying structures, or employ insertion of material not naturally occurring in the body (for a review, see Henry 1971). Hence, it is not quite certain that such experimental thrombi reflect the correct pathophysiologic process of venous thrombus formation. At present, there are between 200 and 300 experimental thrombosis models, which probably reflect some of the uncertainty in drawing conclusions from an animal experimental model of postoperative venous thrombosis in man.

In certain types of trauma and surgical operations, there is a proven direct involvement of nearby veins, sometimes even a vein wall injury. This is particularly the case in fractures of the tibia (Hjelmstedt 1968, Nylander and Semb 1972), and in arthroplasty of the hip joint (Stamatakis et al. 1977b). In the latter, a pronounced distortion of the femoral vein at certain stages of the operation has been demonstrated phlebographically. As mentioned before, both these conditions entail a high incidence of thrombosis within the area of the operation or trauma (see p. 16). Also, in association with venous trauma, the incidence of local thrombosis is high when reconstructions are made without ensuring a simultaneous increase of flow, for instance, by creating a temporary arteriovenous fistula (Bryant et al. 1958, Vollmar 1968, Johnson and Eiseman 1969, Rich and Spencer 1978).

In most cases of postoperative venous thrombosis, however, this serious injury of the venous wall is not present. In an experimental study in rabbits, a thrombus was induced by a combination of transitory stasis and stimulation with an electrical current of low voltage (Day et al. 1977). Electron microscopy examination revealed a normal venous wall, but approximately 5 min after induction of the current a fibrin network formed, and this happened before platelet aggregates were observed. Platelet pseudopodia formed after approximately 30 min, and then the thrombus formation proceeded.

It has been confirmed by phlebography that venous thrombi derive from valve pockets where the blood flow is comparatively stagnant in conditions with impaired venous drainage (McLachlin et al. 1960). In a lightmicroscopic study of valve pocket thrombi, the oldest and most distal parts were composed of erythrocytes and fibrin, while there were platelet aggregates in the growth zones (Sevitt 1974). Diener (1975) also found that the oldest parts were localized in the bottom of the valve pocket.

Lightmicroscopy studies have revealed no endothelial injury associated with such microthrombi in man (Sevitt 1974, Havig 1977). Recent studies have, however, demonstrated a pO_2 decrease under conditions of stasis in venous valve pockets (Malone et al. 1979, Hamer et al 1981). It is theoretically possible to have a minimal endothelial injury which cannot be detected by light microscopy, perhaps not even by electron microscopy, but where thrombus-inducing substances are still being released. Under anoxia gaps are formed between endothelial cells (Morrison et al. 1977). On the other hand, Havig (1977), in his autopsy study, often found that the valve pockets were not affected by the thrombotic process in spite of pronounced changes of the venous system in general. This might be explained by the fact that the valvular endothelium has a higher fibrinolytic activity than the venous wall endothelium in general (Astrup et al. 1971).

It might be possible to go further with the aid of electron microscopy. Studies to that effect have been performed by Stewart (1975, Stewart et al. 1978), who showed an increased vascular permeability and leukocyte migration through the vein wall in an experimental model using dogs, where a combination of stasis and trauma was used. In a similar experimetal situation using rabbits, the incidence of thrombosis was high (about 70%) following partial venous ligature and trauma, but the development of thrombosis appears not to be related to the presence of phlebitis (Bergqvist, Rausing and Åberg, unpublished data).

Neutrophils adhering to an area with transient stasis release proteases capable of activating the coagulation process (Lerner et al. 1977). In contrast, it has not been proven that these changes of the vein wall are a preliminary stage of thrombus formation. On the basis of experimental studies in rabbits with agranulocytosis, it can also be questioned whether or not the granulocytes and their migration through the vein wall play an important role initially in the development of thrombosis (Lerner et al. 1974).

However, ADP-induced platelet aggregation in the microcirculation and in the femoral vein may, in experimental situations, give rise to scattered vascular injuries, with the disappearance of endothelial cells, degeneration of the internal elastic membrane, edema, and aggregation of leukocytes (Vasalli et al. 1963, Inagaki 1968, Jørgensen et al. 1970). Thrombin may also induce damage of endothelial cells (Barnhardt and Chen 1978, Cazenave et al. 1979). At any rate, the absence of more extensive endothelial injuries in venous thrombosis contrasts sharply with the severe damage associated with arterial thrombosis.

The fibrinolytic system is an important part of the body's defense against thrombi and intravascular coagulation. The vein walls, and especially the endothelium, contain plasminogen activators capable of enzymatic transformation of plasminogen into plasmin (Fearnley 1965, Astrup 1966, Pandolfi 1970, Åstedt ct al. 1971). A release of such activators occurs, for instance, in venous stasis and in different stress situations (Nilsson and Pandolfi 1970, Robertson et al. 1972a, b, c, Cash 1975). A reduced content in the vein walls of such activators is an important and not altogether rare cause of venous thrombosis (Pandolfi et al. 1969). In the postoperative period following resection of the rectum, the content of fibrinolytic activators decreases significantly, and low values are more often noted in patients developing postoperative thrombosis (Åberg et al. 1974, Åberg and Nilsson 1978). The activator production also decreases in the majority of patients after transvesical prostatectomy but not after transurethral prostatic resection (Ljungnér and Isaksson 1979, Ljungnér et al 1982b). The decrease occurs during surgery and lasts for at least 2 weeks (Ljungnér et al. 1982b). Experimentally, trauma decreases the amount of activators, which is manifested by a reduced fibrinolytic activity in the blood (Wu and Mansfield 1980). Administration of tranexamic acid (AMCA) — a plasminogen inhibitor, almost routinely used in prostatic surgery — does not affect the plasminogen activator content in the vein wall (Åstedt et al. 1978).

Estrogen therapy, which has been discussed as a risk factor in thrombosis, appears to reduce the fibrinolytic activator content in the vein wall when used after the menopause (Åstedt 1971) and prostatic cancer (Carlsson and Åstedt 1974, Varenhorst 1980).

Patients with a post-thrombotic syndrome have a lower fibrinolytic activator content in their superficial veins than healthy individuals and patients with varicose veins (Wolfe et al. 1979). These patients also run a greater risk of developing a fresh thrombus with a surgical operation.

In cadavers, the fibrinolytic activator content appears to be lower in the soleal veins than in the femoral and popliteal veins (Nicolaides et al. 1972a). This has been suggested as one of the reasons why the postoperative thrombotic process occurs more frequently in this part of the venous system. Recent investigations where vein biopsies were taken at the same level during an amputation have nonetheless shown that the deep veins have a higher content of plasminogen activators (Ljungnér et al. 1981a).

Johnson and Mansfield (1978) found a significantly reduced content of plasminogen activators in the greater saphenous vein with increasing age (20–80 years). Age is probably the most important single risk factor for the formation of postoperative thrombosis. The endothelial cells have also been considered to be a source of fibrinolytic inhibitors (Dosne et al. 1978).

Another factor released from the vein wall endothelium is coagulation factor VIII (Bloom et al. 1973, Jaffee et al. 1973, Holmberg et al. 1974). Its von Willebrand activity is important for initiating hemostasis. In connection with trauma of different origin, e.g., surgical operations, the content of factor VIII-related antigen (VIII:Ag) in the blood rises (Butler et al. 1975, Nilssen 1979). This increase may play a role in the pathogenesis of thrombosis in different stress situations and pathologic conditions (Nilsson 1979). When epidural analgesia is used the postoperative increase of VIII:Ag does not occur (Rem et al. 1981). Not until a few years ago, however, was it possible to understand the various functions of factor VIII. In this field, many new findings are anticipated in the near future. Factor VIII plays an important role in the influence of dextran on the hemostatic system (p. 132).

The content of plasminogen activators and factor VIII rises in the plasma after administration of various so-called vasoactive substances, such as adrenalin, vasopressin, and nicotinic acid, indicating a release from the vascular endothelium (Mannucci et al. 1975). The release of plasminogen activators and VIIIR:Ag has been shown to be closely related (Nilsson et al. 1980a, b).

One more vein wall factor is of potential importance in the pathogenesis of thrombosis. It is probably released by the endothelium and is called prostacyclin or prostaglandin I_2 (PGI_2) (Fig. 3). (For review see Harlan and Harker 1981.)

PGI_2 is synthetized from arachidonic acid via cyclic endoperoxides. The first step (arachidonic acid → endoperoxides) is mediated by the enzyme cyclo-oxygenase, and the second step (endoperoxide → prostacyclin) is mediated by prostacyclin synthetase.

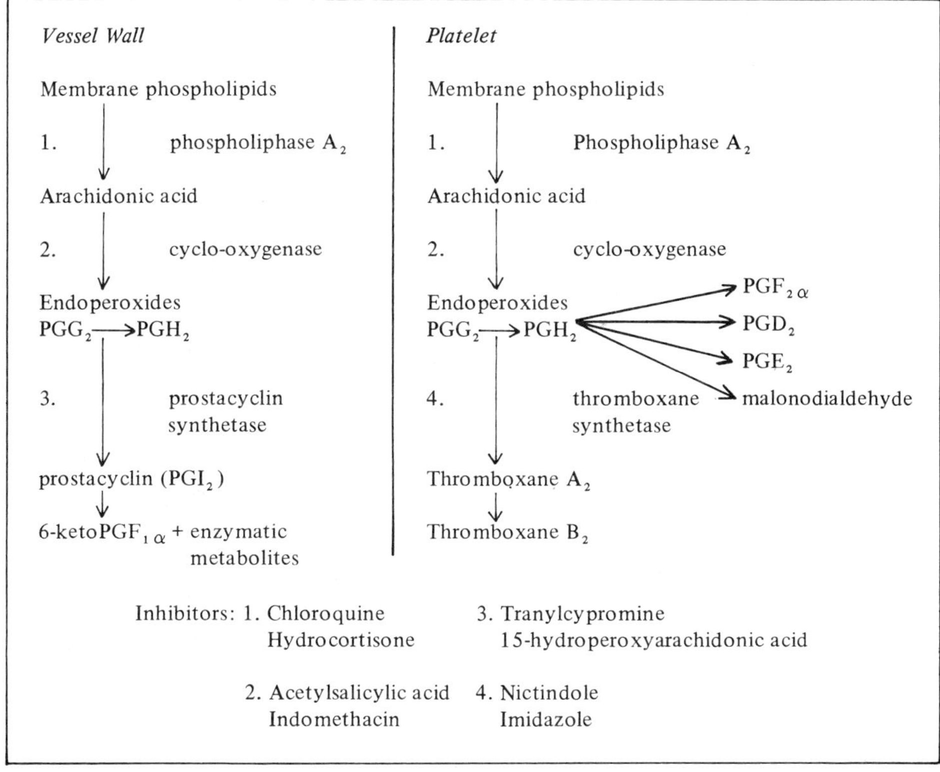

Fig. 3. Prostaglandin metabolism

Cyclo-oxygenase is inhibited by acetylsalicylic acid (see p. 121). PGI_2 is very unstable, with a half-life in plasma of approximately 120 s (Gryglewski et al. 1976, Moncada et al. 1976). Great methodologic difficulties exist in the determination of the PGI_2 concentration. PGI_2 is hydrolyzed to a stable end product: 6-ketoprostaglandin-$F_1\alpha$ (Cho and Allen 1978, Sun et al. 1978, Tansik et al. 1978). Recent findings indicate that PGI_2 is continuously produced in the lungs, and thus should be capable of affecting circulating platelets (Gryglewski et al. 1978, Moncada et al. 1978). This is, however, subject to discussion (Needleman 1979, Kelton and Blajchman 1980).

The exact physiologic role of the substance is still unclear, but it is a very potent inhibitor of platelet aggregation and causes marked vasodilatation (Moncada et al. 1976, Moncada and Vane 1978, Sinzinger et al. 1978). The probable mechanism by which PGI_2 inhibits platelet aggregation is by stimulating adenylate cyclase, thereby increasing the intracellular concentration of cyclic AMP (Tateson et al. 1977, Gorman et al. 1977, Gerrard and White 1978). Both cyclic AMP and PGI_2 inhibit thrombin-induced phospholipase A_2 activity in the platelet membranes, thus preventing thromboxane A_2 synthesis (Lapetina et al. 1977, Minkes et al. 1977). Thromboxane A_2 is a very potent stimulator of platelet aggregation (p. 45).

PGI_2 can also inhibit the adhesion of platelets. The amount necessary to produce this effect is much higher than physiologic concentrations (Higgs et al. 1978). Whether or not a PGI_2 deficiency can give rise to thrombosis is not known, and its postoperative importance has not been studied in detail. Most of the PGI_2 is inactivated in peripheral tissues, which means that the arterial concentration is much higher than the venous concentration (Hensby et al. 1979).

Recently, ADPase activity in the vessel walls from different animals has also attracted attention (Heyns et al. 1974, 1977, Lieberman et al. 1977, Cooper et al. 1979). ADPase degrades ADP to AMP and adenosine in sufficient quantities to induce inhibition of platelet aggregation. So far, this enzyme has primarily been studied on the arterial side of the circulation.

Finally, the presence of different glucosaminoglycans can also contribute to the athrombiogenicity of normal endothelium (see Lindahl and Höök 1978). Endothelial cells contain heparan sulfate, which has a heparin-like effect (Buonassisi 1973, Murata et al. 1975, Kraemer 1977, Wasteson et al. 1977), although this effect is much less pronounced than that of heparin (Teien et al. 1976a). In fact 80% of the glucosaminoglycans of the vascular endothelium consist of heparan sulfate, the rest being hyaluronic acid, chondroitin sulfate, and heparin. Heparan sulfate accelerates inactivation of thrombin by antithrombin III. Dermatan sulfate has a similar effect and is present at least in aortic endothelium (Hatton et al. 1978). Chondroitin sulfate and hyaluronic acid, on the other hand, do not produce this effect (Hatton et al. 1978). SSHA (p. 113), an interesting substance from a thromboprophylactic point of view, possibly acts by releasing heparan sulfate from the vascular endothelium (Thomas et al. 1979). Heparan sulfate may also act as a carrier of negative surface charges, which has been claimed to be an important part of the athrombogenicity of the endothelium (Sawyer and Srinivasan 1973).

Furthermore, antithrombin III has been found in the cells of vascular endothelium (Chan and Chan 1979, Awbrey et al. 1979).

Changes in the Blood Flow

Although Virchow (1856) pointed out the importance of decreased blood flow in the development of a thrombus, Aschoff (1912) further stressed the idea that without a reduced flow no thrombus will form. On the other hand, it is well known that stasis per se does not induce thrombosis. A column of blood between two ligatures in a vein will not clot for more than 3 h (Hewson 1771, Senftleben 1879, Wessler 1952, Marin 1961).

Changes in the intraoperative blood flow have been studied by several methods and the results have been somewhat contradictory. Part of the confusion in this area, other than methodologic differences, is probably because of the fact that "venous stasis" is not always clearly defined and may have different meanings in different contexts. It is important to distinguish at least between volume flow (volume per time) and velocity of fluid (distance per time), and possibly pulsatility.

Jönsson (1951) and Doran et al. (1964), using ^{24}Na, measured the venous circulation time in the lower extremities and found that the time increased in relation to surgery, i.e., the venous flow velocity decreased. Similar results were obtained by Kemble (1971) using ^{125}I-hippuran, and by Becker and Schampi (1973) with xenon. Jansen (1972) nonetheless found a reduced time using different isotope-labeled substances immediately after surgery in patients still under anesthesia. The venous blood flow velocity was thus increased. According to Jansen, previous investigators had chiefly measured changes in the superficial blood flow. He was of the opinion that in an anesthetized patient the blood empties through a few large veins, and that the majority of the crural veins are collapsed; therefore venous reflux does not occur.

By serial phlebography, Hodgson (1964) was able to show that the use of intermittent positive pressure breathing during anesthesia reduced the venous drainage from the crural veins. This was later confirmed by Laaksonen et al. (1974). These authors also showed that the venous return during epidural analgesia, on the other hand, remained unchanged compared to preoperative values. Clark and Cotton (1968), using volume flow measurement with thermodilution technique, found a reduction of about 50% during anesthesia. This, therefore supports the results of investigations which have demonstrated a prolonged flow time. A 100% increase of the arterial flow assessed by plethysmography in surgery of the gallbladder was found by Lindström et al. (1977). This increase of the arterial flow was independent of the position, whereas the venous volume and venous emptying decreased with the patient in a horizontal position as compared to having the legs elevated above the level of the heart. This was still more accentuated with the use of abdominal retractors. Walser et al. (1980) also found an increased intraoperative blood perfusion in the lower extremities but only when using neuroleptic analgesia.

With the aid of a combination of serial phlebography and ^{125}I-fibrinogen clearance measurements it has been shown that venous drainage from the legs occurs in two phases: rapid drainage from the major veins, and slow drainage from the soleal veins (Nicolaides et al. 1972d). The slow phase may extend over several minutes. On occlusion of the aorta, the time of contrast clearance increases markedly, up to 60 min (Lewis et al. 1972). However, when a substance is used which is not recirculating, there is no sign of a biphasic emptying, but it is continuous. Mathematically, the emptying can be expressed as two or at most three exponential functions (Bergqvist et al. 1982c). The use of serial contrast phlebography in such studies is not ideal as the contrast medium has different rheologic properties from that of blood.

Especially the valve pockets exhibit very slow drainage when the legs are in a horizontal position (Stanton et al. 1949, McLachlin et al. 1960). Apart from the slow drainage, turbulence and a concomitant increased interaction between the different blood cells may also develop. A turbulent flow markedly increases the risk of thrombus formation (Smith et al. 1972, Stein and Sabbah 1974). In vitro, Karino and Motomiya (1981) have demonstrated the occurrence of vortices in valve pockets and that blood corpuscles can spend as long as 10 s within the valve under physiologic flow conditions. During anesthesia, the calf muscle pump (Almén and Nylander 1962) does not work, particularly when drug-induced muscle relaxation is used. Also, a reduced flow rate increases blood viscosity (Wells 1969).

Intraoperative reduction of the arterial perfusion could possibly also contribute to the reduced volume flow (Browse 1962). Bird (1972) found that the arterial inflow to the calf is reduced to about 58% of the normal value during the early postoperative period after general anesthesia, whereas epidural analgesia induces a postoperative increase in the arterial flow (Modig et al. 1980b).

The intraoperative slowing down of the drainage of the muscle veins has been clarified. Using the ^{125}I-fibrinogen test, it has also been possible to show both that the majority of postoperative thrombi are located in the calves, and that the onset of thrombosis occurs in very close connection to the operation. These facts lend support to the assumption that an impeded drainage plays an important role (Flanc et al. 1968, Negus et al. 1968, Flute et al. 1972, Nicolaides and Gordon-Smith 1975). Most of these thrombi will remain in the calf or be spontaneously lysed; 78% according to Kakkar et al. (1969b).

Thrombi located in the iliofemoral segment may give rise to extensive pulmonary emboli. Postoperatively, most cases are characterized by a proximal extension of thrombi from the calf veins, whereas isolated proximal thrombi are rarely seen. In 73 general surgery patients, no isolated proximal thrombi were detected by combined fibrinogen test and ultrasound (Bolton and Hoffman 1975). Even thrombi detected postmortem are rarely isolated in the iliofemoral segment (Havig 1977, autopsy; Diener 1975, postmortem intraosseous venography). Yet, as a source of pulmonary emboli, thrombi extending into the iliofemoral segment are of great importance (Mavor and Galloway 1967, 1969, Linder et al. 1967, Bertelsen 1971, Havig 1977).

The venous system in the soles of the feet is another low-flow area, called "the Sargasso sea, where the eels are born" by Ask-Upmark (1963). In Havig's (1977) autopsy study, plantar vein thrombi were relatively common and occasionally gave rise to pulmonary embolism. Still, postoperatively the calf is the most common location of a thrombus, and plantar vein thrombi are then comparatively rare (Bergqvist and Hallböök 1978a). By phlebograms, the most common thrombus locations are the soleal and tibial veins (Nicolaides et al. 1972e).

It is not clear how a thrombus attaches to the venous wall. According to certain authors, one of the factors involved may be a mechanical retention in the valve pockets (Paterson 1969, Hume et al. 1970). However, postoperative thrombi also occur in the valveless soleal veins, suggesting mechanisms of attachment other than purely physical ones. Experimental thrombi have been shown to be so firmly attached that they can withstand a perfusion pressure of 10–20 cm H_2O (Stewart et al. 1973), and electron microscopy has demonstrated that these thrombi appear to be fastened to the vein wall by fibrin threads (Steward 1975).

Proximal venous obstruction will cause distal stasis, e.g., temporarily by the pressure of abdominal retractors during surgery, and for longer periods of time by intrapelvic tumors or hematomas. A special situation occurs toward the end of pregnancy, when the pregnant uterus exerts pressure on the inferior vena cava (Kerr et al. 1964), thus impeding the venous return (A. Bergqvist et al. 1979, Bergqvist and Hallböök 1979a).

Following kidney transplantation, there is at least a theoretical possibility that the transplanted kidney will constitute a mechanical obstruction to venous drainage. Proximal thrombi also appear to be common in these patients (Joffe 1975a). Moreover, the vein is submitted to a surgical trauma.

For anatomic reasons, with a crossing artery isolated iliofemoral thrombi are much more common on the left side (May and Thurner 1956, Cockett and Lea Thomas 1965, Lea Thomas and Browse 1972, Johnsson et al. 1974, Dodd and Cockett 1976). The so-called iliac compression syndrome (Cockett and Lea Thomas 1965) with chronic stasis, venous claudication, and leg ulcers is mainly caused by such isolated iliofemoral thrombi, often combined with considerable lymph stasis. Other causes are various forms of external compression or obstructing fibrous strings inside the vein lumen; these fibrous bands are called venous spurs.

If hernioplasty using Cooper's ligament is made too tightly, a condition is created for an ipsilateral development of thrombosis (Brown et al. 1980). In such cases a direct intraoperative injury of the femoral vein is of course also possible.

A decreased venous blood flow per se probably does not cause thrombosis, but rather in combination with an activation of coagulation factors (Borgström et al. 1959, Wessler 1962, Wessler and Yin 1969). Stasis can certainly, in more than one way, facilitate local intravascular clotting and platelet aggregation. The thrombogenic- and platelet-affecting substances released are not washed away effectively, but are concentrated locally. Circulating inhibitors do not quite reach the target, and thus their concentration is low. On the other hand, the local release of fibrinolytic activators due to stasis will have an antithrombogenic effect.

When the flow is diminished, blood viscosity increases, which may induce thrombus formation (Wells 1969, Dormandy 1975). Surgical trauma increases viscosity, resulting in a decreased flow in the microcirculation, with diminished oxygen consumption (Dawidson et al. 1975). Blood viscosity also depends on the concentration of fibrinogen (Matsuda and Murakami 1976). This is important postoperatively, because the elevation of fibrinogen will augment the viscosity of the blood (see p. 45).

In a few studies, the preoperative blood viscosity was correlated to the postoperative development of thrombosis (Dormandy and Edelman 1973, Humphreys et al. 1976). The viscosity was higher in patients developing thrombosis diagnosed by fibrinogen test and phlebography. This was particularly marked in patients with malignant diseases (Humphreys et al. 1976). Nevertheless, it has not been possible to correlate the pre- and/or postoperative hematocrit to the postoperative development of thrombosis (Dormandy and Edelman 1973, Pletscher and Gruber 1977).

An example which illustrates the importance of stasis very well is the great difference in the incidence of thrombosis between the paralyzed and the healthy leg in hemiplegic patients (Cope et al. 1973, Gibbard et al. 1976, Warlow et al. 1976). Another example is the increased incidence of thrombosis detected at autopsy, when there has been a prolonged period of bed rest before death (Hunter et al. 1945, Havig 1977, Eriksson and Saldeen 1979). The highest risk of thrombosis occurs during the first 14 days of bed rest (Havig 1977). This can be explained by the fact that the fibrinolytic activity of a normally active person is 3 to 4 times greater in the arms than in the legs (Menon et al. 1971a, Robertson et al. 1972b). But after 14 days of bed rest the fibrinolytic activity of the legs increases to the same level as that of the arms (Karaca and Nilsson 1971). This fits with the observation that the frequency of thrombosis is lower if the diagnosis starts with the fibrinogen test after the first 10 days (Miyamoto and Miller 1980).

Changes of Blood Properties

Platelet Changes

The structure of a platelet head and a fibrin tail is not as pronounced in venous as in arterial thrombi (Sevitt 1978). Whether the initial phase of thrombus development consists of platelet aggregation to a damaged vein wall, or whether platelet aggregation develops due to the release of thrombin or ADP, is still unclear. However, platelets as well as other blood cells collect in the "backwater" of the valve pockets. Turbulence phenomena increase the danger of collision between the various corpuscular elements, and ADP may be released from red blood cells as well as from platelets in such an environment. Under low-flow conditions, the platelets do not adhere as easily to a damaged vein wall as when under high-flow conditions (Baumgartner and Haudenschild 1972). This can partly explain the morphologic difference between arterial and venous thrombosis.

The idea that platelets should play a very important role in the initial formation of a venous thrombus is partly contradicted by the fact that various platelet-modifying agents have been shown to have a thromboprophylactic effect only in a few cases (see p. 120). Nor is the platelet turnover particularly affected in venous thrombosis (Harker and Slichter 1972b).

A great deal of attention has been given to the study of platelet changes after trauma, both with respect to their number and their reaction pattern. The latter has mainly been assessed as the aggregating capacity of the platelets employing Born's method (1962), where the physiologic substances ADP, thrombin, and collagen have most often been used to induce aggregation, or their capacity to adhere to foreign surfaces, especially to glass (e.g., Hellem 1960). After trauma, the platelets increase in number and reach a maximum 4–10 days later, often following an initial fall during the first 2–3 days (Warren et al. 1953, Bergentz and Nilsson 1961, Innes and Sevitt 1964, Bennett 1967, Ygge 1970, Hergt 1972, Hedlund and Blombäck 1979). The initial fall is probably due to an accumulation of platelet aggregates in the lungs (Ljungqvist et al. 1971).

Concurrently with the rise in the number of platelets, an increased reactivity has also been shown (Payling Wright 1942, Warren et al. 1953, Emmons and Mitchell 1965, Bennett 1967, Ham and Slack 1967, Cockburn et al. 1973).

Studies have also demonstrated a decreased platelet activity during surgery and immediately postoperatively, leading to a significant prolongation of the bleeding time (Kokores et al. 1977, Yamazaki et al. 1979). ADP-induced platelet aggregation increases during the first postoperative week. In women who underwent hysterectomy, this increased tendency toward aggregation persisted for at least 1 month, whereas in women who underwent both total hysterectomy and total oophorectomy it was normalized after a month, and was significantly lower than in the former group (Yamazaki et al. 1979). This has been ascribed to the fact that estrogen favors platelet activity. In a similar way an increased platelet aggregability has been shown in patients treated with estrogen because of prostatic carcinoma (Eisen et al. 1975).

It has not, however, been possible to correlate the postoperative increase in platelet adhesiveness either to the extent of the surgical trauma (Ardlie et al. 1967) or to postoperative thrombus development (Negus et al. 1969, Becker 1972c). Only in a few cases do patients with idiopathic or spontaneous venous thrombosis have an increased platelet adhesiveness (Isacson and Nilsson 1972a).

Thus, there is at present little proof that an increased number of platelets or an increased reactivity per se causes venous thrombosis. In an experimental model, where arterial and venous thrombi were compared, venous thrombi formed in spite of a very low number of platelets (S. Olsson 1974). On the other hand, fibrinogen was necessary for venous thrombus formation.

β-thromboglobulin – a platelet-specific protein released during aggregation (Moore et al. 1975) – increases in deep vein thrombosis, but in patients developing thrombi detected by fibrinogen test postoperatively, the increase is not significant (Smith et al. 1978a). Plasma-β-thromboglobulin increases with age (Zahavi et al. 1980a).

King and Joffe (1974) have described a platelet function test which measures platelet thromboplastin generation. They found that thrombi rarely occur in patients with a normal test, whereas they occur frequently in patients with a positive test.

Although little is known about the postoperative metabolism of arachidonic acid, a short summary of the prostaglandin synthesis of the platelets should be given, since knowledge of this mechanism is of importance for discussion of the mode of action of acetylsalicylic acid (see p. 121). Figure 3 (p. 39) shows the different steps in the synthesis. Arachidonic acid is formed from phospholipids in the platelet membranes, and then synthesized to cyclic endoperoxides (a cyclo-oxygenase reaction), inducing platelet aggregation on release (Willis and Kuhn 1973, Hamberg et al. 1974, Smith et al. 1974). In the platelets, the endoperoxides are further metabolized to thromboxane A_2, a very unstable product with a half-life of 30 s (Hamberg et al. 1975). Thromboxane A_2 is a very potent platelet-aggregating substance, which is released during the aggregation (Hamberg et al. 1975, Smith et al. 1976a, b, Moncada and Vane 1977). Thromboxane A_2 is spontaneously degraded to a stable thromboxane B_2, which is inactive against the platelets. In knee surgery, when the blood flow is reestablished after tourniquet-induced ischemia, the thromboxane B_2 level in plasma rises significantly (Zahavi et al. 1980b). These results have also been experimentally reproduced in pigs, where platelet aggregation on deendothelialized surfaces could be observed when the leg veins had been ischemic for 1 h.

Proof of a physiologic role in the hemostatic system of prostaglandin endoperoxides and thromboxane A_2 exists in the form of mild hemorrhages in patients lacking cyclo-oxygenase and thromboxane synthetase (Malmsten et al. 1975, Weiss and Lages 1977, Lagarde et al. 1978, Nyman et al. 1979, Pareti et al. 1980). The mild hemostatic defect indicates that platelet arachidonic metabolism is not essential, and the precise role in hemostasis and thrombosis remains to be fully defined.

Changes in Coagulation Factors

It has been known for a long time that the fibrinogen level rises after trauma, reaching a maximum after 3–4 days (Foster and Whipple 1922, Olow 1963). This is a reaction pattern common to many plasma proteins such as orosmucoid, haptoglobin, ceruloplasmin, and antichymotrypsin (Aronsen et al. 1972), as a general response to trauma.

After trauma, other coagulation factors exhibit variations in plasma, in most cases a rise, and a "hypercoagulable" state has also been discussed. It is considered improbable that such a state should be of etiologic importance in venous thrombosis. It could, however, be important for the thrombus growth. Wessler (1975a) is of the opinion that a hypercoagulable state exists when there is an increased acitivation of factor X, possibly through a deficiency in factor Xa inhibitor (see p. 47).

Fibrinogen and factors II, V, VII, and XIII increase postoperatively. This increase largely parallels the increase in the number of platelets (Egeberg 1962, Godal 1962, Ygge 1970), with an initial fall immediately after the operation (Olow 1963, Ljungqvist et al. 1969). After kidney transplantation in patients with uremia, however, no fibrinogen increase is seen (Ljungqvist et al. 1969). Certain data indicate that this can be ascribed to a diminished fibrinogen synthesis secondary to uremia and not to the immunosuppressive therapy these patients receive (Ljungqvist et al. 1970).

After surgery the fibrinogen turnover increases (Hickman 1971, Davies et al. 1970). The synthesis, plasma concentration, catabolism, and possibly also the fibrin formation rate increase (Davies et al. 1970). The biological half-life of fibrinogen is reduced by about 30%.

There are indications that hip arthroplasty induces a local increase of factors II, V, and VII in the operated extremity, which is significantly higher than in the central circulation (Houghton et al. 1978).

Changes in the concentration or activity of the coagulation factors alone do not produce a thrombus. Activation of the coagulation process combined with stasis leads to thrombus formation, but neither of these two factors alone will do so (Botti and Ratnoff 1964). The increase in fibrinogen can also be of importance because of the increased viscosity it produces (Dintenfass 1962, Matsuda and Muramaki 1976).

When Chandler thrombi are formed (Chandler 1958) ex vivo, they increase significantly in size and weight postoperatively. There is a statistically significant correlation between the size of the thrombus and the fibrinogen level (Ardlie et al. 1967). It has not been possible to correlate postoperative changes in the concentration of different coagulation factors to thrombus formation, however (Flute et al. 1972).

Thus, it is not only the quantity of a coagulation factor that is responsible for the thrombogenicity, but whether the factor is activated or not. This has been shown, for instance, with factor X using Wessler's stasis thrombosis model (Wessler and Yin 1968). Stasis thrombosis could not be produced with 630 units of factor X, but a quantity as small as 5 units of activated factor X was thrombogenic. In trauma, factor X activation is possible via the intrinsic as well as the extrinsic coagulation system. Factor X activation is the common step for both, with subsequent formation of thrombin, which induces both platelet aggregation and fibrin formation. A great deal of the discussion on thromboprophylaxis today concerns the activation of factor X and the possibility of influencing it.

Attempts have been made to correlate late steps in the coagulation process to thrombus formation (Fletcher et al. 1972), but no great success is expected. No correlation between fibrinopeptide A (determined according to Nossel et al. 1974, Kockum-Ivemark's modification 1979) and postoperative thrombus formation, as assessed by the ^{125}I-fibrinogen test, has been shown (Törngren et al. 1979b). Nevertheless, the method of analysis is relatively complex, and the sampling procedure is a very critical step. Hence, the patient population in the study mentioned was too small to permit any definite conclusion.

On the other hand, the serum level of fibrinopeptide A rises postoperatively both clinically (Törngren et al. 1979b) and experimentally (Medén-Britth and Rådegran 1980), indicating thrombin activation.

By thromboelastography, a measure of the total coagulability of the blood is obtained (Scott Blair and Matchett 1972). By diluting the blood with physiologic saline in such a test system, the coagulation rate is increased. Heather et al. (1980) found that patients developing postoperative thrombi have a preoperatively significant increase in coagulation rate after dilution.

Inhibitor Changes

The varios inhibitors play an important role in the prevention of thrombus formation in the venous system. The physiologic importance of these coagulation inhibitors has attracted a great deal of interest.

The most important inhibitor is a α_2-globulin which inhibits both thrombin and activated factor X (Xa). It is called antithrombin III or Xa-inhibitor (Yin et al. 1971a). An increased danger of thrombosis in patients with a deficiency of antithrombin III was described for the first time in Norway in the form of a familial deficiency with development of early thrombi (Egeberg 1965). Since then several such families have been described. The antithrombin III defect can also vary as to type (Sas et al. 1974).

Postoperatively, the antithrombin III level falls (Olsson 1963, Stathakis et al. 1973, Åberg et al. 1973, Hedlund and Blombäck 1979, Schipper 1980), but no correlation with postoperative thrombus formation has been shown (Åberg et al. 1973, Ishaka and Morley 1981). Gitel et al. (1979) and Seyfer et al. (1981) were able to show that the decrease of antithrombin III occurred intraoperatively and the greater the trauma the more pronounced the decrease. The postoperative reduction in antithrombin III is especially pronounced in patients with a bacterial infection as a postoperative complication (Schipper 1980, Schipper et al. 1981). This group of patients is particularly prone to postoperative thromboembolism (Törngren 1979b). There are other studies, however, showing no influence on antithrombin III in relation to surgery (Hedner and Nilsson 1973). A Norwegian research group found in a small series of patients that the development of postoperative thrombosis following elective hip surgery was related to a significantly lower preoperative level of antithrombin III than that exhibited by patients without thrombi (95.5% vs. 106.1%; Nilsen et al. 1980).

A method for the determination of Xa-inhibitor (Xa-I) developed by Yin and Wessler (1970) was used by Stamatakis et al. (1977c) to study whether Xa-inhibitor is affected by surgery, and whether preoperative Xa-inhibitor measurement could be used to predict postoperative thrombus formation. Patients taking oral contraceptives exhibited preoperative Xa-inhibitor reduction. Patients undergoing hip arthroplasty who postoperatively developed a phlebographically confirmed thrombus had significantly lower preoperative Xa-inhibitor values than patients with no thrombi. Also in a series of patients undergoing elective abdominal surgery, patients developing postoperative thrombosis had a preoperative decrease in Xa-inhibitor (Kruse-Blinkenberg et al. 1980). This lowered preoperative level in patients prone to thrombosis was not verified in another study (Wallenbeck et al. 1979). In patients developing postoperative thromboembolic complications, however, significantly lower Xa-inhibitor values were seen postoperatively than in patients without such complications. Using the same method for Xa-I determination, Gunn (1979) was not able to show any correlation between the concentration of Xa-I and postoperative thrombus formation.

Three other protease inhibitors — α_2-antiplasmin, α_2-macroglobulin, and α_1-antitrypsin — were studied by Taberner et al. (1979) in relation to surgery. No increased concentration of these inhibitors could be demonstrated postoperatively in patients developing a thrombus. On the contrary, the α_2-antiplasmin level fell. In other studies, the α_1-antitrypsin level rose (Aronsen et al. 1972, Lahnborg and Bergström 1975, Paul and Medén-Britth 1975, Hedlund and Blombäck 1979). In patients undergoing elective hip surgery Bagge and Saldeen (1978), Bagge et al. (1979), and Carlin et al.

(1980) found an increased inhibition of fibrinolysis, reaching a maximum on the third postoperative day. In patients with thromboembolism discovered at autopsy, a higher plasmin inhibitory activity was found in the great saphenous vein than in patients without thromboembolism (Eriksson and Saldeen 1980). An immediate postoperative lowering of the antiplasmin level was noted by Teger-Nilsson et al. (1978), followed by a significant rise.

Changes in Fibrinolysis

The earliest publication on fibrinolysis in connection with surgery probably dates from 1937, when MacFarlane discovered that blood from a cholecystectomized patient showed normal coagulation, but was unclotted on the first postoperative day.

Intraoperatively, and during the first few hours post-trauma, the fibrinolytic activity is increased (Bergentz and Nilsson 1961, Andersson et al. 1962, Leandoer 1968, Macintyre et al. 1976, T.E. O'Brien et al. 1979). There is a significant decrease in fibrinolytic activity in the first postoperative days (Ygge 1970, Mansfield 1972, Knight et al. 1977, T.E. O'Brien et al. 1979). Such a decrease could be demonstrated by Browse et al. (1977) only in patients developing a thrombus or in patients with an underlying malignant disease. Preoperatively, there was no difference between these groups of patients. In a study of patients with fractures of the femur, a reduced fibrinolytic capacity in systemic blood and blood from the unfractured leg was observed 2 and 10 days after the trauma, while fibrinolytic activity in the arm was normal (Rawles et al. 1975).

Becker (1972a) and Reilly et al. (1980) could not correlate the preoperative fibrinolytic status with postoperative thrombus formation, but several authors (Flute et al. 1972, Mansfield 1972, Gordon-Smith et al. 1974, Knight et al. 1977, Åberg and Nilsson 1978) found that patients developing postoperative thrombi had a significantly lower fibrinolytic activity than those without thrombi. Some authors have not detected any difference between patients with and without postoperative thrombosis (Macintyre et al. 1976), while others have identified an increased fibrinolysis (Reilly et al. 1980).

In two prospective studies, a significant correlation was found between a prolonged lysis time during the postoperative period and the development of thrombosis detected with the fibrinogen test (Flute et al. 1972, Comp et al. 1979). An increased concentration of the inhibitor of plasminogen activator means a clearly increased risk of thrombus formation (Nilsson et al. 1961, Pandolfi et al. 1970, Nilsson 1977). This inhibitor was later shown to inhibit activated factor XII (Hedner and Martinsson 1978), and is thus of importance in the intrinsic or factor XII-dependent fibrinolytic system.

Postoperatively, the concentration of immunochemically determined factor XIIa inhibitator falls to a minimum on days 2–4. The decrease appears to be related to the extent of the trauma. Concurrently with this change, factor XII – the Hageman factor – also falls (Hedner et al. 1983). The interpretation of these findings is not easy, but the simultaneous fall in factor XII and factor XIIa inhibitor could be due to a consumption of these factors, indicating an activation of factor XII, with subsequent inhibition of factor XIIa. Whether or not the factor XII-dependent fibrinolysis is of importance for the pathogenesis of postoperative thrombosis is so far unknown.

Of particular interest are the changes in the fibrinolytic system which occur with surgery of the lower extremities in a bloodless area, since tourniquet-induced ischemia has been suggested as a possible thromboprophylactic measure (Klenerman et al. 1977, Lahnborg et al. 1977, Fahiny and Patel 1981). During the tourniquet-induced ischemia for knee surgery, the concentration of plasminogen activator in superficial veins increases (Larsson and Risberg 1977). When the blood returns, the concentration is normalized, and on the second postoperative day a decrease is seen, with a return to normal values on the 5th day. In the extremity not undergoing surgery, no such changes are observed.

The initially increased tissue activator concentration is reflected in an increase in the fibrinolytic capacity of the blood up to 15 min after ischemia is discontinued (Klenerman et al. 1977, Fahiny and Patel 1981). Long periods of ischemia result in a disturbance of the metabolic function and a lowered production of plasminogen activators (Romanus and Risberg 1978). The favorable increase in fibrinolytic activity from a thromboprophylactic viewpoint is then followed by a decrease, which could have a deleterious result.

It has also been stated that the incidence of thrombosis is higher in the leg occluded by a tourniquet than in the other leg (Risberg 1977), but other authors claim the opposite (Fahiny and Patel 1981).

In a recent study in monkeys, it was shown that tourniquet ischemia (400 mg Hg) for 2½ h produced laboratory values in the ischemic leg similar to those in intravascular coagulation and fibrinolysis. The findings showed a decrease in fibrinogen, antithrombin III, and plasminogen levels in the involved extremity and an increase in fibrin degradation products (FDP) and fibrinopeptide A. When the animals were treated with heparin, only the increase in FDP remained (Miller et al. 1979).

Postoperative Thrombosis. A Pathogenetic Hypothesis

Thrombosis is multifactorial, and a combination of different pathogenetic factors is required to produce a thrombus. The changes in circulating blood described above are general, but the thrombi are almost exclusively localized in the lower extremities. The onset of thrombosis occurs in most cases in areas of decreased blood flow, e.g., valve pockets and muscle vein sinusoids, and there is much evidence in favor of an intraoperative onset. In these areas the conditions are favorable for "back water flowing", turbulence, and rheologic changes which might be thrombogenic and also lead to an enhanced viscosity. There is experimental evidence that the turbulence is thrombogenic (i.e., Smith et al. 1972). By histologic examination of thrombi, where it has been possible to trace the origin to valve pockets, the oldest parts of the thrombus were encountered in the bottom of the valve pocket. Corpuscular elements accumulate, and various substances favoring coagulation and platelet aggregation concentrate. Wall injuries, to such a degree that collagen is exposed, occur only rarely in venous thrombosis. Whether the initial procedure in the thrombotic process consists of platelet aggregation or clotting is still an open question. At present, progress toward answers to these questions is limited by considerable methodologic difficulties.

Wall injuries of electron microscopic magnitude have been demonstrated which have resulted in changes in permeability. Local anoxia could possibly contribute to these changes. Local thrombin formation may occur due to an accumulation of activated coagulation factors formed locally or having been transported from some other part of the organism, e.g., a field of operation. Thrombin in quantities small enough not to induce coagulation can, however, lead to platelet aggregation, supporting the hypothesis that platelet aggregation is the primary event (Zucker and Borelli 1955). Moreover, thrombin can cause damage of the endothelial cells. ADP may be released from the red cells under turbulent conditions, inducing momentary platelet aggregation. Such platelet aggregates may in turn damage the vessel wall. The erythrocytes probably play a more active role in hemostasis as well as thrombosis than earlier assumed — possibly by the release of ADP, but possibly also as a rheologic prerequisite for platelet collision (Bergqvist and Arfors 1980, Turitto and Weiss 1980). On the other hand, large doses of ADP resulting in a decrease in circulating platelets have not been capable of inducing thrombi in isolated venous segments (Stuart and Thomas 1967). This speaks against ADP being an important initial stimulator in thrombosis. More thrombin leads to coagulation and growth of the thrombus,which is finally determined by the balance between thrombogenic factors and the fibrinolytic defense. Most postoperative thrombi remain in the calf and are probably dissolved promptly.

Summary

Thrombosis is multifactorial; several different factors are probably implicated in the formation of a thrombus. The development of a thrombus is a complex process, known only in rough outline. Virchow's triad — changes in the blood flow, changes in the vessel wall, and changes in blood properties — still summarizes the most important aspects of the thrombopathogenesis. What initiates thrombus formation is still largely unknown, however, which makes it difficult to fight the disease by rational prophylaxis.

Risk Factors

As stated in the previous discussion of the pathogenesis of thrombosis, there are no general preoperative laboratory tests for platelets, coagulation, or fibrinolysis which can accurately predict whether or not a patient will develop a postoperative thrombus. In some cases a statistical difference has been demonstrated between two groups of patients — those developing thrombosis and those who do not — but in the individual case there is very little to go by. If it were possible to preoperatively identify patients who will develop postoperative thrombosis, selective prophylaxis would be possible. This would lower the costs of prophylaxis and also reduce the number of people being submitted to the risks involved.

It is a known fact, however, that the risk of thrombus formation is considerably increased if the patient exhibits certain specific defects in his hemostatic system, e.g., a low level of fibrinolytic activators, antithrombin III deficiency, or a high level of plasminogen activation inhibitors. Changes occurring postoperatively are of course of pathogenetic interest, but of little importance in the individual patient situation. Patients exhibiting postoperative deviations in laboratory values are rarely given antithrombotic therapy, even though it is a known fact that these changes are often correlated with thrombosis.

On the basis of epidemiologic and clinical investigations and autopsy studies, a number of more or less well-documented risk factors have been identified.

- Age (Borgström 1950, Johansson and Holmdahl 1945, Sevitt and Gallagher 1961, Linder et al. 1967, Flanc et al. 1969, Kakkar et al. 1970, Törngren et al. 1980a, Bernstein et al. 1980, Sikorski et al. 1981)
- Type of operation (see p. 12)
- Trauma (see p. 16)
- Prolonged operation (Forsberg and Törngren 1977, Rakoczi et al. 1980)
- Long immobilization (Hunter et al. 1945, Gibbs 1957, Sevitt and Gallagher 1961, Heatley et al. 1976)
- Previous thromboembolic disease (Kakkar et al. 1970, Schaub et al. 1975, Prescott et al. 1978)
- Varicose veins (Kakkar et al. 1970, Segal et al. 1975, Takkunen 1975)
- Malignancy in general (Coon and Coller 1959, Kakkar et al. 1970, Kohn et al. 1974, Roberts and Cotton 1974, Walsh et al. 1974, Schaub et al. 1975)
- Cancer of the prostate (Kasimis and Spiers 1979)
- Radiotherapy for uterine cancer (Jaswig and Jaswig-Prieme 1973)
- Obesity (Kakkar et al. 1970, Joffe et al. 1973, Kohn et al. 1974, Hume et al. 1976, van Geloven et al. 1977, Havig 1977)
- Cardiac disease (Gallus et al. 1973b, Simmons et al. 1973)
- Cardiac infarction (Nicolaides et al. 1971, Handley 1972, Handley et al. 1972, Warlow et al. 1973, Wray et al. 1973, Cristal et al. 1976, Miller et al. 1976, Emerson and Marks 1977)
- Cardiac insufficiency (Pitt et al. 1980)

- Infection (Nicolaides et al. 1972f, Fossard et al. 1974b, Törngren et al. 1980a)
- Cushing's syndrome (Sjöberg et al. 1976)
- Blood group A (Jick et al. 1969, Talbot et al. 1972)
- Blood group non-O (Jick and Porter 1978)
- Pregnancy and puerperium (Henderson et al. 1972, Bonnar 1975, Henry 1975)
- Use of oral contraceptives (Sagar et al. 1976b, Stamatakis et al. 1977c, Skillman et al. 1978, Vessey and Mann 1978, Böttiger et al. 1980, Tso et al. 1980)
- Estrogen medication (Åstedt et al. 1980, Järhult and Mårtensson 1980)
- Intravenous saline infusions in large amounts during surgery (Janvrin et al. 1980a,c)
- Treatment with substances favoring hemostasis (Vere et al. 1979)

Importance of the Type of Anesthesia

The importance of the type of anesthesia in thrombus formation has been discussed, but only recently have more systematic investigations started to appear. As early as 1943 Bohmansson claimed that patients at risk of thrombosis should be operated on using spinal analgesia.

Venous drainage is quicker in epidural analgesia than in general anesthesia (Laaksonen et al. 1974). This difference increases postoperatively in continuous epidural block (Modig et al. 1980b). Theoretically, therefore, there is evidence that epidural analgesia might have a certain thromboprophylactic effect. That this is the case has been suggested in some uncontrolled studies (Lahnborg and Bergström 1975, Lahnborg et al. 1977, Thorburn et al. 1980). In other studies, no such difference could be demonstrated (Bergqvist and Hallböök 1980).

Rem et al. (1981) compared the effect of general anesthesia and epidural analgesia on different coagulation and fibrinolytic factors. The only obvious finding was the lack of postoperative increase of the factor VIII-related antigen in the group receiving epidural analgesia. In patients who receive epidural block there is a less pronounced depression of the fibrinolytic system postoperatively (Saldeen et al. 1981).

In different prophylaxis studies, as a rule the type of anesthesia in the different groups is not mentioned. According to Carter and Eban (1973, 1974) no difference in the incidence of thrombosis between spinal, epidural, or some other form of anesthesia could be shown. In some studies, the kind of anesthesia used is stated, but no difference could be seen (Table 19).

However, in a group treated with oral anticoagulants for prophylactic purposes, Kunz et al. (1977) found a much lower incidence of thrombosis in the general anesthesia group versus the epidural analgesia group (0 of 16 vs 9 of 65). In a study with scintigraphically diagnosed pulmonary emboli, Nillius (1978) found no difference in the incidence between patients with neuroleptic analgesia or epidural analgesia (22.9% and 16.7%, respectively). Similar findings have also been encountered in a general surgery population (Allgood et al. 1970).

Bernstein et al. (1980) found no difference in the incidence of thrombosis between gynecologic patients receiving general anesthesia or epidural analgesia. A comparison between spontaneous and controlled respiration and between intermittent positive pressure ventilation and intermittent positive and negative pressure ventilation yielded no difference in the postoperative incidence of thrombosis (Laaksonen et al.

Table 19. Incidence of thrombosis following different types of anesthesia
Diagnosis of thrombosis by the ^{125}I-fibrinogen text, except by Barnes, who used ultrasound

Author	Type of surgery	Number of thrombi/ number of patients (%)	
		General anesthesia	Epidural/ spinal analgesia
Hirsjärvi et al. (1974)	Hip	7/12 ⎱ (50)	35/ 61 ⎱ (56)
Barnes et al. (1978)	Hip	3/ 8 ⎰	5/ 10 ⎰
McCarthey et al. (1974)	Gynecologic	8/65 ⎱	10/ 67 ⎱
Ballard et al. (1973)	Gynecologic	12/65 ⎭ (15)	6/ 45 ⎭ (12)
Kunz et al. (1977)	Gynecologic	5/39 ⎰	14/139 ⎰
Hassan et al. (1974)[a]	Urologic	8/77 (10)	2/ 27 (7)

[a]Sudanese patients.

1973, Takkunen 1975), although the flow rate in the femoral vein showed great variation between different types of respiration (Nicolaides 1975).

In the few studies performed using multivariate analysis of possible risk factors, no correlation between the form of anesthesia and the incidence of thrombosis could be shown using the ^{125}I-fibrinogen test (Hedlund 1975, Nicolaides and Irving 1975), nor could thromboembolic complications be detected at autopsy (Havig 1977).

In order to settle with greater certainty whether epidural analgesia is effective in thromboprophylaxis, a randomized study in an otherwise similar patient population would be required, where a choice could be made between epidural analgesia and general anesthesia. Suitable for such a study would be patients undergoing gynecologic, prostatic, or hip surgery. Such a study was recently performed by Modig et al. (1980a) in 30 patients undergoing elective hip surgery. The total incidence of detected thrombi by phlebography did not differ between the epidural analgesia and the general anaesthesia groups, but in the former the number of proximal emboli was significantly lower. The number of scintigraphically diagnosed pulmonary emboli was also significantly lower in the epidural analgesia group. Also Davis et al. (1980) found less fibrinogen test-detected thrombi in patients with hip fracture operated on in epidural analgesia than in patients receiving general anesthesia. The study was randomized, but objections could be raised against the use of Armitage's sequential analysis. In a randomized study on transvesical prostatectomy, the frequency of thrombosis was significantly lower in the epidural analgesia than in the general anesthesia group (Hendolin 1980).

Muscle relaxants affect several factors of possible importance in thrombus formation. The venous return to the heart is reduced, for instance. Theoretically, alcuronium should be preferable to curare, with less pronounced ganglion-blocking and no histamine-releasing effect (Stovner and Lund 1970, Feldman 1973). There is no difference, however, in the postoperative incidence of thrombosis between patients receiving these two agents (Takkunen 1975).

Geographic Factors

It has been stated that the incidence of thrombosis is lower outside Europe and the United States, and certain studies indicate that this is the case. In an autopsy comparison between Kyushu, Japan, and Boston, United States, of patients with comparable ages, the difference was obvious both regarding venous thromboembolism and myocardial infarction (Gore et al. 1964). A study of 782 344 autopsy reports including 18 090 cases of pulmonary embolism from different pathology departments showed an incidence of 2.5%–5% in Europe, the United States, and Canada, whereas South America and Asia had less than 0.5% (Sandritter and Felix 1967, Hwang 1968). In South Africa the incidence was 2.8% among Europeans, and 0.6% among Bantu blacks, while in the United States the incidence was approximately the same in black and white people. This fact, together with the reduction of thromboembolic complications in Germany and Norway during the two World Wars (Adelsten-Jensen 1952, Linder et al. 1967) led to the assumption that the nutritional state is a more important underlying factor than geographic factors and race. However, blacks as a group are much more poorly nourished than whites in the United States.

The incidence of fatal pulmonary embolism in connection with hip fractures has proved to be very low among Chinese (Bong and Chow 1977). Also postpartum thromboembolism is said to be much lower in nonoccidental societies (seven cases in 41 056 deliveries in Thailand; Chumnijarakij 1974). Nevertheless, very few studies have been performed in which firm conclusions have been possible, and in recently published

Table 20. The incidence of thrombosis in studies on non-Western patients
Diagnosis of thrombosis using the ^{125}I-fibrinogen test. All studies are based on a mixed general surgery population except Tso et al. (gynecologic surgery). The majority of patients are older than 40 years, mean age about 60 years

Author	Country	Number of patients	Incidence of thrombosis (%)
Baker and Houlder (1973)	South Africa[a]	72	11
Baker and Prajapat (1976)	South Africa[a]	125	16
Chumnijakakij and Poshya-chinda (1975)	Thailand	169	2.4
Cunningham and Young (1974)	Malaysia	68	13
Hassan et al. (1973)	Sudan	100	12
Joffe (1974)	South Africa, Europeans	50	48
	South Africa, non-Europeans	50	56
Latto (1979)	Nigeria	50	22
Nandi et al. (1980)	Hong Kong	150	2.6
Osime (1978)	Nigeria	112	30
Shead and Narayanan (1980)	South India	50	28
Tso et al. (1979)	Hong Kong	145	2.8
Williams et al. (1973)	Queensland	75	12

[a]Indians and Africans.

Nigerian investigations the incidence of thrombosis is similar to that of a Western population composed of the same type of patients (Table 20). Approximately the same incidence was also found by Joffe (1974) among European and non-European South Africans.

Tso et al. (1979) studied the incidence of thrombosis after gynecologic surgery. As appears in Table 20, the total incidence in this study is 2.8%. Among women taking oral contraceptives it was 5.4%, and in patients with malignancy 6.9%.

Among 53 Chinese from Hongkong with hip fractures, the phlebographically confirmed incidence of thrombosis in the fractured leg was 53%, in the healthy leg 14%. Eighty-five percent of these thrombi were localized to the calf (Mok et al. 1979). The incidence is of the same magnitude as in Westerners (Table 7).

The natural history of thrombosis does not appear to differ between occidental patients and what has been reported from Kenya, for instance (Colin et al. 1975).

In a few studies geographic differences have been shown, even within industrialized societies. Thus, a significantly higher postoperative incidence of thrombosis was found by Sripad et al. (1971) in London compared to some rural hospitals in Essex. The ^{125}I-fibrinogen test was used for diagnosis in this study. A higher incidence of thrombosis, as confirmed by phlebography, in Borås than in Ulricehamn, Sweden, was found by Kierkegaard (1980), but these figures are much less reliable than those in the English study. The difference may be related to different procedures in handling patients with suspected thrombosis.

Seasonal Variation

Seasonal variation in the incidence of thrombosis was reported in the mid-1940s (Allen et al. 1945), but the problem has not been further studied to any great extent. Publications from Australia suggest a possible variation with season, with a higher incidence during the cold months (Lawrence et al. 1977, Xabregas et al. 1978). In a South African study, however, the incidence of thrombosis was not found to vary with season (Groote Schuur Hospital 1979), whereas Smyrnis and Kolios (1973) from Athens found the highest incidence of thrombosis in summer.

An American analysis based on deaths due to venous disorders shows a statistically significant cyclic course with death peaks in December — January and lower figures for June — July during the years 1962–1967 (Feinleib 1972). Moreover, these deaths increased in number during the 6-year period studied.

In Oslo, Havig (1977) found more fatal pulmonary emboli in spring and autumn than in winter and summer, while in a Danish study the incidence of pulmonary embolism varied quite randomly (Andreasen and Kriger Lassen 1965).

Other Factors

Sex may be important in the formation of postoperative thrombosis. Most studies give information about the sex of the patients, stating that different prophylactic groups do not differ in this respect. Mention of the incidence of thrombosis divided by sex is, however, markedly rare. In the majority of studies where this information is given, the incidence of postoperative thrombosis did not differ between men and women (Pinto 1970, Williams 1971, Sagar 1974, Lahnborg and Bergström 1975, Soreff et al. 1975, Strand et al. 1975, Takkunen 1975, Hutter et al. 1976, Joffe 1976, Kelsey et al. 1976, Lawrence et al. 1977, Barnes et al. 1978, Jackaman et al. 1978, Bergqvist et al. 1979, Bergqvist and Hallböök 1980). In two studies the incidence of thrombosis is approximately twice as high in women, but because of the small number of patients, there is no statistically significant difference (Kakkar et al. 1972, Carter and Eban 1973). In an autopsy study it was found that pulmonary emboli were more common in female patients (Vollmar and Rüdiger 1972).

As to the prophylactic effect of different methods, a possible sex difference has been discussed in a few cases. Thus, acetylsalicylic acid was shown to be effective only in men in one study (Harris et al. 1977), something that has also been suggested by Soreff et al. (1975). In some studies it has also been suggested that dextran should be more effective in women, but in all cases the tendency was nonsignificant (Becker and Schampi 1973, Stephensen et al. 1973, Hutter et al. 1976, Bergqvist et al. 1979, Bergqvist and Hallböök 1980).

In various epidemiologic studies since the beginning of the 1960s, oral contraceptives have been considered to carry a risk of thromboembolism (Vessey and Doll 1968, Inman et al. 1970, Böttiger and Westerholm 1971). Sagar et al. (1976b) showed a significantly higher incidence of postoperative thrombosis and a lower preoperative level of antithrombin III in women taking oral contraceptives. In a group of women undergoing dental extraction the intraoperative antithrombin III level fell to lower values in patients taking oral contraceptives. This decrease could be prevented by preoperative administration of 2500 IU heparin subcutaneously. The incidence of thromboembolic complications in association with oral contraceptives can apparently be reduced by use of a lower estrogen pill (Böttiger et al. 1980). In a prospective randomized study the factor Xa inhibitor activity decreased significantly after administration of contraceptive pills, but there was no difference between pills containing 30 and 50 μg estrogen, and the values were stable for 1 year (A. Bergqvist et al., to be published b). In elective surgery it seems reasonable to stop contraceptive medication 1 month preoperatively. If for some reason surgery is to be performed in patients taking oral contraceptives, some kind of prophylaxis is required.

Previous thromboembolism is a risk factor for the formation of postoperative thrombosis. Since the diagnosis is difficult and used to be still more so, the clinical history is not easy to assess. A way of objectively identifying changes in the post-thrombotic extremity by performing a so-called after exercise thermography (*AET*) was described by Henderson et al. (1978). In chronic venous insufficiency AET has been claimed to exhibit a special pattern. Patients with such changes preoperatively formed a high-risk group for the development of postoperative venous thrombosis. However, only one risk factor is studied by this method. In a prospective study of 112 patients it was not possible to find a correlation between a positive AET and the development of postoperative thrombosis (Lindhagen et al. 1982b).

Phleboliths are calcified thrombi in the pelvic veins, a finding that is quite common in survey radiography of the pelvis. A high incidence of periprostatic thrombi were found in an autopsy study by Ljungerud et al. (1973). Janvrin et al. (1980b) studied whether or not phleboliths, as a sign of a previous pelvic vein thrombus, are a risk factor for postoperative thrombus formation. The risk of developing a thrombus verified by the fibrinogen test increased with the number of phleboliths.

The importance of smoking in venous thrombosis is much less clear than in arterial disease (Feinleib 1972). It has even been considered that smoking supplies a certain protection against thrombus formation (Clayton et al. 1978, Pollock and Evans 1978, Prescott et al. 1978, Hendolin 1980, Ishak and Morley 1981, Hendolin et al. 1981). Smokers developing postoperative thrombosis appear to be seriously overweight (Clayton et al. 1978).

Risk Factor Assessment

Studies of clinical risk factors are of importance, since our objective is to identify patients at risk during the preoperative period in order to give them prophylactic treatment or to observe them for possible development of thrombosis. The factors listed previously (p. 51) provide information about the individual risk factors for thrombus formation. In the clinical situation, though, the risk factors are seldom isolated, and there is a cumulative effect of several factors. An early effort to give selective prophylaxis on the basis of a risk factor analysis was made by Bergqvist in 1940. He measured coagulation time daily postoperatively and found that there was a parallelism between decrease in this time and the debut of thrombosis. In a small series he gave heparin to patients with preoperative decrease in coagulation time and found no clinical thrombi in these patients.

An assessment of the relative importance of the different factors would be of value. In the seventies some studies were published on this issue, employing different statistical methods. Statistical methods had been used long before then, however, as an aid in the assessment of risk factors. One of the pioneers was Lister (1927), who found that age of the patient, intra-abdominal operations, and fractures of the femur were of the greatest importance for the development of pulmonary embolism detected at autopsy.

The first more thorough analysis of a long series of coagulation and fibrinolytic factors pre- and postoperatively was made by Gallus et al. (1973a), by comparing patients who developed postoperative thrombosis with those who did not. Of the preoperative measurements, partial thromboplastin time was the only value that differed between the two groups. On the first postoperative day, the thrombosis patients exhibited a lower antiplasmin level and a higher FDP level. These statistical differences were small and not useful in a practical sense.

Several coagulation factors were measured preoperatively by Nilsen et al. (1980) in a group of patients undergoing elective hip surgery and being followed postoperatively by the ^{125}I-fibrinogen test. The patients developing postoperative thrombosis had significantly higher preoperative fibrinogen and lower antithrombin III levels than those not developing thrombosis. The authors constructed a quotient between fibrinogen and antithrombin III, and this was significantly higher preoperatively in patients who later developed thrombosis. The authors proposed that this quotient be used as an additional aid in the assessment of risk patients.

As early as 1963, Breneman developed a risk assessment tool and had the foresight to base it on discriminant analysis. He created a formula where the different factors

Table 21. Prognostic grading of risk factors for postoperative thrombus formation. (After Laaksonen et al. 1973)

Risk factor	Points
1. Age: 30 years	2
40 years	3
50 years	4
60 years	5
70 years	6
2. Obesity: $<$10 kg overweight	3
$\geqslant$10 kg overweight	4
3. Varicose veins or previous thromboembolism	3
4. Cardiac/vascular disease	3
5. Diseases of the liver or kidneys, anemia	2
6. Cachexia	2
7. Malignancy, suspected infection	3
8. ESR $\geqslant$ 20 mm	2
9. Surgical trauma:	
Gastric resection, hip surgery, mastectomy	4
Urologic surgery	2–4
Cholecystectomy, explorative laparotomy, excision of herniated disc	3
Hemorrhoidectomy, herniorrhaphy	2
Other major operations	4
Other minor operations	2

were balanced against each other (Breneman 1953, 1965). He found, for instance, age, weight, duration of anaesthesia, and duration of postoperative immobilization to be of importance. The study was retrospective and entirely based on the clinical diagnosis of the thromboembolic complications, and was soon forgotten.

Tammisto et al. (1970) and Laaksonen et al. (1973) awarded points to various clinical factors and were thus able, by the sums obtained, to separate high-risk from low-risk patients. The assessment was made retrospectively, the diagnosis of thrombosis clinically. The factors assessed are presented in Table 21. High-risk patients have a sum of more than 12 points. The definition is perhaps somewhat diffuse, particularly with respect to surgical trauma. Later studies on the incidence have shown that some other kind of grading is required; nonetheless, this is one of the first attempts with a prognostic purpose to balance different risk factors against each other.

A similar prognostic index for the development of postoperative venous thrombosis was used by Clayton et al. (1976). In 124 patients a series of clinical and laboratory data were recorded preoperatively. ^{125}I-fibrinogen tests were performed in the usual way, and patients developing thrombosis were compared with those who did not. On the basis of discriminant analysis five factors were chosen which exhibited the largest difference between groups, and a formula for a prognostic index (I) was constructed:

$$I = -11.3 + 0.0090 \times X_3 + 0.22 \times X_4 + 0.085 \times X_5 + 0.043 \times X_7 + 2.18 \times X_8$$

X_3 = euglobulin clot lysis time
X_4 = fibrinogen-related antigen
X_5 = age
X_7 = percent overweight (correlated to height)
X_8 = varicose veins (0 no, 1 yes)

High positive values for I are combined with a high risk of postoperative thrombus formation, whereas high negative values indicate little danger.

These findings and views have later been confirmed in two investigations in patients undergoing gynecologic surgery (Rakoczi et al. 1978, Crandon et al. 1980a). The true value of such an index, however, can only be proven by a prospective comparative study of risk patients given prophylactic treatment and others receiving no prophylaxis. How the two groups differed with respect to thromboembolic complications would then be analyzed. Attempts in this direction have begun (Clayton et al. 1979), and recently a limited study of 105 patients was published (Crandon et al. 1980b). Thirty-one patients obtained an index classifying them as high-risk patients. They received the usual low-dose heparin prophylaxis, while the others were not given any treatment. The incidence of thrombosis was reduced to the level expected if the whole patient group had been treated.

In recent years multivariate models have been developed which can be used in medical prognosis (Cornfield et al. 1961, Walker and Duncan 1967, Lange 1977). The first multivariate analysis dealing with the formation of postoperative venous thrombosis was performed by Nicolaides and Irving (1975). They studied 535 patients undergoing various surgical, orthopedic, urologic, and thoracic surgery operations. The ^{125}I-fibrinogen test was employed as diagnostic method, and a series of high-risk factors were recorded, as had been judged by previous authors. Factors significantly correlated with postoperative venous thrombosis were age, premedication with morphine, varicose veins, infection confirmed by culture, previous deep-vein thrombosis, difficulty of the operation (minor or major), urologic operations, and thoracic surgery. The last two factors exhibited a negative correlation, i.e., the risk of thrombosis was diminished. Factors such as obesity, malignancy, icterus, and vascular surgery were not significantly correlated with postoperativ thrombosis.

On the basis of these findings a prognostic index was created:

$$I = -6.00 \text{ (age} \times 0.0617) \times \text{(varicose veins} \times 1.26) + \text{(previous thrombosis} \times 1.38)$$
$$+ \text{(complexity of operation} \times 0.79) + \text{(premedication with morphine} \times 0.97)$$
$$+ \text{(infection} \times 0.84) - \text{(urologic operation} \times 1.94) - \text{(thoracic operation} \times 1.15).$$

Even though this index overlaps considerably between patients with and without thrombosis, it can be used for the individual patient in order to express the probability of his/her developing a postoperative thrombus. According to this model, the relative risk of thrombosis thus rises dramatically with an age of more than 40–50 years (Fig. 4). This agrees well with the risk of thrombosis in the general population (Nylander and Olivecrona 1976). Postoperative thrombosis in children is very rare, but has been reported (Joffe 1975c).

Table 22 also presents the postoperative risk of thrombosis in certain types of patients. These figures agree well with Buttermann's findings (1977), using a similar statistical model (Siegerstetter and Neiss 1977).

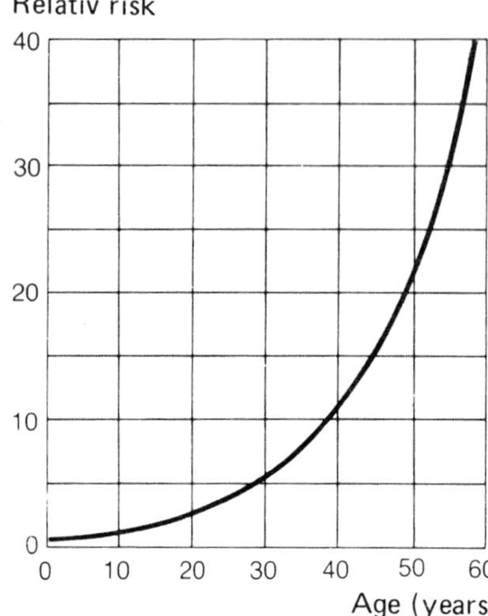

Fig. 4. Relative risk of postoperative thrombosis in relation to age. (After Nicolaides 1975, courtesy of MTP Ltd., Lancaster, England)

In his thesis on postoperative thrombosis diagnosed by the fibrinogen test and occurring in association with prostatic surgery, Hedlund (1975) performed a similar multivariate analysis of 201 patients with respect to risk factors assumed on both clinical and laboratory grounds. In this analysis there were surprisingly few significant correlations between the different risk factors and thrombosis. The most important risk factor was the duration of the operation, with a time limit of 50 min. Surprisingly enough, the amount of time using a leg support was of no importance. Nor did age turn out to be a significant predictor of risk. It should be kept in mind, however, that this study was composed entirely of patients who underwent prostatic surgery, and that the mean value of the duration of the operation includes transvesical as well as transurethral prostatectomy. Also, the age of prostate patients is high, with relatively little scattering, which might explain why age in this population does not appear to be a risk factor.

A few other studies employing the multivariate analysis procedure shall be mentioned, although they do not concern postoperative thromboembolism. In Havig's (1977) study of 503 fatal cases, pulmonary embolism detected at autopsy was significantly correlated with age, duration of bed rest, acute and chronic cerebrovascular disease, leukemia, infarction, and postoperative state.

A similar study was performed by Sigel et al. (1979) in 6527 patients with pulmonary embolism which led to death within a month. Pulmonary embolism was diagnosed in 278 patients by angiography of the pulmonary artery, by autopsy, or by perfusion scintigraphy. The most important individual risk factor was previous history of thromboembolism. Other significant risk factors were right-sided heart failure, venous occlusion diagnosed by ultrasound, and race.

Since thrombosis, as pointed out earlier, is multifactorial, weighing the different risk factors against each other is probably the right way to attack the problem. As previously mentioned, the results vary a great deal, but the studies performed are very few, comprising not very homogeneous groups of patients. For these reasons it is doubtful whether a single preoperative laboratory test will ever be found that is capable

Table 22. Risk of thrombosis in eight hypothetical patients. (After Nicolaides and Irving, 1975)

Patient	Risk (%)
1. 20 years old, minor surgery	0.8
2. 40 years old, minor surgery	2.9
3. 40 years old, major surgery	6.3
4. 60 years old, minor surgery	9.1
5. 60 years old, major surgery	18.3
6. 60 years old, major surgery, previous thrombosis	47.0
7. 80 years old, major surgery	43.0
8. 80 years old, major surgery, previous thrombosis, varicose veins, infection	96.0

of predicting which patients will develop postoperative thrombosis. The methods of analysis mentioned are of course of interest for scientific purposes, but it is not expected that clinicians will use such complex formulas to help them decide which patients are to receive preoperative thromboprophylaxis.

For the time being we are thus dependent on relatively coarse clinical parameters such as age, previous thromboembolism, type of surgery, etc. In a critical survey of different tests intended for the diagnosis of prethrombotic conditions, Sixma (1978) concludes: "No reliable test is available for identifying a prethrombotic tendency in individual patients."

The thrombosis-antithrombosis balance of the individual patient is, to a frightening degree, still unknown to us.

Summary

Certain defects in the hemostatic system will with a high degree of certainty lead to thrombosis after trauma, e.g., antithrombin III deficiency or a reduced concentration of fibrinolytic activators in the vein walls. In the majority of cases, where a postoperative thrombus forms, laboratory changes are of little help in predicting whether a thrombus will form or not. Statistical differences can possibly be demonstrated between the patient group developing thrombosis and the group which does not, but in the individual case there is very little guidance to be expected. Thus, at present there exists no preoperative screening test capable of accurately predicting the risk of postoperative thrombosis.

Since thrombosis is multifactorial, multivariate analysis has been employed in some studies to identify risk patients. Still, these studies are too few as yet to permit any firm conclusions. In some cases risk formulas and prognostic indices have been worked out, but they are of scientific interest only.

In the practical patient situation, comparatively coarse but simple clinical factors still form the basis of assessment of whether there is risk of thrombosis or not: age, type of surgery, previous thromboembolism, prolonged immobilization, malignancy, and obesity. The assessment of risk factors should be of guidance in the decision as to which patients or groups of patients should receive thromboprophylactic treatment.

Prophylaxis of Thromboembolism

Introduction

Compilation and comparison of thromboprophylactic studies can be difficult for several reasons, e.g., different groups of patients, different criteria for inclusion and exclusion, differences between diagnostic principles, differences in follow-up time, etc. In the comparison between different studies using the same prophylactic method there are also differences in dosage, route of administration, duration of prophylaxis, etc.

In the following analysis almost exclusively prospective studies will be discussed, where objective diagnosis of thromboembolism has been performed. The demands on the design of such studies are becoming heavier, if the results are to be accepted and relevant conclusions possible (Genton et al. 1975, Gruber et al. 1975a, b, Harker et al. 1975, Verstraete 1976b, Gent and Sackett 1979, Kakkar 1979a, Turpie and Hirsh 1979, Vessey 1979).

When such studies are planned, current biostatistical viewpoints should also be taken into consideration (e.g., Schoolman et al. 1968, Burdette and Gehan 1970, Shaw et al. 1974, Byar et al. 1976, Feinstein 1977, Freiman et al. 1978). If a study indicates that the different therapeutic alternatives do not differ as to effect, it is of particular importance to be aware that the true effect might have been missed because the population was too small. Whether such a slight difference in effect is of clinical importance is of course another question, often requiring that additional factors be considered in the assessment.

After a period of thrombodiagnostic and thromboprophylactic enthusiasm, some critical views and questions have appeared. Firstly, there is some confusion and disagreement over the clinical importance of a positive fibrinogen test (Blaisdell 1978); secondly, it is questionable whether thromboprophylaxis is necessary at all (Pachter and Riles 1977, Bell and Zuidema 1979); and thirdly, there is doubt as to what degree the established methods for thromboprophylaxis do in fact prevent thromboembolic complications (Blaisdell 1979, Groote Schuur Hosp. 1979). Two other important questions are whether the thromboprophylactic effect is obtained at the price of serious adverse effects, and whether the overall mortality can be influenced (Pachter and Riles 1977, Morris and Mitchell 1978, Mitchell 1979).

It is of course important that these questions be continuously studied. Nonetheless, there are sufficient data showing that effective prophylactic methods do exist. It is the responsibility of the clinician in charge to define the patients at risk and provide adequate prophylaxis.

Thromboprophylactic methods can be divided into *general* and *specific* methods. The general ones include an adequate supply of fluids and shock prophylaxis. On loss of blood and fluids, substitution should be continuous in order to avoid dehydration with subsequent hemoconcentration and increased blood viscosity. A careful and atraumatic surgical technique is of great importance. Large tissue traumatization should be avoided. The patients should be encouraged to do early postoperative leg movements, and this is an important task for our physiotherapists. Early mobilization is vital, and it is not enough to place the patient in a chair beside the bed, with legs dangling. The patient should be properly mobilized, including walking exercise. Oral contraceptive medication should be stopped 1 month before elective surgery.

The specific prophylactic methods can be divided into mechanical and drug therapy methods. A possible analytic approach is to follow the various steps in Virchow's triad. However, several methods may have an effect on more than one level of this triad. Hence, in the following, each method will be discussed separately.

Mechanical Methods

Elevation of the foot of the bed, electric calf muscle stimulation, and active ankle flexion increase the clearance rate of the radiopaque agent from the soleal veins in approximately the same way as normal muscular contraction (Almén and Nylander 1962, Kemble 1971, Nicolaides et al. 1972e). Leg elevation reduces the incidence of thrombosis in patients undergoing hip surgery (Hartman et al. 1970), but not in patients undergoing elective general surgery (Rosengarten and Laird 1971, Browse et al. 1974b, Takkunen 1975). Intensified physical therapy with the aid of a physiotherapist has not been shown to have any thromboprohylactic effect (Flanc et al. 1969, Browse et al. 1974b).

Compression Stockings

Table 23 shows that there is disagreement about the thromboprophylactic effect of compression stockings. In the studies where an effect was noted, a stocking with

Table 23. Thromboprophylactic effect of compression stockings

Author	Number of Patients	Type of Stocking	Method[a]	Incidence of Thrombosis		Significance
				Controls	Treatment	
Barnes et al. (1978b)[c]	18	TED	A	50	0	$P = 0.029$
Bolton (1978)	142	TED	A	38	12	$P < 0.05$
Browse et al. (1974b)	90	Tubigrip	B	29	24	NS
Holford (1976)	95	TED	A	49	23	$P < 0.025$
Ishak and Morley (1981)	76	TED	A	54	20	$P < 0.01$
Moser and Froidevaux (1976)	35	?	A	13	25	NS
Nillius et al. (1979a)[c]	56	Ortha-wear[d]	A	49	38	NS
Rosengarten et al. (1970)	50	Tubigrip	A	32	32	NS
Scurr et al. (1977)	76	TED	B	37	11	$P < 0.01$

[a]*Method A:* The study included two groups of patients: one treated group and one control group. *Method B:* The study included one group of patients. One leg was used as control. Armitage's sequential analysis was employed for the statistical calculations.
[b]Ultrasound diagnosis.
[c]Barnes et al. and Nillius et al. have studied hip surgery.
[d]available in four sizes with graded compression.

graded compression gradually decreasing in a proximal direction was used (TED antiembolism stocking, thromboembolism deterrent).

In Bolton's study (1978), no effect was noted in patients with malignant diseases, where only palliative surgery could be performed. No effect of a graded compression stocking could be shown in a study in patients who underwent elective hip surgery (Nillius et al. 1979). Barnes et al. (1978) were able to demonstrate an effect in a small series of patients, using ultrasound to establish the diagnosis. Also Ishak and Morley (1981) found that TED stockings reduced the frequency of thrombosis after elective hip surgery. Phlebography was used for diagnosis. However, the patients received dextran 70 in an uncontrolled manner. These patients, however, constitute a high-risk group which is always difficult to influence prophylactically irrespective of the method employed.

For the emptying of the venous system, the degree of compression is probably of great importance, which might partly explain the large differences between the studies where flow measurements have been performed with continuous elastic compression. With a gradual decrease of compression proximally, the clearance rate of the radiopaque agent increases significantly in the whole venous system of the leg (Lewis et al. 1976). Several other authors have also shown that the venous flow rate increases with the use of elastic compression stockings (Meyerowitz and Nelson 1964, Makin et al. 1969, Sigel et al. 1973, 1975, Tillberg 1974, Arnoldi 1976).

A combination of elastic stockings, raising the foot of the bed, and passive leg movements has been shown to have a thromboprophylactic effect in major abdominal surgery (Tsapogas et al. 1971, Papadimitriou et al. 1977). Kunz et al. (1979) used compression stockings as a routine for all patients in a study where the primary aim was to investigate the effect of low-dose heparin, low-dose heparin in combination with dihydroergotamine, and peroral anticoagulation in patients undergoing gynecologic surgery.

Motorized Foot Mover

A foot mover with rhythmic dorsal and plantar flexion doubles the flow rate (Wrigth and Osborn 1952) and increases the maximum flow in the femoral vein (Roberts et al. 1971, Cotton et al. 1972). It also empties the soleal sinusoids effectively (Nicolaides et al. 1972d). A frequency of 50 flexions/min and an amplitude of $\pm 20°$ give optimal conditions. By this means a thromboprophylactic effect was demonstrated by Sabri et al. (1971c) and Scurr et al. (1981). In addition, the blood flow of the skin is stimulated (Goldsmith 1966).

With the aid of a bed bicycle (of the kind that the patient drives himself as well as the motorized type) for 5 min 3 times a day, the postoperative incidence of thrombosis was significantly reduced (Mühe 1977). Dorsal flexion alone also has a thromboprophylactic effect (Scurr et al. 1979).

Electric Calf Muscle Stimulation

The flow-improving effect of electric calf muscle stimulation was shown by Doran et al. in 1964, and was later confirmed by several authors (Becker and Schampi 1973, Nicolaides et al. 1972d). Whether or not the coagulation and/or fibrinolytic system is influenced by electric calf muscle stimulation is still largely unknown. Electroconvulsive therapy in psychiatric practice activates the fibrinolytic system. This seems to be related to muscular activity, since it can be blocked by muscle relaxants (Worowski et al. 1970).

In Table 24 thromboprophylactic studies employing electric calf muscle stimulation are presented. In 50% of the studies no effect could be demonstrated. The great variation in results may be due to differences in contraction frequency, which may give rise to flow differences. On the whole, the optimal stimulation conditions are unknown, but impulse groups of short duration are said to counteract stasis better than single impulses (Lindström et al. 1979).

In the studies reported, voltage, type of stimulation, frequency, electrode size, and site of application varied (Bernhard and Gruber 1976).

The patients were too few to permit any conclusion as to the prophylactic effect on pulmonary embolism. Out of 300 elderly patients undergoing major surgery with intraoperative electric stimulation, Powley and Doran (1973) found one fatal pulmonary embolus. Unfortunately, there was no reference group in this study.

This method is not very practical and can hardly be used in conscious patients.

Intermittent Calf Muscle Compression

Most studies of mechanical thromboprophylactic methods have employed intermittent calf muscle compression, a method proposed by Brush et al. (1959) and Breneman (1963) among others.

Table 24. Thromboprophylactic effect of electric calf muscle stimulation

Author	Number of patients	Method[a]	Incidence of thrombosis (%)		
			Control	Treated	Significance
Becker and Schampi (1973)	74	A	31	5	$P < 0.01$
Browse and Negus (1970)	110	B	21	8	$P < 0.01$
Dejode et al. (1973)	64	B	15	13	NS
Lindström (1982)	77	A	30	14	NS
Nicolaides et al. (1972d)	116	A	22	2	$P < 0.0003$
Pollock et al. (1976)	229	A	41	32	NS
Pollock (1977)	194	A	35	16	$P < 0.05$
Rosenberg et al. (1975)	139	A	44	28	NS

[a]*Method A.* The study included two groups of patients: one treated group and one control group. *Method B.* The study included one patient group, one extremity being used as control. Armitage's sequential analysis was used for the statistical evaluation.

Mode of Action

In 1949 Stanton et al. were able to show that the venous flow rate in the human femoral vein increased on local calf compression to 20–35 mm Hg. Ashton (1966) and Ginsberg et al. (1967) measured the volume flow by mercury strain gauge plethysmography, finding a clear reduction on compression to 30–40 mm Hg with a duration of 10–45 min. Similar results were shown by ^{133}Xe-clearance technique (Campion et al. 1968). Spiro et al. (1970) and Sabri et al. (1971a), using electromagnetic flow measurement, found that the flow in the femoral vein decreased after 5 min of compression to a pressure between 15 and 140 mm Hg. A shorter compression time and a pressure of 30 mm Hg, on the other hand, resulted in an increased maximum flow in the femoral vein, whereas the average flow remained the same (Sabri et al. 1972). The maximum flow reached its highest level at a compression interval of about 1 min (Roberts et al. 1972).

By contrast clearance technique (according to Nicolaides et al. 1972e) Harris et al. (1976) were able to show that the venous system could be effectively drained using a calf muscle pump, and that optimal conditions existed at inflation to 40–50 mmHg for 1 s, maintaining the pressure at this level for 12 s, and deflation for 45 s (III in Fig. 5, p. 72).

Ah-see et al. (1976) compared an alpha bed pump (Calnan et al. 1970; II in Fig. 5) with one of their own construction (IV in Fig. 5) at different inflation pressures, finding that the latter was more effective with regard to the flow, and that optimal conditions were obtained at a pressure of 40 mm Hg (Table 25). The conditions were similar for dogs and humans when electromagnetic volume flow measurement was employed. With the slower cycle (II in Fig. 5) even a reduced arterial flow was obtained during a certain phase of the pump inflation. In spite of differences in flow pattern, both pump types had a similar thromboprophylactic effect in an experimental thrombosis model in the dog.

Thus, the flow-increasing effect obtained with certain pump types is not very impressive. In certain cases there is even a reduction of the net flow. Nevertheless, these pumps have a thromboprophylactic effect (see below). For this reason alternative explanations of the prophylactic effect will be briefly discussed.

Table 25. Percentage changes in volume flow in the femoral vein on intermittent calf muscle compression

Pump pressure (mmHg)	Alpha bed pump (type II)	Pump type IV
15	98 ± 2	106 ± 5[a]
30	95 ± 2	116 ± 9[a]
40	91 ± 4	121 ± 8[a]
60	88 ± 4	123 ± 7[a]
100		120 ± 7

[a]$P < 0.03$ (significant differences between pump types II and IV in Fig. 5). Electromagnetic flow measurement of the femoral vein was performed in surgery for varicose veins.

Firstly, during a certain phase of the pump inflation there may be an increase in the volume flow, with elimination of various thrombogenic substances, e.g., from valve pockets. Phlebographic results indicate that stasis is more pronounced inside the valve pockets (McLachlin et al. 1960, Harris et al. 1974) and that intermittent calf muscle compression can effectively eliminate contrast medium from them (Harris et al. 1976). Moreover, Paterson and McLachlin (1954) showed that the histologically oldest parts of a thrombus are usually found in the valve pockets. During stasis hypoxia develops in the valve pockets and it can be prevented by intermittent calf compression (Hamer et al. 1981). Using $^{99}Tc^m$-macroaggregated albumin clearance it was, however, possible to show that the elimination rate in intermittently compressed legs was slower than in noncompressed (Bergqvist et al. 1982c). From a prophylactic point of view the most important thing thus would be to keep the blood in motion, the direction of the motion being of less importance.

Secondly, activation of the fibrinolytic system may occur. This system has attracted much attention in recent years in the discussion of the pathogenesis of thrombosis. Patients with a reduced concentration of fibrinolytic activators in the vein walls are predisposed to thrombosis (Pandolfi et al. 1969, Nilsson 1977). The release of fibrinolytic activators is stimulated by venous stasis (Robertson et al. 1972c, Shaper et al. 1975). Allenby et al. (1973) found that intraoperative pneumatic calf muscle compression stimulated fibrinolysis during the postoperative period, when it was lowered in the control. Knight and Dawson (1976) showed that the fibrinolytic activity decreases during surgical operations and that this decrease can be prevented by intermittent muscle compression.

Furthermore, it has been shown that intraoperative pumping of the arms prevents the development of thrombi in the lower extremities (Knight and Dawson 1976). Also in this case, the normal postoperative decrease in fibrinolytic activity was prevented. The fibrinolytic activity in the arms is normally higher than in the legs (Nilsson and Robertson 1968). Increased fibrinolysis has also been demonstrated in healthy volunteers, in whom it was higher in blood draining the compressed extremity than in mixed venous blood (Stevenson et al. 1977, Tarnay et al. 1980).

However, O'Brien et al. (1979) and Browse (1978) found no difference in the fibrinolytic response in patients with or without calf compression. This is in agreement with our own findings (Ljungnér et al. 1981b). The fibrinolytic activity of the blood measured by means of euglobulin lysis time and the lysed area on fibrin plates is the same before and after pumping, and the plasminogen activator level in the vein wall does not differ between compressed and uncompressed extremities. Inflation time, deflation time, and pump pressure appear to play no role in this connection (Ljungnér et al. 1981b). Pumping of the arm does not differ from pumping of the leg. The results are the same whether or not the analysis is performed on blood from the pumped extremity or from the general circulation. As the release of plasminogen activators is closely related to the release of factor VIII-related protein (VIIIR:Ag) (Nilsson et al. 1980a,b), the concentration of this substance has also been studied in intermittent calf muscle compression without showing any effect (Ljungnér et al. 1981b). The assumption that fibrinolytic activity should play an essential role for the thromboprophylactic effect of intermittent calf muscle compression is thus disproved.

Different Pump Models

There are different models for intermittent calf muscle compression available today. All of them have a "stocking" that is fitted on to the foot and leg. This stocking can then be pumped cyclically. What differs between the models is the pumping pattern.

Figure 5 shows the four most common types and their principle with respect to the pumping function.

A recent pump type used by Turpie et al. (1979) consists of a series of isolated segments which are inflated, starting distally. The inflation is rapid, and when all segments have been filled (50 mm Hg), the pressure remains for 5 s, followed by rapid deflation. The next inflation follows 60 s later. A similar sequential pump but with other times has been used by Zelikovski et al. (1981).

Another model has different pressures in the segments, with the highest pressure distally (Nicolaides et al. 1980). Optimal flow conditions are obtained with inflation for 12 s and deflation for 60 s, with an ankle pressure of 35 mm Hg and a thigh pressure of 20 mm Hg.

Clinical Documentation

In Table 26 the studies are listed where objective diagnosis has been employed. It has been established that the incidence of deep vein thrombosis has decreased markedly following intermittent calf muscle compression in nonorthopedic patients undergoing surgery for nonmalignant diseases.

Hull et al. (1979a) studied the effect of intermittent calf muscle compression in 61 patients undergoing knee surgery, all in a bloodless field, the majority of cases

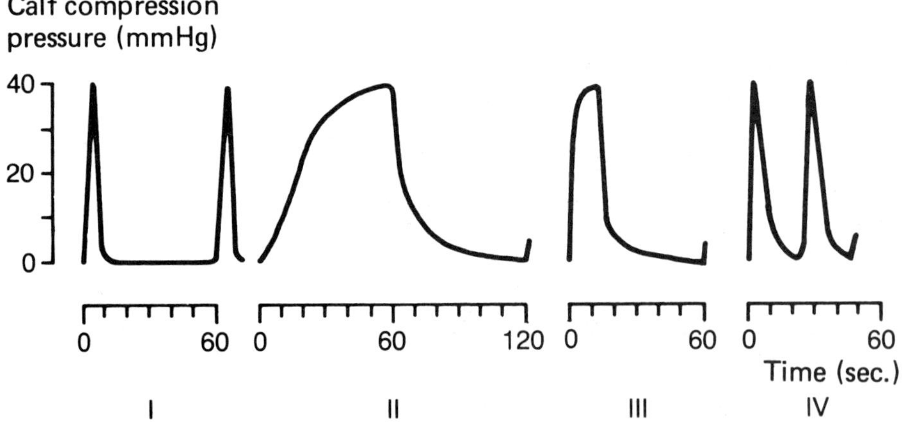

Fig. 5. The principal compression pattern of four different calf muscle pumps. **I** Inflation at 8 mm Hg/s to 40 mmHg, followed by abrupt deflation. Parke, Davis and Co. (Sabri et al. 1971b). **II** Gradual inflation to 40 mmHg for 1 min, followed by deflation for 1 min. Flowtron-Aire Ltd. (Hills et al. 1972). **III** Inflation to 40 mmHg for 12 s, followed by deflation for 48 s (PED-90). (Cranley et al. 1976). **IV** Inflation at 7.7 mmHg/s to 10 mmHg, followed by inflation at 22 mmHg/s to 40 mmHg. Deflation for about 20 s. (Ah-see et al. 1976)

having plaster casts postoperatively. Bilateral phlebography was performed 14–17 days postoperatively. The reference group showed 66% thrombosis, the compression group 6.3% (P <0.01). A follow-up for 2 months showed no evidence of pulmonary embolism. Similar results were reported by McKenna et al. (1980) in a much smaller series of patients who underwent knee arthroplasty.

Roberts and Cotton (1975) failed to reduce the incidence of thrombosis still further by an additional supply of low-dose heparin. A significant improvement of the prophylactic effect was found by Smith et al. (1978b) if dextran 70 and intermittent calf muscle compression were combined instead of compression alone. Almost the same decrease in the incidence of thrombosis was obtained also in a group given only dextran, and no conclusions can therefore be drawn about the combination effect. Harris et al. (1976), comparing compression with warfarin in elective hip surgery, found that anticoagulation therapy was superior to compression. In hip arthroplasty patients, Gallus and Darby (1981) were able to show that the frequency of calf thrombi was reduced by intermittent compression, while the number of proximal thrombi was uninfluenced. But all thrombi were of a smaller size in the treatment group. In elective abdominal surgery intermittent compression equals low-dose heparin in effect (Moser et al. 1981). In two studies where intermittent pneumatic compression had no effect in general surgery, the frequency of thrombosis in the control group was extremely low (Takkunen 1975, Butson 1981). With a sequential pumping device continued until the patient was fully ambulant the prophylactic effect was equal to that of low-dose heparin (Ellis and Scurr 1982).

Nicolaides et al. (1980) performed a comparative study between conventional intermittent calf muscle compression (pump II in Fig. 5), compression of sequential type with graded pressure (described on p. 72), and low-dose heparin. After the 2nd day, heparin was more effective. The sequential pump prevented thrombi proximally to the calf more effectively than the conventional pump model.

The study by Browse et al. (1976) is interesting because the incidence of pulmonary embolism was studied using a combination of perfusion and ventilation scintigraphy. The incidence of thrombi of the calf was not influenced as measured by the ^{125}I-fibrinogen test, whereas the incidence of pulmonary embolism was significantly lowered (from 24% to 8%). From a methodologic viewpoint it is regrettable that untreated controls were compared with a group of patients who had received prophylactic treatment in the form of a combination of dextran 70 and calf muscle compression. Since dextran has a documented prophylactic effect on pulmonary embolism, it is impossible to draw any conclusions on the role of calf muscle compression in this study.

In a study by Lee et al. (1976), of 42 patients who underwent elective hip surgery, there were three fatal pulmonary emboli in the reference group and none in the compression group. Some other studies indicate a reduced incidence of embolism (Cranley et al. 1976, Pedegana et al. 1977).

However, the prophylactic effect on pulmonary embolism remains to be studied using intermittent calf muscle compression in an extensive prospective investigation employing adequate diagnostic methods with regard to pulmonary embolism.

The duration and type of compression varies with the studies, making comparison rather difficult. Also the time when the thrombi were diagnosed varies. It is mainly intraoperative thrombi and thrombi forming immediately postoperatively that can be

Table 26. Thromboprophylactic effect of intermittent calf muscle compression

Author	Number of patients	Pump type (Fig. 5)	Start of pumping	Duration of pumping	Incidence of thrombosis (%)		Signi-ficance	Comments
					Control	Treated		
Browse et al. (1976)	100	II	Preop.	Approx. 1 h postop.	34	24	NS	General surgery, test group both dx 70 and pump
Butson (1981)	119	III	Intraop.	24–48 h	7.0	9.7	NS	General surgery
Calnan and Allenby (1975)	100	II	Intraop.	Intraop.	30	12	S	General surgery, no effect on malignancy
Clark et al. (1974)	37	II	Intraop.	17–23 h	20	0	S	General surgery
Coe et al. (1978)	53	III	Intraop.	Hospitalization	25	7	S	Urology
Collins et al. (1977)	94	III	Intraop.	→ 17 days	29	15	S	Neurosurgery
Cranley et al. (1976)	195	III	Postop.	?	12	9	NS	Elective hip surgery, uncontrolled heparin administration
Gallus and Darby (1981)	78	III	Intraop.	7 days	33	32	NS	Elective hip surgery
Harris et al. (1976)	56	III	Intraop.	4–5 days	30	50	NS	Elective hip surgery, control group warfarin
Hills et al. (1972)	73	II	Intraop.	Incl. day 1	39	3	S	General surgery, benign diseases
Knight and Dawson (1976)	128	II	Preop.	24 h	32	14	S	General surgery
Lee et al. (1976)	42	III	Intraop.	Until ambulation	39	0	S	Hip joint surgery
Pedegana et al. (1977)	100	III	Intraop.	4 days	17	0	S	Elective hip surgery, control group, elastic stocking
Roberts and Cotton (1974)	99	I	Intraop.	Intraop.	26	6	S	General surgery, effect on malignancy
Roberts and Cotton (1975)	84	I	Intraop.	Intraop.	26	18	NS	General surgery, control group both heparin and pump
Sabri et al. (1971b)	39	I	Intraop.	Intraop.	28	5	S	General surgery
Skillman et al. (1978)	95	III	Intraop.	Hospitalization	25	9	S	Neurosurgery

Table 26 (continued)

Author	Number of patients	Pump type (Fig. 5)	Start of pumping	Duration of pumping	Incidence of thrombosis (%)		Signi-ficance	Comments
					Control	Treated		
Takkunen (1975)	70	a	Intraop.	Intraop.	13	14	NS	General surgery
Turpie (1976)	128	III	Postop.	5 days	19	2	S	Neurosurgery
Turpie et al. (1979)	129	b	Postop.	14 days	23	6	S	Neurosurgery
Zelikovski et al. (1981)	43	d	Intraop.	24 h	50	4.3	S	Neurosurgery
Mean incidence					*26[c]*	*11[c]*		

[a]Angiomat. Each cycle 10 s with a frequency of three min. Rapid inflation and rapid deflation. Pressure 40 mmHg.
[b]Rapid sequential inflation of a series of isolated segments. Maximum pressure 50 mmHg maintained for 5 s. Rapid deflation.
[c]If hip surgery patients are excluded, the incidence of thrombosis is 27% in the control groups and 9% in the treated groups.
[d]Sequential pump with four segments and a pressure of 50 mmHg.

avoided by calf muscle compression (Roberts and Cotton 1974, Nicolaides et al. 1980). In a study of neurosurgical subjects (Turpie et al. 1977), intermittent calf muscle compression was employed for 5 days, resulting in a significant reduction of the incidence of thrombosis during this period. On days 6-14 the incidence was the same in the controls as in the treated patients.

Using the patient as his own control and pumping only one extremity has the statistical advantage that other factors are identical (provided that randomization between the legs is performed). Armitage's sequential analysis can be used for the assessment. The disadvantage, which is greater, is that it is impossible to judge whether there is any prophylactic effect on pulmonary embolism. Moreover, the extremity that has not been pumped may be affected. Also, comparison with studies employing pharmacologic prophylaxis becomes more difficult.

Complications

Contrary to drug prophylaxis, intermittent calf muscle compression has a low frequency of complications. Slight pain and a sensation of heat (Cranley et al. 1976) are relatively common. A few cases of skin blisters have been reported (Holt and Bennett 1972, Cranley et al. 1976, Harris et al. 1976) as well as one case of paresthesia in the peroneal region (Bechtol et al. 1976).

Comments

Intermittent calf muscle compression is a possible alternative in thromboprophylaxis. The controlled studies are few, however, and exhibit great differences in pumping time and diagnostic principles. Whether or not a prophylactic effect against pulmonary embolism exists is difficult to establish, the patients being very few. Comparison with other prophylactic methods is rare.

Patients with malignant disease appear not to profit from this type of prophylaxis, but this is a group of patients with a considerable resistance also against other prophylactic methods. Nevertheless, in one study a significant reduction of the incidence of thrombosis was obtained in patients with malignant disease (Roberts and Cotton 1974).

The method is unsuitable for hip surgery and is of course quite unsuitable for any type of surgery involving the lower extremities.

Which compression conditions (cycle pattern, time, and duration of treatment) are optimal from a prophylactic point of view remains to be studied. The veins of the extremities are embedded in tissue of varying density, and the dynamics of flow are complex during external compression. The venous flow and venous collapse in different types of pumping are not known in detail (Kamm and Shapiro 1976). Sequential and graded compression seem to have certain advantages. At least theoretical studies on model systems point in that direction.

The pumping cycle pattern appears not to be of great importance for the prophylactic effect, a similar decrease in the incidence of thrombosis being obtained in spite of considerable differences in pumping function. This observation also agrees with experimental results (Ah-see et al. 1976).

In a recent study in urologic patients intraoperative compression and compression during the waking-up period (about 7.2 h) was compared with compression until complete mobilization or at least for 3 days (about 54,7 h). No differences in the incidence of thrombosis could be demonstrated (Salzman et al. 1980a). According to Scurr et al. (1981), however, a prolonged compression time appears to reduce the incidence still further.

In conditions where not even minimal bleeding can be tolerated, e.g., in neurosurgical operations, this prophylactic method seems to be preferable.

Vena Caval Interruption

Ligation or different methods for interruption of the vena cava have been employed in patients at risk of developing pulmonary embolism, particularly recurring emboli. This method is not performed to any great extent except in the United States. In the 1940s a less extensive method was used: division of the superficial femoral vein, which was considered protective against pulmonary embolism (Allen 1947, Colby 1948). The method was described by Homans (1934).

Ligation of the caval vein entails a very high incidence of edema of the legs (Mozes et al. 1966, Wheeler et al. 1966). Due to a drastic reduction of the venous return to the heart, shock may also ensue, with a relatively high mortality (Wheeler et al. 1966, Gazzaniga et al. 1967). Techniques have therefore been developed which do not interrupt the vena cava completely, and these methods are now being discussed in regard to thromboembolic prophylaxis. Plication and clips also give a high frequency of edema. The frequency of fatal pulmonary embolism is around 2% with all the different interruption methods (Donaldson et al. 1980).

Carmichael and Edwards (1967) used prophylactic caval plication in 36 patients undergoing aortoiliac or colonic surgery. One patient died of pulmonary embolism, while four developed iliofemoral thrombi. The authors used a historical reference population, and the three (out of 41) patients in this group who died were not subjected to autopsy.

In another uncontrolled study, Fuller and Willbanks (1971) used partially occluding caval clips in patients undergoing various surgical operations with a high risk of thrombosis. No fatal pulmonary emboli were observed in any of the groups.

Rosenthal et al. (1979) made a retrospective survey of 160 unrandomized patients who underwent different reconstructive operations in the aortoiliac system, where half of the patients were provided with a partially occluding caval clip (Adams and DeWeese 1966). The incidence of pulmonary embolism was 10% in the untreated group (one fatal case) compared to 0% in the clip group.

With the arrival of transvenous caval filters, the technique has become simpler (Mobin-Uddin et al. 1969). One study has been reported where the postoperative prophylactic effect of such filters against emboli was studied under controlled conditions (Fullen et al. 1973). Patients with hip fractures were randomized to a group with caval filters or to another group with no prophylaxis. The incidence of definite pulmonary emboli (based on clinical findings and a combination of pulmonary X-ray and pulmonary scintigraphy) as well as mortality was lower in the filter group (pulmonary embolism 0% vs 12%, mortality 10% vs 24%). No complications that could be directly ascribed to the filter were observed.

Even though the effect was thus undeniable in this single study, the method is too laborious to warrant more extensive use. The 10% mortality in the filter group is comparable to mortality figures reported in other studies where different types of chemoprophylaxis were used (Hamilton et al. 1970, Bergqvist et al. 1972, Edwards 1975, Bergqvist et al. 1979).

Summary

Various mechanical methods for the prophylaxis of thrombosis have been developed in order to obtain an improved blood flow. This effect varies a great deal with the method, however. Electric calf muscle stimulation is probably effective, but the optimal conditions have not yet been elucidated. Elastic stockings with a gradually decreasing compression in a proximal direction are effective in general surgery.

Most studies of mechanical thromboprophylaxis have employed intermittent calf muscle compression. There are several pump types with different principles of pumping cycle pattern. The thromboprophylactic effect does not appear to differ very much between tnese different models, however, and must be considered as firmly established in general surgery and neurosurgery. The method is somewhat laborious and cannot be used in surgery of the limbs. It has no effect in hip surgery. A combination with various drug prophylactic methods apparently does not increase the effect. The risk of adverse effects is naturally insignificant, and in neurosurgery, where even a slight hemorrhage may be deleterious, intermittent calf muscle compression is ideal. Whether or not the method has any prophylactic effect on pulmonary embolism remains to be shown.

Oral Anticoagulants

As mentioned previously, the first actually modern study on thromboprophylaxis was based on the effect of oral anticoagulants which were shown to reduce significantly the incidence of fatal pulmonary embolism following hip fracture surgery (Sevitt and Gallagher 1959).

Long before that, however, coumarin anticoagulants had been introduced into clinical practice. Initially, these were isolated from spoiled sweet clover (*Melilotus alba*), which often caused fatal internal hemorrhages (sweet clover disease) in cattle in North Dakota in the American middle west, and in Alberta in Canada (Butt et al. 1941, Bingham et al. 1941, Allen et al. 1942, 1947, Lehmann 1942a, 1943, 1959, Link 1943, 1959). The general bleeding tendency was well known as a pathologicoanatomic entity in cattle (Schofield 1924, Roderick 1929). The condition was soon shown to be reversible if spoiled clover was removed from the food and fresh blood from healthy cattle was transfused. This conditon was described as "prothrombin deficiency."

The original substance was 4-hydroxycoumarin or dicoumarol, which was later to give rise to a great number of derivatives counteracting vitamin K (acenocoumarol, phenprocoumon, warfarin).

As anticoagulants with a similar mechanism of action, inandione preparations are also used. They are derivatives of indan-1,3-dione (anisindione, diphenadione, phenindione).

Mode of Action

Vitamin K is necessary for the final step in the hepatic biosynthesis of coagulation factors II (prothrombin), VII, IX, and X, factors in the so-called prothrombin complex. Vitamin K does not influence the polypeptide synthesis per se, but modifies a precursor to make it work as a coagulation factor (Hemker et al. 1963, Suttie et al. 1974).

The nature of the vitamin K molecule makes it feasible that it participates in an oxidation reduction reaction. An important reaction of this kind is the transformation of glutamic acid groups in the precursors of factors II, VII, IX, and X into γ-carboxyglutamic acid, a reaction which is probably necessary for the calcium-binding capacity of prothrombin (Nelsestuen and Suttie 1972, Stenflo and Ganrot 1973, Nelsestuen et al. 1974, Stenflo et al. 1974. For review, see Stenflo and Suttie 1977). The calcium-binding capacity separates the coagulation factors dependent on vitamin K from the otherwise closely related serine proteases from the pancreas.

Administration of anticoagulants produces an even inhibition of the synthesis of the biologically active component of the four factors, but the factors have a different biologic half-life (II: 60 h, X: 40 h, IX: 20 h, and VII: 5–7 h; Loeliger et al. 1963, van der Meer et al. 1968, Hemker 1977).

If the vitamin K-dependent mechanism is blocked, the precursors mentioned reach the circulation in the form of "proteins induced by vitamin K absence or antagonists" (PIVKA). PIVKA are immunologically identical to the coagulation factors, but biologically they do not participate in the coagulation process (Veltkamp et al. 1971, Nelsestuen et al. 1974, Brozovic and Howarth 1975, Stenflo 1975).

At present, anticoagulants are supposed to interfere with the vitamin K-dependent carboxylation of the prothrombin complex precursors in the microsomes of the liver by preventing the regeneration of vitamin K from 2,3-epoxide (vitamin K oxide) (Suttie 1979). This results in a high concentration of vitamin K oxide in relation to vitamin K in the liver.

Clinical Documentation

Most studies of thromboprophylaxis with oral anticoagulants have been performed in patients undergoing hip surgery (Table 27).

A number of methodologic objections can be raised against Sevitt and Gallagher's (1959) now classic study. This was also the case in Eskeland's paper (1962). Thus several controls exhibited transtrochanteric fractures, several controls did not undergo surgery, and the general condition of the controls was not comparable to that of the treated patients. Moreover, eight patients who had been excluded from the treatment group because the operation had been postponed were transferred to the control group. However, it is improbable that the result would have been different using a better method, and the main conclusion about the prophylactic effect is still valid.

Against the study by Borgström et al. (1965) it can be objected that Armitage's sequential analysis was used for statistical assessment. The method necessitates the choice of "identical" patients in pairs, one receiving treatment and the other none. In the assessment, which is based on relatively complex mathematical methods, only patient pairs with different results of treatment are included.

From these studies it can be concluded that oral anticoagulants have a prophylactic effect in hip surgery. In studies where a comparison with dextran has been made, the effect is equal for both methods (for more details, see p. 136).

The effect seems to be better the earlier the anticoagulant treatment is started (Bronge et al. 1971, Bergqvist et al. 1972, Myhre et al. 1973). The only study showing no effect (Pinto 1970) does not have fully comparable groups, since elective and post-traumatic surgery were pooled. These two groups should be studied separately (Bergqvist et al. 1979).

In other forms of surgery, the documentation is much more scarce. Lambie et al. (1970a) found that warfarin introduced 36 h postoperatively as thromboprophylaxis had a significantly inferior effect compared with dextran 70 in gynecologic surgery. Davidson et al. (1972) reported that introduction of warfarin 36 h prior to surgery was equal to dextran 70 in the same population of patients. However, none of these studies included an untreated reference group.

An investigation was performed in 100 general surgery patients, showing that acenocoumarol medication started on the first postoperative day was significantly less effective than low-dose heparin (5000 IU × 3 for 8 days): 18% vs 2% ($P < 0.025$; van Vroonhoven et al. 1974).

Baertschi et al. (1975) found that low-dose heparin was significantly superior in gynecologic surgery to oral anticoagulants introduced on the second postoperative day (107 patients; 7% thrombosis in the heparin group and 21% in the anticoagulants

Table 27. Oral anticoagulants as thromboprophylaxis in hip surgery
The studies concern hip fracture surgery with the exception of Barber et al. and Hume et al. (elective hip surgery)

Author	Method of Diagnosis	Number of Patients	Incidence of Thrombosis (%)			
			Control	Anti-coagulant	Dex-tran	Others
Barber et al. (1977)	Fibrinogen test	128	–	58[d]	51	52[a]
Bergqvist et al. (1972)	Phlebography	138	–	30[e]	33	–
Bergqvist and Dahlgren (1973)	Fibrinogen test	75	–	50[e]	44	–
Borgström et al. (1965)	Phlebography	58	52	9[f]	–	–
Bronge et al. (1971)	Phlebography	135	–	34[f]	42	–
Eskeland et al. (1966)	Autopsy	200	16	8[f]	–	–
Hamilton et al. (1970)	Phlebography	76	48	19[f]	–	–
Harris et al. (1974)	Phlebography	157	–	20[g]	25	36[b]
Hume et al. (1973)	Fibrinogen test	36	42	59[k]	–	–
Morris and Mitchell (1976b)	Fibrinogen test	149	68	31[h]	–	–
Myhre and Holen (1969)	Phlebography	160	48	18[i]	20	–
Pinto (1970)	Phlebography Fibrinogen test	50	32	36[j]	–	–
Sevitt and Gallagher (1959)	Autopsy	300[c]	83	14[k]	–	–

[a] Low dose heparin.
[b] Acetylsalicylic acid.
[c] Based on autopsy in 56 patients.
Anticoagulation principles:
[d] Introduced 36 h after surgery.
[e] Introduced on establishing the diagnosis.
[f] Introduced immediately after the operation.
[g] Introduced the night before operation.
[h] Introduced 24 h after admission.
[i] Introduced on the second postoperative day.
[j] Introduced at the operation.
[k] Introduced on the first postoperative day.

group; $P < 0.05$). Taberner et al. (1978) started treatment with anticoagulants 5 days preoperatively in a study of patients undergoing gynecologic surgery. The incidence of thrombosis was significantly reduced from 23% in the reference group to 6% in the anticoagulant group ($P < 0.05$). This study also included a low-dose heparin group, and the incidence of thrombosis in this group was also 6%. Also, a study of general surgery patients (van der Linde 1975) and chest surgery patients (Storm 1958) supports preoperative introduction of anticoagulants.

In a large investigation in Tübingen, the 11 739 patients were divided into a reference group and a coumarin group on the basis of their date of birth (Matis 1968). The incidence of fatal pulmonary embolism was significantly reduced from 0.41% to 0.07% ($P = 0.03$). Similar figures can also be found in compilations of uncontrolled studies (Clagett and Salzman 1975, Loeliger 1976).

Practical Aspects

Although it has not been investigated in controlled studies with objective diagnosis of thrombosis, the effect of oral anticoagulants appears to be better, the earlier the prophylaxis is introduced. Ideally, the patient should be on anticoagulant therapy when the operation is performed.

Rustad's (1970) study dealt with this problem both experimentally and clinically. The clinical investigation comprised 800 patients, and, although randomized, it was based on clinical diagnosis. It clearly indicated that preoperative anticoagulation is of prophylactic value. The increased tendency toward hemorrhage was considered of little importance.

Nevertheless, the effect of early introduction of anticoagulants is not so pronounced as might be expected (Sturm and Gruber 1974). To attain an effective therapeutic level, approximately 5 days of treatment are required, making it impossible to use the method in association with emergency surgery.

Oral anticoagulants are contraindicated in all severe hemorrhages, in malignant hypertension, acute damage or surgery within the craniocerebral space or the eye, recent biopsy of the liver or kidneys, and severe hepatic or renal disease.

An undeniable drawback of this type of prophylaxis is that relatively frequent laboratory tests (P&P, thrombotest, normotest, or Simplastin A) are necessary to check the effect. Tolerance is variable, and the doses for obtaining an anticoagulant effect may vary at least fivefold between different individuals. Moreover, different preparations have different half-lives. For phenindione it is 5 h, for warfarin 42 h, and for dicoumarol it may range from 24 to 100 h (Fenech et al. 1979). An operation should not be performed if the thrombotest is less than 20%. In surgery on such patients it is important for the surgeon to be particularly careful with regard to hemostasis.

In patients on oral anticoagulant therapy who require surgery, the anticoagulant effect can be utilized for thromboprophylactic purposes, provided that the prothrombin complex level is not too low or decreasing. If some other chemoprophylaxis is planned, the oral anticoagulation therapy should be stopped 4–5 days prior to elective surgery. In emergency surgery, and when there is a risk of hemorrhage, 10–25 mg vitamin K_1 is administered intravenously, or plasma where the vitamin K-dependent factors are stable.

Oral anticoagulants interact with several preparations which may be used in association with surgery and trauma (Table 28). These drugs may act according to different principles (Gallus and Hirsh 1976a): lowered vitamin K resorption (e.g., cholestyramine), reduced (e.g., cholestyramine) or increased (e.g., nortriptyline) coumarin resorption, reduced albumin binding (e.g., sulfonamides, phenylbutazone, chloral hydrate), increased (e.g., barbiturates, rifampicin) or decreased (e.g., allopurinol, chloramphenicol) inactivation through the microsomal enzyme system of the liver, influence on the hepatic synthesis or degradation rate of the vitamin K-dependent coagulation factors, impaired platelet function leading to potentiation of the hemostatic defect (e.g., salicylates, phenylbutazone, oxyphenbutazone). The interaction between warfarin and sulfinpyrazone is complex. A biphasic interaction has been reported with an initial potentiating effect followed by antagonism (Nenci et al. 1981).

The tolerance of the patient may also vary, e.g., as a result of changes in the intestinal flora, changes of the liver function, cardiac failure and thyroid disturbances, through changed food habits and changes in the resorption of the bowel, or through the influence of infections or fever.

Table 28. Interaction between oral anticoagulants and various drugs

---

1. Agents increasing the anticoagulant effect (increased risk of hemorrhage)

Allopurinol	Nortriptyline
Amitriptyline	Oxyphenbutazone
Chloral hydrate	Phenfuramidol
Chloramphenicol	Phenylbutazone
Chlorpropamide	Quinidine
Cimetidine	Salicylic acid derivatives
Clofibrate	Steroids
Disulfiram	Sulfonamide
Ethacrynic acid	Sulfinpyrazone
Indomethacin	Thiouracil
Metronidazole	Thyroxine
Nalidixic acid	Tolbutamide
Neomycin	Trimethoprim sulfamethoxazole

---

2. Agents reducing the anticoagulant effect (lowered effect)

Barbiturates	Diuretics
Carbamazepine	Glutethamide
Chlorovinylpentynon	Griseofulvin
Chlorthalidone	Haloperidol
Cholestyramine	Heparin
Clopoxide	Meprobamate
Diazepam	Phenazone
	Rifampicin

Adverse Effects

A potentially serious risk in an operated patient, which is obviously a result of successful anticoagulation, is hemorrhage. Several authors have reported increased bleeding in the anticoagulant group versus untreated controls or patients given some other kind of prophylaxis (Dick et al. 1959, Neu et al. 1965, Salzman et al. 1966, Myhre and Holen 1969, Hamilton et al. 1970, Bergqvist et al. 1972, Hume et al. 1973, Harris et al. 1974, Morris and Mitchell 1976b).

Although mainly the number of small hemorrhages is increased, there were two fatal hemorrhages in 63 patients in a study where preoperative therapy was given. Another four patients developed serious hemorrhage (Bergqvist et al. 1972).

According to a compilation by Sturm and Gruber (1974) the total frequency of bleeding complications appears to decrease, the later the prophylaxis is introduced. In a gynecologic population where the patients had received complete anticoagulation therapy intraoperatively (TT on average 16%), there was no increased intraoperative blood loss, but in five cases out of 59 considerable postoperative hemorrhages occurred (Pyörälä and Lampinen 1970).

Anticoagulation entails a risk of spontaneous bleeding especially retroperitoneally, quite often with a fatal outcome (Hodin and Dass 1969, Macon et al. 1970, Bergqvist et al. 1976b, Lowe et al. 1979b). Also cases of "spontaneous" organ ruptures have been reported (Weseley et al. 1957, Amados 1965, Seltzer and Quarantillo 1973, Roberts and Johnston 1975, Dizadji et al. 1979). Hemorrhage induced by anticoagulants may occasionally involve the nervous system (brain, spinal canal, and peripheral nerves). Because of the difficulty in interpreting the neurologic picture, these hemorrhages often cause considerable diagnostic difficulties (Chiu 1976, Silverstein 1979).

Another bleeding complication, which is rare, however, and as a rule does not appear until after a long period of treatment, is intramural small bowel hematomas resulting in obstructive ileus (Herbert 1968).

A difficult and also rare complication is skin necrosis induced by anticoagulants. Warfarin is responsible for many of these cases (Kipen 1961, Nalbandian et al. 1965, Moses and Warren 1973, Faraci et al. 1978), but the condition has been reported after all types of oral anticoagulant therapy.

Necrosis of the skin is most often seen in females. It usually involves parts of the body where there is an abundance of subcutaneous fatty tissue, such as the thighs, hips, and breasts (Jipp 1962). In most cases the changes occurred 4–7 days after the introduction of anticoagulants, and the development did not seem to be related to an attained therapeutic anticoagulant level or to hematoma formation. The process begins with redness over an area of skin, which is excessively tender, resembling "peau d'orange". After a day or two central blisters containing a violet fluid appear. In this area necrosis will develop, with a long healing process. The origin is still unclear. A direct toxic effect on the vessel wall has been suggested as a possible mechanism (Koch-Weser 1968, Faraci et al. 1978), and a certain resemblance to the Shwartzman-Sanarelli phenomenon has been shown (Lieb 1964). Histologically, vasculitis is seen, and also thrombosis of capillaries and venules (Nudelman and Kempson 1966, Shnider and D'Souza 1976, Faraci et al. 1978). Heparin has been reported to have a favorable effect (Nalbandian et al. 1971), but the process appears to be self-limiting, even if medication is not stopped. In several cases of breast involvement ablation had to be performed.

Oral anticoagulants are made of small molecules and therefore pass the placental barrier. This may induce a risk of intrauterine fetal hemorrhage. Moreover, a teratogenic effect has also been reported. It is a malformation syndrome called chondrodysplasia punctata (Conradi-Hunerman's syndrome), characterized by nasal hypoplasia, skeletal deformity, and optic atrophy (Kerber et al. 1968, Palacios-Macedo et al. 1969, Bloomfield 1970, Becker et al. 1975, Pettifor and Benson 1975, Schaul et al. 1975, Stevenson et al. 1980). The syndrome has frequently also been called warfarin embryopathy (Hall et al. 1980). So far, 10–70 cases have been described (Bonnar 1979, Hall et al. 1980).

The pathogenesis of this malformation syndrome is not quite clear. It has been suggested that intrauterine microhemorrhages may be responsible, but there are also data indicating a direct effect of the anticoagulant substance or possibly an effect of the vitamin K deficiency per se (Barr and Burdi 1976).

There is limited experience with administration of oral anticoagulants during the second trimester; however, deterioration of the mental function as well as growth disturbances and visual defects have been reported (Quenneville et al. 1959, Carson and Reid 1976, Sherman and Hall 1976). Anticoagulant therapy during the third trimester may cause fetal and placental hemorrhage, quite often fatal for the fetus (von Sydow 1947, Sachs and Labate 1949, Gordon and Dean 1955, Mahairas and Weingold 1963).

In a review of published cases of pregnancies in which coumarin derivatives had been used, one-sixth of the pregnancies resulted in abnormal liveborn infants, one-sixth in abortion or stillbirth, and two-thirds in apparently normal infants (Hall et al. 1980).

Although the molecule is small, there is no inhibition of the coagulation mechanism in normal full-term infants when they are breast-fed by mothers who are therapeutically anticoagulated with warfarin sodium (McKenna et al. 1981). Breast-feeding has also earlier been practiced by mothers on oral anticoagulants without bleeding complications from the child (Brambel and Hunter 1950, Orme et al. 1977).

In rare cases, oral anticoagulant medication has caused reversible icterus secondary to intrahepatic stasis (Renschler et al. 1963, Hargreaves and Howell 1965, von Kreiter and Fink 1967, Orning et al. 1967, Rehnqvist 1978).

When a hemorrhage occurs, the anticoagulant substance is stopped and vitamin K is administered, whereupon a good hemostatic effect can be expected within 6 h. Still, a normal prothrombin value is not attained until after 12–36 h (Clagett and Salzman 1975). If an immediate effect is desired, for instance in large hemorrhages, plasma or possibly a commercial concentrate of factors II, VII, IX, and X (Preconativ contains factor II and factor IX) can be administered. The latter is much more expensive than plasma, but plasma must be administered in a quantity of 1–1.5 liters (Cade et al. 1979), which in some cases may be too heavy a load for the heart.

When there is an adequate therapeutic anticoagulant level, spontaneous hemorrhages from the gastrointestinal or genitourinary tract are so rare that some authors recommend an investigation with respect to an underlying organic disease, such as tumors (Zweifler 1962, Clagett and Salzman 1975).

Summary

Oral anticoagulants inhibit the transformation of inactive precursors of coagulation factors II, VII, IX, and X to biologically active factors by blocking a vitamin K-dependent process, where glutamic acid groups are transformed to γ-carboxyglutamic acid. Treatment with oral anticoagulants is an effective thromboprophylactic method, provided that the patient receives anticoagulation therapy during the surgical operation. This requires an adjustment time of a few days preoperatively. The majority of the documentation concerns hip surgery.

An undeniable disadvantage of the method is the need for relatively frequent laboratory tests. Another drawback is the interaction with a great number of drugs, several of which may be used in association with surgery or trauma. The risk of hemorrhage is greater in therapeutically adequate oral anticoagulant treatment than in any other method employed in postoperative prophylaxis of thromboembolism.

Ancrod

A bite of the Malayan viper *Agkistrodon rhodostoma* (Boie) produces a form of coagulopathy in at least one-third of the patients (Reid et al. 1963a, b). The poison — ancrod — was purified in 1967, and its effect on the coagulation system was described as resembling thrombin (Regoeczi et al. 1966, Esnouf and Tunnah 1967).

After administration of ancrod, the fibrinogen level rapidly falls without affecting any other coagulation factors (Bell et al. 1968a) or prothrombin metabolism (Bell et al. 1978). At the same time, peptides with antithrombin action are formed (Ashford et al. 1968). The effect of thrombin on fibrinogen is to split off fibrinopeptides A and B, whereupon polymerization to fibrin occurs with a subsequent stabilization by factor XIII. Thrombin activates factor XIII, which ancrod does not (Kiesselback and Wagner 1966, Barlow et al. 1970).

Ancrod only splits off fibrinopeptide A (Ewart et al. 1970, Holleman and Coen 1970, Mattock and Esnouf 1971, Edgar and Prentice 1973, Aronson 1976). The result is a differently polymerized fibrin, which is lysed more easily by the normal fibrinolytic activity of the body (Kwaan and Barlow 1971). Coagulable fibrinogen as well as immunoreactive fibrinogen falls (Bell 1974). Fibrin degradation products with small molecules are more quickly formed than if fibrinolysis of thrombin-coagulated fibrin takes place (Kwaan et al. 1973). The fibrin-stabilizing factor XIII or the fibrinolytic system per se is not influenced by ancrod (Turpie et al. 1971, Pizzo et al. 1972), but the plasminogen concentration quickly falls (Pitney et al. 1969a, Silberman et al. 1973, Bell 1974). The low plasminogen level persists during treatment.

During the early phases of defibrinogenization, the concentration of fibrin and fibrinogen degradation products (FDP) is high, and they are probably responsible for the influence on the platelets reported by several authors (Pitney et al. 1969a, Prentice et al. 1969, Kwaan et al. 1973, McKenzie et al. 1973, Slade et al. 1976). Concurrently with the fibrinogen decrease a decreased plasma viscosity develops (Ehrly 1973, 1975, Gustafsson et al. 1977), resulting in an increased blood flow (Gustafsson et al. 1977).

Some studies have indicated that it should be possible to use ancrod in the treatment of venous thrombosis because of its "defibrinogenizing" property (Bell et al. 1968b, Sharp et al. 1968, Bowell et al. 1970). Experimentally, it was shown by Olsen and Pitney (1969) that ancrod induced histologic changes in pulmonary emboli, which also disappeared more quickly from the pulmonary vessels than emboli in control animals.

In the few controlled studies reported, ancrod was not shown to be superior to heparin, and in the acute phase of thrombosis it is rather less effective than streptokinase (Kakkar et al. 1969a, Davis et al. 1972, Tibbutt et al. 1974).

Considering the mechanism of action of ancrod, treatment introduced preoperatively can be assumed to have a prophylactic effect. In a small series of patients with hip fractures, Barrie et al. (1974) found no difference in the incidence of thrombosis between ancrod-treated and untreated patients, but suspected that there were fewer extensive thrombi in the treated group. Ancrod was administered in a dose which lowered the fibrinogen level approximately by half compared with that of the controls. Treatment was started 4–12 h preoperatively in the form of continuous intravenous infusion and was continued for 72 h postoperatively.

A few basic studies on administration and dosage were performed by Lowe et al. (1978) in patients with hip fractures. The authors consider this to be a simple model for thromboprophylaxis. Lowe (1978) and Lowe et al. (1979a) studied 105 patients with hip fractures (53 ancrod, 52 controls). The incidence of thrombosis confirmed by phlebography was 73% in the control group and 45% in the ancrod group ($P < 0.01$). The difference was still greater if the estimation was made on "large" thrombi (65% vs 30%; $P < 0.001$). The same group also made a study on elective hip surgery with similar results, that is a reduction in the frequency of phlebographic thrombi larger than 5 cm (Belch et al. 1981).

Ancrod can be administered intravenously, intramuscularly, or subcutaneously. The effect has to be followed by checking the fibrinogen level. A relatively simple plan for subcutaneous administration without any fibrinogen measurement has been worked out by Ehrly and Köhler (1976).

Injection of ^{131}I-ancrod showed that the ratio of extravascular/intravascular ancrod is 1.7 in man (Bell 1974). Ancrod is degraded intravascularly and excreted in the urine. Only very small quantities are excreted in the active form. Ancrod does not influence central hemodynamics (Klein et al. 1969) or renal function (Marshall and Esnouf 1968).

The initial hemostatic mechanism is influenced by ancrod, probably by FDP influence on the platelets (Bergqvist and Arfors 1974). This hemostatic effect causes a certain increased tendency toward bleeding (Slade et al. 1973), which was not significant in clinical studies (Bell et al. 1968b, Davies et al. 1972, Tibbutt et al. 1974). It occurs in less than 5% of patients (Bell 1971). On excessive hemorrhage, antivenom can be used to neutralize ancrod and, preferably, fibrinogen should also be administered.

Resistance to ancrod has been described in a few cases (Pitney et al. 1969b).

In principle, the contraindications are the same as in conventional anticoagulation therapy, i.e., mainly various hemorrhagic conditions. Moreover, ancrod is contraindicated when the fibrinolytic or the reticuloendothelial systems are blocked. Pregnancy is another contraindication, both with regard to the risk of hemorrhage and from a teratologic point of view where knowledge is still limited. Ancrod probably does not pass the placental barrier, however (Martin et al. 1971).

Defibrinogenization using ancrod is a relatively new and interesting principle, but further studies employing objective methods of measurement are required to establish its place as a thromboprophylactic agent. At present, ancrod does not seem to superior to heparin. Optimal dosage and duration of treatment have not been studied in detail.

Summary

Ancrod is a poison with a thrombin-like effect, derived from a Malayan viper. It causes defibrinogenization with a subsequent increase of fibrinogen degradation products, and influences the platelets, leading to a decreased plasma viscosity.

A simplified plan for subcutaneous administration of ancrod has been established, eliminating the need for frequent fibrinogen determinations. This plan was used in a study on patients with hip fractures, with good thromboprophylactic effect. However, ancrod cannot be recommended yet for general clinical use, but is of interest exclusively for research purposes.

Low-Dose Heparin

Low-dose heparin refers to the prophylactic subcutaneous administration of heparin prior to trauma in doses which do not affect the usual coagulation tests.

Heparin was discovered in 1916 and has been used clinically since the 1930s (Jorpes 1936). From a chemical viewpoint, heparin is an acid-sulfated polysaccharide with three cyclic hexose derivatives (hexopyranosides): D-glucosamine, D-glucuronic acid, and L-iduronic acid. The molecule consists of a simple chain constructed of repeating disaccharide units, all of which contain glucosamine and uronic acid. The uronic acid may be glucuronic acid or iduronic acid. The disaccharide units are sulfated to a varying degree (one to three sulfate groups per disaccharide unit), and the position of the sulfate groups varies (Fig. 6). The sulfur content is about 10%. Because of its large number of acid groups, heparin is a strong acid. A combination of chemical properties is required for anticoagulation activity: free carboxyl groups, 0-sulfate ester groups from hexuronic acid, and sulfamino groups on glucosamine (Jorpes et al. 1950, Cifonelli 1974, Danishefski 1975).

Commercial heparins are very heterogeneous, containing at least 21 components with molecular weights ranging from 6000 to 30 000, and with varying electrophoretic mobilities, nuclear magnetic spectra, and anticoagulation activites (Jaques and Kavanaugh 1973, Kiss 1973, Nader et al. 1974, McDuffe et al. 1975, Andersson et al. 1976, Johnson et al. 1976, Thomas 1978b). There are probably many more components. Heparin from rat blood has a very high molecular weight — about one million (Horner 1971) — and commercial heparin from only one source may vary between 4000 and 16 000 (Lasker and Stivala 1966).

The anticoagulant effect is dependent on the molecular weight (Cifonelli 1974, Laurent et al. 1978). Low molecular weight heparin potentiates the inhibition of activated factor X, whereas heparin of a higher molecular weight influences the coagulation system as a whole (Andersson et al. 1976, 1979). For prophylactic purposes more low molecular weight fractions are therefore desirable, and theoretically, the risk of hemorrhage would then be reduced. This is also the reasoning behind the development of various heparin-like substances for thromboprophylaxis (see p. 113).

It is now known that a certain monosaccharide sequence of 12—16 units is responsible for the strong heparin binding to antithrombin III (Hopwood et al. 1976, Lindahl et al. 1979). Approximately one-third of the heparin molecules possess the mono-

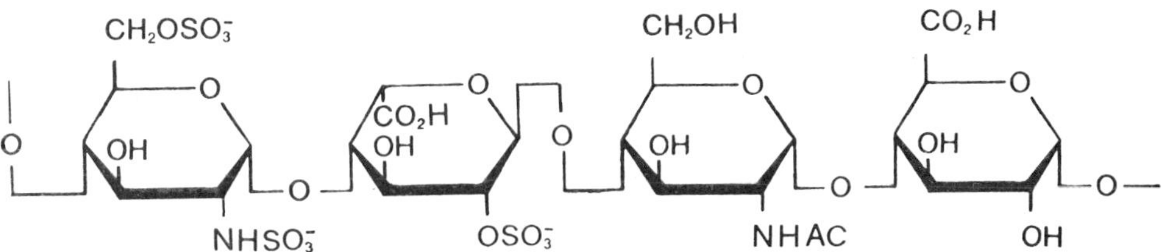

Fig. 6. Structure of heparin

saccharide sequence required for the binding, and this is the heparin part responsible for the anticoagulant activity. Using pure antithrombin III, this active third (high affinity heparin) can be separated from a heparin preparation. The negatively charged heparin binds to positively charged amino acids on the antithrombin molecule (Rosenberg and Damus 1973).

The relation between the Xa-inhibitor effect and antithrombotic effect seems to be dependent on the molecular weight, but experimental data are in part discrepant (Holmer et al. 1981, Ockelford et al. 1981, Thomas et al. 1981, Choay et al. 1981). Clinical investigations on the thromboprophylactic effect of low molecular weight heparin have started (Kakkar et al. 1981b), and although no controlled studies have been carried out so far, preliminary data indicate a very low frequency of thrombosis after abdominal surgery with low molecular weight heparin administered once daily (Kakkar et al. 1982).

More and more concentrated and purified heparin preparations have been produced, but absolute purity has not yet been attained. It has been discussed whether such an adverse effect as thrombocytopenia (see p. 109) might be caused by contamination (Genton 1974).

The great differences between various commercial heparin preparations obviously make comparison between studies somewhat difficult. Hence, Jaques (1976) suggestion that heparin be identified in publications (by manufacturer, batch number, nature of tissue, animal species, mode of extraction) should be adopted.

The heparin used commercially today is manufactured from porcine intestinal mucosa or, in a few cases, from bovine lungs. At present it is not known if there is any great clinical difference between these two heparins (Wessler and Gitel 1979). In a comparative study of mucosal heparin from pigs, sheep, and cows, and bovine lung heparin, differences in potency were shown. These differences were not large enough, however, to justify a recommendation for separate international standards (Bangham and Woodward 1970). Primarily the Xa-inhibitor activity may vary considerably, depending on the origin of the heparin (Barrowcliffe et al. 1977, Thomas et al. 1980b). European heparin is for the most part manufactured from intestinal mucosa.

The mast cells seem to be the main storage place for heparin, since the distribution of tissue heparin is similar to the distribution of mast cells (Jaques 1967, Raich et al. 1974). Jorpes et al. (1937) were able to show that the metachromatic staining reaction in certain granules of the mast cells was due to the presence of heparin. It is also probable that heparin is synthesized in the mast cells (Engelberg 1978). In the metachromatic granules of the mast cells, heparin is covalently bound to protein (Lindahl 1966). In most vessels, there is a great number of mast cells immediately beneath the endothelium (McGovern 1956). Moreover, heparin is present in basophilic granulocytes (Behrens and Taubert 1952). Heparin can easily be diffused to the blood from these sources. The total concentration of heparin in man has been estimated to about 20 000 IU.

One unit of heparin activity is defined as the activity in 1/30 mg of the first international heparin standard (1943). The heparin activity in commercial preparations is decided either by the United States Pharmacopeia (USP) or the British Pharmacopeia (BP), with an international standard as reference. The potency of a commercial heparin depends on whether the USP or BP is used; the BP determinations are as a rule 7%–10% higher than those of the USP.

When heparin is prepared, protein is first removed using alkali, phenol, or enzymatic degradation (Charles and Scott 1933, Homan and Lens 1948, Jeanloz 1965). Continued selective purification can be performed by precipitation with quaternary ammonium compounds, electrophoresis, chromatography, ethanol precipitation, and isoelectric focusing (Wessler and Gitel 1979). It was recently shown that it is possible either by affinity chromatography on antithrombin III agarose or dissolution with binding to antithrombin III to produce heparin with a considerably stronger anticoagulant activity than previously so-called high-affinity heparin (Andersson et al. 1976, Lam et al. 1976).

Apart from its effect on hemostatic system (see p. 93), heparin has an antilipemic activity (Ehrlich and Stivala 1973) and a complement-inhibiting function (Ecker and Gross 1929, Cofrancesco et al. 1979). Small quantities of heparin administered intravenously result in an increased lipoprotein lipase activity (Ham and Slack 1969, Negus et al. 1971, Heaf et al. 1977). This activation is believed to induce the increase in free fatty acids observed on heparinization (Nelson 1970, Russo et al. 1970).

In patients with coronary infarction there is a correlation between high levels of free fatty acids and the incidence of ventricular arrhythmia (Oliver et al. 1968), which could be a risk factor in postoperative patients who develop an infarct while on low-dose heparin prophylaxis. Arnesen et al. (1979a) were able to show that patients with coronary infarction who received low-dose heparin showed no increase in free fatty acids. They had exactly the same levels as patients receiving warfarin. Also, the incidence of ventricular arrhythmia was identical in both groups (Arnesen et al. 1980).

Furthermore, heparin has the ability to complex-bind a series of proteins and peptides (e.g., γ-globulin, β-lipoprotein, Waldenström's macroglobulin, protamine, peptone, histone, hemoglobin, casein, thromboplastin, trypsin), biogenous amines (e.g., histamine, 5-hydroxytryptamine), organic bases (e.g., benzidine, quinine, piperidine), and basic stains (e.g., methylene blue, pyronine, thionin, toluidine blue) (Coon and Willis 1966, Jaques 1979).

Heparin can be administered intravenously or subcutaneously. Intramuscular injection should be avoided: firstly, the risk of hematoma is great and, secondly, the absorption from depots in the muscles is often irregular (Bauer et al. 1950, MacMillan and Brown 1953, Genton 1974, Raich et al. 1974, Jaques and Mahadoo 1978). For prophylaxis against postoperative thromboembolism only subcutaneous administration can be contemplated as yet.

Intrapulmonary administration is a theoretically interesting possibility. This mode of application was suggested in the mid-1960s, but it was concluded that heparin is not resorbed from the lungs, probably because too low a dose was given (Windsor and Freeman 1964, Rosner 1965, Youngchaiyud et al. 1969).

By a single administration of a relatively high dose of heparin in aerosol form, Jaques et al. (1976) were able to show that healthy volunteers and different laboratory animal species responded with moderate hypocoagulability. In man it persisted for 14 days, and the heparin level was equal to that following subcutaneous low-dose heparin prophylaxis. Possibly, heparin is taken up by macrophages in the lungs or the peritoneum and is followed by a slow release (Oh et al. 1973). Another possibility discussed is that heparin is taken up by the vascular endothelium, where it can be concentrated several hundred times more than the plasma level. It is then continuously released into the circulation at a low dose (Hierbert and Jaques 1976, Glimelius et al. 1978).

No toxic effects were observed in spite of very high heparin doses over a long period of time in some cases (Sutherland and Klein 1973, Wright and Mahadoo 1980).

The results were later confirmed by Swedish scientists (Hellgren et al. 1979, 1981). With a dose of 1300 IU/kg body wt. the patients still had measurable heparin levels in the plasma after 3 weeks, as measured according to Teien et al. (1976b). The pulmonary function is not influenced by this mode of administration (Hellgren et al. 1981). In a controlled study in dogs (Wright et al. 1979), the effect of 1500 IU/kg of intrapulmonarily administered heparin was studied on different bleeding parameters, both after small bowel resection and after muscular resection. The operation was performed within 3 h of heparin administration. The intraoperative hemorrhage was the same in the control group as in the heparin group for both types of surgery. After muscular resection, the postoperative hemorrhage was significantly larger in the heparin-treated dogs.

Nevertheless, it is too early to recommend this route of administration.

Haparin is eliminated from the circulation mainly via the reticuloendothelial system, especially in the spleen and liver (Hierbert and Jaques 1976, Mahadoo et al. 1977, Dawes and Pepper 1979), but also in the lungs and kidneys (Dawes and Pepper 1979). Heparin absorbed by endothelial cells can be released again into the circulation (Glimelius et al. 1978, Jaques and Mahadoo 1978). Part of the heparin is metabolized in the reticuloendothelial system and is released again into the blood stream as a biologically inactive metabolite of the same molecular weight as the original heparin. This metabolite is largely desulfated (Dawes and Pepper 1979). Part of it is then degraded and excreted via the kidneys, which probably contain an as yet unknown glycosidase. Heparin at a low dose also affects the reticuloendothelial system, with subsequently increased phagocytic activity (Lahnborg et al. 1976a, Saba and Antikatzides 1979). Heparin does not pass the placental barrier (Flessa et al. 1965).

Heparin elimination is mainly exponential (Olsson et al. 1963). The mean half-life of heparin has been reported to be 90 min in healthy volunteers (Estes 1975, Estes and Poulin 1975), but large variations have been described in the literature (23–360 min). To a large extent this can be explained by methodologic differences when analyzing the heparin concentration (McAvoy 1979). As to the influence of various pathologic conditions on the half-life of heparin, scarce but variable or conflicting information is given in the literature (Wessler and Gitel 1979). Also, the half-life seems to be dose dependent; it is prolonged when the dose is increased (Olsson et al. 1963).

By measuring plasma heparin, Kakkar et al. (1972) were able to show that plasma contains on average 0.120 IU/ml 2 h after subcutaneous injection of 5000 IU. The half-life was considerably shorter in association with elective surgery than in healthy unoperated volunteers. In the former group, only insignificant heparin quantities could be demonstrated after 4 h; in the latter the same low level was attained after 7 h. Lahnborg and Bergström (1975) still found satisfactory heparin levels 7 h later in surgical patients, employing the method for heparin determination described by Yin et al. (1973). However, the individual variation appears to be great, just as is the variation due to different heparin preparations (Brozovic et al. 1973, Giacommetti et al. 1975, Johnson et al. 1976, Thomas et al. 1976, Kakkar 1978, Low and Briggs 1978). The heparin half-life is shorter in smokers than in nonsmokers (Cipolle et al. 1981). In uremic patients, subcutaneous low-dose heparin gives a lower plasma heparin concentration, probably due to a diminished net absorption from the subcutaneous depot (Andrassy et al. 1981).

To 43 patients undergoing elective hip surgery, 5000 IU (1 ml) heparin was administered subcutaneously 48 h preoperatively, and plasma heparin determinations (Denson and Bonnar 1973) were made after 2 and 8 h (Brozovic et al. 1975). Thirty-seven patients had levels ranging from 0.05 to 0.15 IU/ml, three had more than 0.2 IU/ml, and three only trace amounts. Thus, three patients might be at risk with respect to hemorrhage, and just as many were without any prophylaxis. The plasma heparin level was not correlated with age, sex, weight, or intake of analgesics.

No differences in heparin level were shown by Kruse-Blinkenberg et al. (1977a) between patients developing postoperative thrombosis and patients without thrombosis. In a later study the same authors found a lower heparin level in patients who developed postoperative thrombosis (Kruse-Blinkenberg et al. 1980). Nor was it possible to show any correlation between the plasma heparin level and the extent of bleeding or need of transfusion in thoracic surgery (particularly pulmonary surgery) (Kruse-Blinkenberg et al. 1977b). Postoperatively, a higher heparin level than intraoperatively was shown in this particular type of surgery, which is difficult to explain and calls for confirmation. The authors assume that heparin is released from the intraoperatively traumatized pulmonary tissue.

Gurewich et al. (1978) studied the same problem, but measured partial thromboplastin time instead of the heparin level, finding that it was at least doubled in 10%–15% of the 100 general surgery patients. Neither was this value correlated to sex, age, or weight. Two of the three patients requiring more than two transfusion units of blood had prolonged partial thromboplastin time (the third took aspirin daily). The degree of activation of the coagulation system in the individual patient is probably of greater importance for the low-dose heparin effect than the weight of the patient. In most studies, no weight correlation could be shown. There are a few exceptions, and Tilsner et al. (1980) found that dosage according to body weight was superior to routine dosage. Beermann and Lahnborg (1981) found a higher plasma heparin level in overweight patients who also had a prolonged half-life.

Mode of Action

The principal role of heparin as an anticoagulant is due to the fact that the serine protease-neutralizing capacity of antithrombin III is accelerated. The proteases inhibited in this way are thrombin, plasmin, kallikrein, C1-esterase, urokinase, and the active forms of coagulation factors VII, IX, X, XI, and XII (Abildgaard 1968, Biggs et al. 1970, Yin and Wessler 1970, Yin et al. 1971a, Damus et al. 1973, Godal et al. 1974, Highsmith and Rosenberg 1974, Burrowes et al. 1975, J. Rosenberg et al. 1975, Vennerød and Laake 1975, Rosenberg 1976, 1977, Stead et al. 1976, Østerud et al. 1976, Clemmesen 1978). The inhibition of thrombin and activated factor X (Xa) by only antithrombin III is a slow process, but in the presence of heparin it is almost instantaneous, and in this acceleration reaction heparin acts as a catalyst (Brinkhous et al. 1939, Abildgaard 1968, Yin and Wessler 1970, Björk and Nordenmann 1976, Barrowcliffe 1978, Holmer 1980). Antithrombin III is therefore also called heparin cofactor. When the inhibition reaction is completed, the heparin molecule is released from the antithrombin III-thrombin complex, and can be utilized again. The remaining antithrombin III-thrombin complexes are removed by the reticuloendothelial system (Holmer et al. 1979, Rosenberg et al. 1980). Clinically used heparin has recently been separated into molecules with high and low affinity for antithrombin III (Andersson et al. 1976, Rosenberg and Jam 1979). Clinical heparin consists of 30%–50% high affinity heparin.

The coagulation system is considered to be a multiplying cascade, meaning that relatively few molecules of factor XIIa activate a great number of thrombin molecules. Similarly, fewer antithrombin III molecules are required to inhibit factor Xa than to inhibit thrombin. This phenomenon is considered of importance for the mechanism of action of low-dose heparin (Han and Ardlie 1974). The potential formation of 1600 NIH units of thrombin is indirectly inhibited by 32 units of factor Xa (Yin and Wessler 1970, Yin et al. 1971b). This line of thought is the reason why heparin is administered prior to a surgical trauma, i.e., prior to the trauma, giving rise to activation of factor X and later to thrombin. This reasoning is indirectly supported by the fact that low-dose heparin is comparatively inactive as a prophylactic in hip fracture surgery, when patients are already traumatized on admission (see also p. 97).

That the Xa-inhibitor effect is of importance is also supported by the fact that low molecular weight heparinoids with a relatively high Xa-inhibitor effect have a thromboprophylactic action (p. 113).

Theoretically, it is feasible that smaller amounts of heparin than required for Xa-inhibition may block the activation of factors IX, XI, and XII. As mentioned previously, there are indications that heparins of different molecular weights have a different potency. The inhibition of factor Xa in plasma is strongly potentiated by the low molecular weight heparin fractions which have no effect on thrombin (Andersson et al. 1976, Holmer 1979, Lane et al. 1979, Holmer et al. 1980).

The effect of low-dose heparin on different parameters within the coagulation-hemostatic system has been studied by several authors. Antithrombin III measured immunologically and using a chromogenic substrate is not influenced (Bergström and Lahnborg 1975). Hedlund and Blombäck (1979) studied a series of factors, finding no difference compared to controls with respect to the number of platelets, APT time, normotest, fibrinogen, factor VIII, antithrombin III (determined by coagulation technique, by chromogenic substrate, as heparin cofactor using chromogenic as well as immunologic substrate), α_1-antitrypsin, α_2-macroglobulin, thrombin time, reptilase time, factors II, VII, and X, ethanol gelation test, and FDP.

Wu et al. (1977) and Törngren et al. (1979b) obtained similar results, but their analyses included fewer parameters. In the latter study there are certain indications that low-dose heparin prevents the increase in fibrinopeptide A which occurs postoperatively. Fibrinopeptide A is a sensitive test which can also detect thrombin activation (Kockum-Ivemark 1979). Covey et al. (1975), however, found no differences in ethanol gelation tests between controls and patients treated with low-dose heparin, indicating different fibrin monomer levels. Loew and Vinazzer (1974) found an increased thrombin time and recalcification time in patients with thrombosis. Similar findings were noted preoperatively by O'Brien et al. (1972), but postoperatively the difference between heparin and control patients disappeared. A slight but significant prolongation of the APT time up to 5 h following subcutaneous administration of 5000 IU heparin to patients undergoing hip surgery was found by Gallus et al. (1973a). Rem et al. (1975) found a prolonged thrombin time also postoperatively in general surgery and urology patients.

Kruse-Blinkenberg and Gormsen (1980) found plasma changes in general surgery patients on low-dose heparin (5000 IU × 3), indicating that low-dose heparin could enhance thrombolysis: antiplasmin decreased peroperatively and the postoperative increase was not as high in the heparin as in the control group.

No difference has been shown in the plasma half-life of ^{125}I-fibrinogen between untreated patients and patients treated with low-dose heparin (Törngren et al. 1979, 1980b). Nor has any difference been demonstrated for analysis of coagulable fibrinogen and noncoagulable degradation products (Covey et al. 1975).

The effect on platelet function is complex and incompletely known. In the presence of Ca^{++} eight different commercial heparin preparations caused platelet aggregation, which was inhibited by EDTA, apyrase, and adenosine (Eika 1972). Loew and Vinazzer (1974) found that platelets aggregated spontaneously on administration of low-dose heparin, and Gormsen et al. (1974) found that ADP aggregated platelets quicker after low-dose heparin injection. Heparin also increased the embolization rate from laser-induced platelet thrombi in the ear chamber microcirculation of rabbits (Esquivel et al. 1982a). Heparin-induced platelet aggregation might be explained by the recently published findings that heparin neutralizes the inhibiting effect of prostacyclin (PGI_2) on platelet aggregation (Eldor and Weksler 1979, Saba et al. 1979). Other studies have shown that the heparin-induced aggregability increases after a burn (Mims et al. 1977).

Other authors, however, found an inhibition of platelet aggregation (Han and Ardlie 1974). O'Brien et al. (1972) were able to show that low-dose heparin prevented the immediate postoperative decrease in platelet aggregation as a response to ADP and thrombin. Economopoulos et al. (1977) performed different platelet function tests in association with low-dose heparin prophylaxis, without finding any difference between the prophylaxis group and untreated patients. Recent studies have shown that the effect on platelet aggregation is also due to the molecular weight of heparin. Fractions with a higher molecular weight are more reactive than fractions with a low molecular weight (Holmer et al. 1980, Salzman et al. 1980b). The effect on platelets and the anticoagulant effect are not parallel. This fact may partly explain the apparently contradictory effects of heparin on platelet function. The adhesiveness of the platelets diminishes on heparin administration, and this happens even at as low a dose as 1 IU/kg body wt. (Negus et al. 1971).

Low shear values ($0.77 \ s^{-1}$ and $2.62 \ s^{-1}$) result in a reduced blood viscosity on administration of low-dose heparin, with an optimal effect 4–6 h after the subcutaneous injection (Erdi et al. 1976). This observation has not been confirmed, however (Girolami et al. 1978).

An interesting observation with possible clinical implications is the potentiation of PGI_2 by heparin (Bunting and Moncada 1980, Moncada and Vane 1981).

It was shown in a study that arterial pO_2 falls significantly after surgery of the gallbladder. This decrease is more quickly normalized in patients receiving low-dose heparin (Lahnborg et al. 1976b). The pCO_2 value did not differ between the groups. The authors were of the opinion that the shortened hypoxia period in association with low-dose heparin could be ascribed to a reduced incidence of macro- and microemboli in the lungs. However, pulmonary scintigraphy was normal in all patients.

In healthy volunteers, low doses of heparin produce increased serum aminotransferase levels (ALAT and ASAT; Olsson et al. 1978).

Clinical Documentation

Prophylactic use of therapeutic doses of heparin postoperatively (Bergqvist 1940, Crafoord and Jorpes 1941, Wetterdal 1941, Strömbeck 1942, Nielsen 1942, Murray 1947) has never been practiced to any great extent, primarily because of the considerable risk of hemorrhage. In a study of coronary infarction patients, no difference in prophylactic effect on thromboembolism could be shown between a full dose of heparin and low-dose heparin (Pitt et al. 1980).

De Takats (1950) was the first to suggest that a lower dose of heparin was required to prevent thrombosis than to treat it, but Strömbeck had already similar thoughts in 1942. Jaques et al. (1938) had already shown that subcutaneous administration was possible. The general idea of what was later to be known as low-dose heparin was introduced by Sharnoff et al. (1962), who started prophylaxis by supplying 10 000 IU 10 h preoperatively and continued postoperatively with administration of 2500 IU every 6 h. It was vital to maintain a normal coagulation in these patients, and this was achieved by various coagulation tests (Sharnoff 1963, 1966, 1975). An effect on the incidence of fatal pulmonary embolism was shown. Sharnoff continued using this prophylactic method (Sharnoff and DeBlazio 1970), but his results have been questioned for various reasons (Benson 1970).

It was not until strictly controlled studies appeared in the 1970s, employing the ^{125}I-fibrinogen test to establish the diagnosis that the method was evaluated to any great extent. In general surgery, gynecology, and possibly in urology and neurosurgery it has been established that low-dose heparin significantly reduces the incidence of postoperative thrombosis as measured by the ^{125}I-fibrinogen test. A number of surveys have been published over the years (Kakkar 1973, Gallus and Hirsh 1976a, b, Kakkar 1975a, b, Rem et al. 1975, Wessler 1975b, 1976, Sherry 1976, Matt and Gruber 1977, Kakkar 1978, Lahnborg 1978, Thomas 1978b, Törngren 1979b, Wessler and Gitel 1979). Table 29 shows the effect of low-dose heparin in various nonorthopedic operations. In all studies, the ^{125}I-fibrinogen test was used to establish the diagnosis, and in the great majority of cases the effect was very good.

In two of the studies, where no effect was shown, the controls had an uncommonly low incidence of thrombosis (Abernathy and Hartsuck 1974, Covey et al. 1975). The third study concerned patients undergoing urologic surgery (Coe et al. 1978). It was also not possible to demonstrate any effect in the relatively few urologic cases in William's (1971) study, but as appears in the table, other urologic studies showing an effect have been published.

Hedlund (1975) was not able to show any effect of heparin in association with prostatic surgery. It should be pointed out, however, that his study does not deal with low-dose heparin in a proper sense, as claimed in some reviews (Rem et al. 1975, Matt and Gruber 1977). The patients in fact received their first heparin dose on the first postoperative day, i.e., after the activation of factor X in connection with surgery, and were then given 10 000 IU × 2. In a later study, Hedlund and Blombäck (1981) found that when prophylaxis was begun preoperatively, low-dose heparin halved the incidence of thrombosis following transvesical prostatic surgery (from 46% to 21%; 59 patients). If only thrombosis with onset during ongoing prophylaxis is taken into account (5 days), the effect is still more marked (from 39% to 7%; $P < 0.0005$).

In a few studies, diagnostic methods other than the ^{125}I-fibrinogen test were employed. Ribaudo et al. (1975) used nucleide venography with ^{99}Tc^m-macroaggregated albumin, finding 50% thrombi in the reference group compared with 21% in the heparin group. In the latter group all nine thrombi were located in the calf, while two out of 19 in the reference group were found in the femoral veins. No thrombi of the pelvic veins were found. The incidence of scintigraphically demonstrated pulmonary emboli was reduced from 5.3% to 0% in the low-dose heparin group. Arbeit et al. (1981) used phlebography in patients who underwent groin lymph dissection because of malignant melanoma and found no difference in thrombosis frequency between a low-dose heparin and a control group in a double-blind study.

From the Groote Schuur Hospital (1979; Immelman et al. 1981) in Cape Town results have recently been published which question the effect of low-dose heparin on proximal thrombi. Although the incidence of thrombosis was reduced by low-dose heparin as assessed both by the ^{125}I-fibrinogen test and by phlebography, closer analysis showed that the reduction only concerned thrombi of the calf veins. The number of phlebographically demonstrated iliofemoral thrombi was the same in the reference group as in the heparin group. The results of pulmonary perfusion scintigraphy were classified using a special scoring system. Nor did the groups differ in what were considered to be definite emboli. Although the population was small, the study has attracted attention and given rise to some discussion (Adiseshiah 1979, Kakkar 1979b, Norgren 1979, Prentice et al. 1979, Stubbs 1979).

Nevertheless, some previous studies employing the fibrinogen test have shown that the number of proximal thrombi decreases on administration of low-dose heparin (Corrigan et al. 1974, International Multicentre Trial 1975, Rem et al. 1975, Rosenberg et al. 1975, Gallus et al. 1976, Nicolaides et al. 1972b, Bergqvist and Hallböök 1980). This effect of low-dose heparin is less pronounced in hip surgery (Gallus and Hirsh 1976b).

An undeniable prophylactic effect in association with neurosurgery was shown by Cerrato et al. (1978), but the risk of hemorrhage, however slight, makes low-dose heparin unsuitable for this purpose. It was only recently shown that these patients are in need of thromboembolic prophylaxis (Holmgren 1980), which may explain the low number of studies.

Table 30 shows the thromboprophylactic effect of low-dose heparin in orthopedic surgery. It is apparent that the effect is much less pronounced in these high-risk patients than in general surgery, and many authors have been unable to demonstrate any prophylactic effect whatsoever. This applies primarily to fracture surgery, and, as mentioned previously, there are theoretical grounds for expecting considerably less effect in this group of patients. The dramatic reduction of the incidence of thrombosis in the study by Lawrence et al. (1977) appears somewhat difficult to explain. The same patients are probably included in the investigation by Xabregas et al. (1978). Svend-Hansen et al. (1981), using Armitage's sequential statistical analysis, was not able to show an effect of low-dose heparin in patients undergoing hip fracture surgery. In a rather small study (150 patients) the frequency of fatal pulmonary embolism was not reduced after hip fracture surgery (Kiviluoto et al. 1979). However, when using an individual dose depending on the plasma heparin level, Lowe (1981) found that it was possible to improve the prophylactic effect. As mentioned previously, there are also methodologic difficulties in establishing the diagnosis in patients undergoing hip sur-

Table 29. The thromboprophylactic effect of low-dose heparin in general surgery, urology, neurosurgery, and gynecologic surgery Diagnosis employing the ^{125}I-fibrinogen test

Author	Patient population	Number of patients	Incidence of thrombosis (%)		
			Controls	Low-dose heparin	Significance
Abernathy and Hartsuck (1974)	General surgery	125	5	6	NS
Ansay et al. (1977)	General surgery	50	63	26	$P < 0.05$
Ballard et al. (1973)	Gynecology	110	29	4	$P < 0.01$
Bergqvist and Hallböök (1980)	General surgery	97	27	13	$P < 0.05$
Cerrato et al. (1978)	Neurosurgery	100	34	6	$P < 0.005$
Coe et al. (1978)	Urology	52	25	21	NS
Covey et al. (1975)	General surgery	105	10	8	NS
Gallus et al. (1973b)	General surgery	104	15	1	$P < 0.001$
Gallus et al. (1976)	General surgery	782	16	4	$P < 0.05$
Gordon-Smith et al. (1972a)	General surgery	150	42	14[a]	$P < 0.003$
				8[b]	$P < 0.001$
Groote Schuur Hosp. (1979)	Abdominal surgery	199	27	12	$P < 0.007$
Gruber et al. (1977b)	General surgery	194	36	13	$P < 0.005$
Hedlund and Blombäck (1979)	Urology	59	46	21	NS
Int. Multicentre Trial	General surgery	1292	25	8	$P < 0.005$
Jackaman et al. (1978)	Thorax surgery	183	51	28	$P < 0.005$
Joffe (1976)	General surgery	120	51	9	$P < 0.0005$
Kakkar et al. (1972)	General surgery	78	42	8	$P < 0.001$
Kettunen et al. (1972)	General surgery	200	41	8	$P < 0.001$
Kraytman et al. (1976)	General surgery	50	63	26	$P < 0.05$
Kutnowski et al. (1977)	Urology	47	36	9	$P < 0.05$
Lahnborg et al. (1974)	Abdominal surgery	112	11	3	$P < 0.05$
Lawrence et al. (1977)	Abdominal surgery	242	17	7	$P < 0.05$

Table 29 (continued)

Author	Patient population	Number of patients	Incidence of thrombosis (%)		
			Controls	Low-dose heparin	Significance
Multi-unit Contr. Trial (1974)	General surgery	160	43	15	$P < 0.05$
	Gynecology	55	14	0	$P < 0.05$
	Thorax surgery	38	44	15	$P < 0.05$
Nicolaides et al. (1972b)	General surgery	251	24	1	$P < 0.0000003$
Plante et al. (1979)	General surgery	108	21	7	$P < 0.05$
Rem et al. (1975)	General surgery urology	178	36	13	$P < 0.001$
Rosenberg et al. (1975)	General surgery	154	44	7	$P < 0.001$
Sebeseri et al. (1975)	Urology	65	58	12	$P < 0.01$
Strand et al. (1975)	General surgery	100	20	6	$P < 0.05$
Taberner et al. (1978)	Gynecology	57	23	6	$P < 0.05$
Törngren and Forsberg (1978)	Abdominal surgery	124	33	16	$P < 0.05$
Williams (1971)	Abdominal surgery	44	33	0	$P < 0.02$
Wu et al. (1977)	Abdominal surgery	88	14	0	$P < 0.01$

[a]In total three doses of low-dose heparin.
[b]Low-dose heparin for five days.

Table 30. Thromboprophylactic effect of low-dose heparin in orthopedic surgery
Diagnosis of thrombosis by the ^{125}I-fibrinogen test except for Galasko et al., who used a combination of clinical diagnosis and phlebography

Author	Number of patients	Incidence of thrombosis (%)		Significance
		Control	Low-dose heparin	
Hip fracture surgery				
Bergqvist et al. (1979)	50	91	63	$P < 0.05$
Checketts and Bradley (1974)	51	50	68	NS
Galasko et al. (1976)	100	46	16	$P < 0.001$
Gallus et al. (1973b)	46	48	13	$P < 0.012$
Lawrence et al. (1977)	50	48	0	$P < 0.0005$
Morris and Mitchell (1977b)	48	67	50	NS
Moskovitz et al. (1978)	51	39	41	NS
Schöndorf (1978)	45	60	33	NS
Xabregas et al. (1978)	100	48	0	$P < 0.0005$
Elective hip surgery				
Bergqvist et al. (1979)	143	63	48	NS
Dechavanne et al. (1975)	40	40	5	$P < 0.025$
Dechavanne et al. (1974)	54	48	7	$P < 0.01$
de Mourgues et al. (1979)	158	59	12	$P < 0.001$
Hampson et al. (1974)	100	54	46	NS
Hume et al. (1973)	23	73	50	NS
Lowe (1981)	94	33	14	$P < 0.05$
Manucci et al. (1976)	143	49	20	$P < 0.005$
Morris et al. (1974)	59	50	11	$P < 0.005$
Moskovitz et al. (1978)	67	59	23	$P < 0.003$
Sagar et al. (1976a)	57	69	32	$P < 0.01$
Venous Thromb. Clin. Study Group (1975)	64	37	7	$P < 0.0046$
Other orthopedic surgery				
Abraham-Inpihn and Vreeken (1975)	25	46	8	$P < 0.05$
Gallus et al. (1976)	38	25	0	$P < 0.05$
Protoulis et al. (1976)	80	53	25	$P < 0.01$

gery. Moreover, it is possible that many thrombi have their onset quite late in the process (Hampson et al. 1974, Bergqvist et al. 1976a, Cooke et al. 1977b).

A study of the effect of low-dose heparin in hip surgery, employing phlebography as the method of diagnosis, is still lacking, although in a study by Galasko et al. (1976) phlebography was used in patients with clinical signs of thrombosis, showing that low-dose heparin was significantly superior to no treatment at all. However, the diagnostic procedure cannot be accepted, and the results cannot therefore be considered as proof of the effect of low-dose heparin in hip fracture surgery.

Morris et al. (1974) administered dextran during the operation to a certain number of patients in both groups. Hence, the conclusions in this study are somewhat dubious.

De Mourgues et al. (1979) compared the usual low-dose heparin with heparin in the same dose, but introducing prophylaxis on the evening of the day of operation in patients undergoing hip joint prosthesis surgery. The incidence of thrombosis was significantly lower (33%) in the latter group than in the reference group (59%), but higher than for low-dose heparin prophylaxis (12%).

Heparin in combination with aspirin did not further reduce the incidence of thrombosis compared with heparin alone in total hip replacement (Flicoteaux et al. 1977). Schöndorf (1978), using a combination of heparin and aspirin, was nevertheless able to obtain an additional reduction, but his population was probably too small to permit any firm conclusions. Nor does a combination of low-dose heparin and sulfinpyrazone (see p. 125) further reduce the incidence of postoperative thrombosis following either elective or fracture hip surgery (Rogers et al. 1978).

According to Bygdeman et al. (1970) data from randomized studies can be added in order to obtain a larger group for analysis, e.g., the frequency of such an unusual complication as fatal pulmonary embolism. This is possible, provided that each partial study is acceptable from a statistical point of view. Gruber (1975) used this procedure, and Bergqvist (1978) extended the analysis to include also the total number of deaths. Such an addition of studies of low-dose heparin prophylaxis is presented in Table 31. The total decrease in the number of deaths is only barely significant, but the reduction of the number of fatal pulmonary emboli is beyond doubt ($P < 0.0005$).

In order to make it possible to establish with more certainty a prophylactic effect on fatal pulmonary embolism, a large multicenter study headed by Kakkar was performed (International Multicentre Trial 1975). After exclusion of 350 patients, there remained 2076 in the reference group and 2045 in the heparin group. Pulmonary embolism was considered as the cause of death if the autopsy showed a massive recent embolus in the pulmonary trunk, the main stem of the pulmonary artery, or at least in two lobar arteries, in the absence of other causes of death. According to these criteria, there were 16 fatal pulmonary emboli in the controls and two in heparin-treated patients ($P < 0.005$).

For reasons of the relatively low autopsy frequency (72% in the reference group and 66% in the heparin group) this study has been criticized. There are also deficiencies in the material and the presentation of the results, the postoperative follow-up time, for instance, being unclear. One of the main objections is thus the low frequency of autopsies, and it has even been discussed whether or not the patients autopsied had been specially selected. However, in a leading article in the *New England Journal of Medicine*, Sherry (1975) pointed out that since the autopsy frequency was more than two-thirds, the principal conclusion of a prophylactic effect upon fatal pulmonary embolism is still reasonable.

One of the strongest critics of the multicenter study was Gruber of Basel, who stated that he had delivered results other than those presented in the study (Gruber 1977). The Basel group published their data separately (Gruber et al. 1977b), resulting in a new version of the multicenter study, but the results were such that the conclusions of the previous version were still completely valid (Kakkar et al. 1977). If the figures from the multicenter study are excluded from Table 32, the incidence of fatal pulmonary embolism in the low-dose heparin group increases to 0.52%.

Kakkar (1979) later countered the objections to the multicenter study, saying that most of the viewpoints were at fault. His discussion primarily concerned the selec-

Table 31. Prophylactic effect of low-dose heparin on fatal pulmonary embolism (FPE) and total mortality

Author	Control			Low-dose heparin		
	Number of patients	Number of fatal cases	Number of FPE	Number of patients	Number of fatal cases	Number of FPE
Abraham-Inpijn and Vreeken (1975)	13	0	0	12	0	0
Ballard et al. (1973)	55	0	0	55	0	0
Bergqvist et al. (1979)	93	5	2	100	4	1
Bergqvist and Hallböök (1980)	51	7	0	46	2	0
Coe et al. (1978)	24	0	0	28	0	0
Covey et al. (1975)	52	1	0	53	1	0
Gallus et al. (1973b)	141	0	0	131	0	0
Gallus et al. (1976)	412	0	0	408	0	0
Gordon-Smith et al. (1972a)	50	0	0	100	0	0
Groote Schuur Hosp. (1979)	99	9	0	100	5	1
Gruber et al. (1977b)	100	8	4	94	7	6
Int Multicentre Trial (1975)	2076	100	16	2045	80	2
Joffe (1976)	101	0	0	54	0	0
Kakkar et al. (1971)	27	0	0	26	0	0
Kakkar et al. (1972)	39	0	0	39	0	0
Kiil et al. (1978)	653	50	7	643	45	5
Kroese and Doblaug (1976)	91	2	1	100	1	0
Kutnowski et al. (1977)	18	0	0	19	0	0
Lahnborg et al. (1974)	54	0	0	58	0	0
Multi-unit Contr. Trial (1974)	128	2	1	125	1	0
Nicolaides et al. (1972b)	122	0	0	122	0	0
Rosenberg et al. (1975)	121	0	0	79	0	0
Sagar et al. (1975)	236	38	8	264	28	0
Sebeseri et al. (1975)	31	0	0	34	0	0
Strand et al. (1975)	50	0	0	52	0	0
Taberner et al. (1978)	48	0	0	49	0	0
Williams (1971)	29	0	0	27	0	0
Wu et al. (1977)	44	0	0	44	0	0
Total	*4958*	*222*	*39*	*4907*	*176*	*17*
Mean incidence		*4.4%*	*0.8%*		*3.5%*	*0.3%*

tion of the centers participating, the design of the study, the number of patients, and definition of endpoint.

Sagar et al. (1975; interim report on 300 cases, Sagar 1974) studied the incidence of fatal pulmonary embolism in 500 patients who underwent abdominal, thoracic, or urologic surgery. In the reference groups 38 deaths occurred, eight as a result of pulmonary embolism; in the heparin group there were 28 deaths but no fatal pulmonary embolism (the difference in pulmonary embolism mortality being significant with $P < 0.01$). A defect in Sagar's study is the fact that fatal pulmonary embolism was not defined. The incidence of 3.4% in the reference group was much higher than in other studies of corresponding types of surgery (see p. 25). Gruber et al. (1977b) had a similarly high incidence of fatal pulmonary embolism in the controls (4%), finding no effect of low-dose heparin in their study.

Later a comprehensive Danish study was also published (Kiil et al. 1978). Participating in the study were 653 placebo patients and 643 heparin patients, and the autopsy frequency was slightly higher than in the aforementioned multicenter study (82%). The authors presented the total frequency of thromboembolic complications, employing different diagnostic methods. The number of complications during the first postoperative week was 16 in the reference group compared with four in the heparin group ($P < 0.05$). The number of emboli detected at the autopsy were four and one, respectively. There was no difference after the seventh postoperative day, however (eight versus eight), which should be kept in mind. Fifty of the patients (24 in the heparin and 26 in the control group) underwent phlebography on the 5th–7th postoperative days and no difference in frequency of thrombosis could be shown (Kiil and Møller 1979). Another subgroup from the main study was investigated with ventilation perfusion scintigraphy, and no difference between the prophylactic methods was found (Kiil and Taagehøj Jensen 1978).

Heparin Salt

As previously discussed, the anticoagulant action of heparin depends on a series of factors, and intensive research is being dedicated to establishing to what part of the heparin molecule this effect is bound.

Today two heparin salts are used in clinical practice, i.e., the sodium and calcium salts. Segesser and Gruber (1977) have made a survey of the literature to see if there is any difference between the two salts from a thromboprophylactic viewpoint. This appears not to be the case. Similar findings were made by Nicolaides (1978b). In a leading article in *British Medical Journal* (Editorial, 1975a), sodium heparin was recommended for practical reasons. In the large international multicenter study (Int. Multicentre Trial 1975) calcium heparin was used.

A few studies have been published in which the heparin salt was specifically discussed. These studies have followed two lines, studying the plasma level of heparin, and the clinical effect, i.e., prophylaxis against thromboembolism and bleeding complications.

Johnson et al. (1976) and Bonnar and Ma (1979) found that sodium heparin caused significantly higher plasma heparin levels in healthy volunteers than did calcium heparin of the same lot. Nicolaides (1978b) found no difference in healthy volunteers on administration of 5000 units subcutaneously. These authors employed the Denson and Bonnar method (1973) for Xa determination. In patients with myocardial infarction, the plasma heparin concentration was higher after administration of the sodium salt than of the calcium salt up to 6 h after subcutaneous injection (Turpie et al. 1978).

Using Denson and Bonnar's method for heparin determination in healthy volunteers, Lahnborg and Bergström (1975) found that the maximum concentration of sodium and calcium heparin from different manufacturers was equally high, but that the plasma maximum for sodium heparin occurred significantly earlier than that of calcium heparin. The elimination rate and the molecular weight distribution did not differ. Nevertheless, when calcium and sodium heparin from the same manufacturer were compared, the plasma heparin concentration was significantly higher for sodium heparin. Similar results were obtained by Thomas et al. (1976), the results thus indicating that the form of salt in which heparin is presented has an influence on its resorption. After subcutaneous injection of 15 000 IU heparin no difference could be shown between calcium heparin and three sodium heparin preparations from different manufacturers (Bender et al. 1980). Yet, this is a dose which is higher than the usual low-dose heparin used for thromboprophylaxis.

The studies discussed were performed as single-dose studies with subcutaneous administration. Thomas et al. (1976) found no difference when both salts were administered intravenously, but Vagher et al. (1979) found a prolonged APT time, an increased FDP, and a decrease in the plasminogen level 15 min after injection in the sodium heparin group. The differences were slight, however.

Whitehead and McCarthy (1976) found more injection hematomas induced by sodium heparin, but this study was uncontrolled and contains several possible systematic errors. In another uncontrolled study, Abou-Abdallah et al. (1975) found no difference in injection hematomas, and neither did Cade (1977) in a double-blind study.

Törngren (1979a) compared the two salts from the same heparin manufacturer in a sequentially designed study, showing that there were significantly more patients with injection hematomas and patients requiring transfusion in the sodium heparin group. No differences with respect to the size of blood loss could be shown, nor in the incidence of thrombosis as assessed by the ^{125}I-fibrinogen test. If the high-risk patients in this study — the colonic and rectal surgery cases — were excluded, sodium heparin was, however, significantly more effective as thromboprophylaxis.

In a prospective, randomized double-blind study, Bergqvist and Hallböök (1978c) found no difference between the two salts from the same heparin batch with respect to the incidence of thrombosis, intraoperative blood loss, need of transfusion, and injection hematomas, as assessed by photography or by the patient's subjective sensation of pain. By measuring the ^{125}I-fibrinogen activity over the injection hematoma, an objective measure of the local hematoma was obtained. Measured in this way, calcium heparin induced significantly larger hematomas.

Neither Arendrup and Toftgaard (1979) nor Allen et al. (1979) were able to establish any difference between the sodium and calcium salt in double-blind studies with respect to the frequency and size of hematomas, and the patient's subjective discomfort. In a double-blind crossover investigation, 77% of the patients preferred sodium heparin (Arendrup and Toftgaard 1979).

In the comparative studies of sodium and calcium heparin presented, no clinically important differences between the two salts could be demonstrated, even if the resorption conditions are definitely different.

Dosage

Low-dose heparin has been administered mainly according to two regimens, either 5000 IU every 12 h, or 5000 IU every 8 h.

In the first studies, dosage every 12 h was practiced, but after plasma heparin determinations, every 8 h was considered to be prefereable (Kakkar et al. 1972). Also in later studies, administration every 8 h has given a higher plasma heparin level in patients undergoing gynecologic surgery (Levesque et al. 1981). Corrigan et al. (1974) were of the opinion that the more frequent dosage more effectively prevents thrombi above the knee. In the International Multicentre Trial (1975) heparin was administered every 8 h, which was also practiced by Gallus et al. (1973b). In the latter study, the incidence of proximal thrombosis was not reduced, however, in spite of the shorter dosage interval, which agrees with other studies (Groote Schuur Hosp. 1979). On the other hand, Nicolaides et al. (1972b) found a reduction of the number of proximal thrombi although heparin was injected only twice in 24 h.

It is thus not clear which regimen is better. In a nonrandomized study no difference was found between the two regimens either with regard to prophylactic effect or to adverse effects (Törngren 1979a). This is in agreement with the results of a randomized study (Gallus and Hirsh 1976b).

An analysis of the available literature shows that no greater difference in prophylactic effect is to be anticipated (Bergqvist 1979). This is also valid for the incidence of both proximal thrombi and fatal pulmonary embolism. More hemorrhagic complications with more frequent dosage were reported, however. The conclusions included both general and orthopedic surgery. Seglias and Gruber (1979) also arrived at the same conclusion in a compilation of published investigations.

At present there is no reason for administering low-dose heparin more frequently than every 12 h. This agrees with the recommendations given by Wessler (1976).

A new principle for the administration and dosage was introduced by Negus et al. (1980). Heparin is continuously supplied intravenously at a dose of 1 IU/kg body wt. per hour during the period that the patient is in need of intravenous fluid (48 h–5 days in this study), i.e., at a considerably lower dose than conventional low-dose heparin. The study was performed in general surgery patients and was randomized and double-blind, with placebo in the reference group. The incidence of thrombosis, as measured by the ^{125}I-fibrinogen test, was significantly reduced in both patients with benign and with malignant diseases (in the whole patient population from $22\% - 4\%; P < 0.01$). No difference in blood loss or need for transfusion was found. The calculated plasma heparin concentration is lower than is possible to measure by most methods for heparin analysis. Very low heparin doses release lipoprotein lipase (Negus et al. 1971, Heaf et al. 1977), which might possibly explain why low-dose heparin prevents the normal postoperative increase in platelet adhesiveness. Another explanation for the effectiveness of heparin in such low doses is that it seems to release heparin sulfate from the vascular endothelium (Kraemer 1977).

Tanner et al. (1980) investigated the effect of heparin on local thrombotic complications after intravenous infusion. The incidence of superficial thrombophlebitis and the frequency of positive bacterial cultures from the infusion catheter were significantly lower in a low-dose heparin group (5000 IU every 8 h) than in a reference group. The incidence could be still more reduced if 1000 IU heparin was added to each liter of infusion solution, i.e., almost an "ultra-low" dose.

As for the duration of heparin administration, it is difficult to form an opinion for several reasons. This is not entirely due to the varying duration of treatment in the different studies, but also to the great variations in the diagnostic follow-up time. For fatal pulmonary embolism a follow-up time of at least 30 days is required.

Gordon-Smith et al. (1974) compared heparin administration during 1 day and 5 days postoperatively. The groups were too small for any statistically significant differences, but the group receiving heparin for 1 day only exhibited almost twice as many thrombi. This indicates that only 1 day of low-dose heparin administration is too short. LeQuesne (1978) arrived at the same conclusion, but the design of this study was not presented in detail.

In a literature survey, no correlation between the total heparin dose and the incidence of thrombosis could be demonstrated (Bergqvist 1979). Some authors were able to show that the prophylactic effect ceases when the heparin supply is stopped (Hampson et al. 1974, Gallus et al. 1976, Kiil et al. 1978, Hedlund and Blombäck 1979). In the study by Hampson et al. (1974) it was shown that heparin also seems to postpone the onset of thrombosis.

At present continuation of the treatment with low-dose heparin for 1 week can be recommended, or as long as the patient remains in the hospital if less than 1 week.

Practical Aspects of Heparin Administration

Individual sensitivity to subcutaneous injection of heparin is great, but there is no simple laboratory test at present by which the effect can be followed. Neither has dosing according to body weight improved results. The most important factor for an optimal effect is probably adjustment of the dose to the degree of activation of the coagulation system, and there is no simple way of determining this today.

The subcutaneous injection is performed in the skin of the abdomen or in the thigh. A very fine needle must be used to avoid hematoma. The technique employed in subcutaneous heparin administration was described in detail by Griffith and Boggs (1964). Today microjet injectors are available for injection of heparin subcutaneously, particularly when such an injection is to be given to many patients in the same ward (Black et al. 1978).

In most studies of low-dose heparin, a concentration of 25 000 IU/ml has been used. The volume injected is then 0.2 ml. Other studies employing other concentrations have been reported, however.

10 000 IU/ml (Gallus et al., 1973b, 1976, Lahnborg et al. 1974, Bergqvist and
Hallböök 1978c, Bergqvist et al. 1979)

5 000 IU/ml (Strand et al. 1975, Törngren 1979a)

1 000 IU/ml (Covey et al. 1975)

Wijnja (1976) has drawn attention to the fact that the highest concentrated solution is difficult to handle and is easily underdosed. This is supported by a randomized study comparing 25 000 IU/ml with 5000 IU/ml (Törngren and Forsberg 1978). Such a tendency toward underdosage was also found by van Geloven et al. (1977), who changed the injected quantity to 0.3 ml in the course of the study.

Low-dose heparin should be avoided in patients with hemorrhagic disturbances (Bergqvist 1980a).

An important question from a practical viewpoint is whether or not low-dose heparin can be given to patients receiving epidural analgesia. The American Heart Association (Special Report 1977), Bonnar (1979), and Stanton-Hicks (1981) recommend that this combination be avoided. As mentioned previously, the method of anesthesia is not very often stated in publications on thromboprophylaxis, but in four studies a total of 113 patients were treated with epidural analgesia concurrently with low-dose heparin prophylaxis with no ensuing hemorrhage (Ballard et al. 1973, McCarthy et al. 1974, Bergqvist et al. 1979, Bergqvist and Hallböök 1980). Schöndorf and Weber (1979) mentioned that about 85% of the 162 patients undergoing elective hip surgery in a prophylactic study had received epidural analgesia. All subjects received low-dose heparin prophylaxis every 8 h, and no complication due to this combination was observed. Should such complications occur, it is very important that they are reported. Moreover, it is of great value when the method of anesthesia is mentioned in prophylactic studies.

Some antibiotic preparations interact with heparin (monomycin, streptomycin, neomycin, polymycin, gentamycin, erythromycin, cephaloridine), resulting in a reduced antibiotic as well as anticoagulant effect. Penicillins do not possess this property. Phenothiazine derivatives, however, have an antagonistic effect on heparin, and salicylics have a synergistic effect, acting both as an antiplatelet substance and as an anticoagulant (Colburn 1976).

In hemorrhages ascribed to the heparin effect, heparin can immediately be neutralized by protamine sulfate (1 mg/100 IU heparin). If 60 min have passed after the heparin injection, 50% of the protamine dose will suffice, and 25% after a lapse of 120 min. Nevertheless, protamine per se is a toxic substance, inducing for instance thrombocytopenia and histamine release (Jaques 1949). Hence, it should be administered only when a hemorrhage is due to the presence of heparin in the plasma.

A clinically important question is to what degree dextran and low-dose heparin can be combined, especially in situations where a more general low-dose heparin prophylaxis has been supplied, and dextran is employed due to its plasma volume expanding effect. The mode of action for the two substances differs markedly, and when combined, two different hemostatic defects will thus ensue. In a thromboelastographic study, a synergistic effect has been demonstrated (Bloom and Brewer 1968). For these reasons it has been recommended not to combine the two substances (Bergentz 1978, Nicolaides 1978a).

Morrison et al. (1976) found an obvious increase in hemorrhagic complications after femoropopliteal venous bypass surgery for arterial insufficiency, when heparin was administered intraoperatively in combination with infusion of dextran 70 (500 ml immediately postoperatively, and on the 1st and 2nd days). Regrettably, the heparin dose was not stated.

In a thromboprophylactic study in association with elective hip surgery, Schöndorf and Weber (1979) found no increased hemorrhagic complications in a group of patients receiving a combination of low-dose heparin (every 8 h) and dextran 40 (500 ml intraoperatively and postoperatively on the 1st and 3rd days) compared with patients receiving only low-dose heparin or low-dose heparin in combination with dihydroergotamine. Nor was any improved thromboprophylactic effect obtained compared with low-dose heparin only.

This problem has not been systematically studied, and in the absence of such studies, there is good reason to be restrictive in using a combination of low-dose heparin and dextran.

Adverse Effects

Hemorrhage

The adverse effect that has attracted most attention and is a logical consequence of the mode of action is hemorrhage. It is to be regretted that the reporting on the quantity of blood and on hemorrhagic complications varies a great deal between studies. Hence, no such summaries as for thromboembolism prophylaxis can be performed.

Out of 25 studies with heparin administration every 12 h, the hemorrhagic problem is discussed in 23. Gordon-Smith (1972a), Kakkar et al. (1972), and Taberner et al. (1978) found a certain increase in hemorrhagic complications, while the other authors stated that no hemorrhage occurred or that the different parameters related to hemorrhage did not differ from those of the reference group.

In the 22 studies where heparin was administered every 8 h, the bleeding problem is mentioned in every paper. In seven of the studies there was an increased tendency toward bleeding measured in different ways (Gallus et al. 1973b, Hampson et al. 1974, International Multicentre Trial 1975, Gallus et al. 1976, Mannucci et al. 1976, Gruber et al. 1977b, Moskovitz et al. 1978).

The large international multicenter study with heparin dosage three times daily reported significantly more patients with wound hematomas in the heparin group (as analyzed in 1475 subjects). There was no difference in the need of transfusion or decrease in hemoglobin, although a few centers considered the hemorrhagic complications a problem (Gruber et al. 1977b, Kroese and Doblaug 1976), and for this reason the Oslo group (Kroese and Doblaug) withdrew from the study. It was especially after surgery of the prostate that increased bleeding was observed. This has also been reported by other authors (Allen et al. 1978).

In another large study (Kiil et al. 1978) from Denmark, including 1296 patients receiving heparin twice daily, no difference in fatal hemorrhage, need of reoperation due to hemorrhage, or intra- or postoperative need of transfusion was noted.

Pachter and Riles (1977) performed a prospective study for the purpose of studying hemorrhagic and wound complications in association with low-dose heparin prophylaxis. They randomized 175 patients to one of three groups: reference, 5000 IU heparin $\times$ 2, starting 3 h preoperatively, and 5000 IU $\times$ 2, starting postoperatively. In the reference group a wound hematoma (1.4%) developed, and in the group receiving heparin postoperatively two infected wound hematomas and one macroscopic hematuria (7.5%) were observed. In the low-dose heparin group, the incidence of hemorrhagic complications was 27% (15 wound hematomas and three cases of hematuria). On the basis of these results in combination with the fact that no cases of clinical pulmonary embolism were observed, the authors arrived at the conclusion that low-dose heparin prophylaxis should be reserved for high-risk patients.

String and Barcia (1975) also found an increased bleeding tendency when low-dose heparin was administered every 8 h or every 12 h, 14% in the reference group versus 22% in the heparin group ($P < 0.05$).

Gjønnaess and Abildgaard (1976) were also interested in the hemorrhagic problem and performed a double-blind study in 95 patients undergoing gynecologic surgery. The need of transfusions and the postoperative hemoglobin decrease were identical in the reference and heparin groups (5000 IU $\times$ 2). Hematomas in the area of operation were observed more often in the heparin group (15% versus 5%, $P > 0.05$, however).

Hemorrhagic complications were studied in another prospective study (Dommering 1979). Eighty-six patients who underwent surgery for inguinal hernias were randomly selected to receive either prophylaxis with low-dose heparin or oral anticoagulants (from the first postoperative day on). Wound hematomas (requiring aspiration or debridement) were noted in 36% of patients in the low-dose heparin group, and in 7% in the anticoagulant group.

In aortic bifurcation surgery, where the patients constitute a high-risk group with regard to bleeding, hemorrhagic complications are significantly increased also at a dosage of 5000 IU every 12 h (49 patients; 33% versus 4% in the reference group, $P < 0.05$; Belch et al. 1979).

In operations for carcinoma of the breast a large raw wound surface ensues, and to judge from one report, the hemorrhage from this wound surface increases on low-dose heparin prophylaxis at a dose of 5000 IU every 8 h (Mosley 1978).

In a controlled prospective study Nicolaides (1978b) analyzed the incidence of wound hematomas, finding a significant increase for heparin levels exceeding 0.2 IU/ml plasma. Hedlund and Blombäck (1979) did not succeed in showing any correlation between blood loss following transvesical prostatectomy and plasma heparin concentration, but most patients in this study had heparin levels below 0.2 IU/ml.

Cerrato et al. (1978) used low-dose heparin three times daily in neurosurgical patients, finding one postoperative hematoma in the reference group, and two in the heparin group. In this study the heparin dose was established by plasma heparin measurements after an initial dose of 5000 IU. If the plasma concentration was lower than 0.18 IU/ml plasma 3 h after the injection, the dose was considered safe; otherwise it was reduced. Only four of the 50 patients had to be given a lower dose (3750 IU).

Barnett et al. (1977) administered 5000 IU heparin every 12 h to 150 neurosurgical patients in order to test the safety of this form of prophylaxis. Four seromas and two hematomas were observed. This study did not include a reference group, however. In another uncontrolled study on 983 neurosurgical patients, low-dose heparin was given with no bleeding complications (van Dulken and Thomeer 1977).

The frequency of hemorrhagic complications is not dependent on the weight of the patient (Seglias and Gruber 1979), a clinical observation agreeing with the findings on plasma heparin levels (p. 93), but elderly women have been said to be more sensitive than others for bleeding complications (Jick et al. 1968).

Injection hematomas have been touched upon previously in this work (p. 104). They occur with a relatively high incidence, but seldom induce any actual symptoms (Arnesen et al. 1979b, Bergqvist and Hallböök 1978c, Törngren and Forsberg 1978).

In patients undergoing inguinal lymph node dissection because of malignant melanoma, the amount of drained serous fluid was larger in patients on low-dose heparin than in control patients (Arbeit et al. 1981).

Thrombocytopenia

It is known that heparin in rare cases may induce thrombocytopenia, particularly with intravenous administration. This was first reported in animals (Copley and Robb 1941) and later in humans (Fidlar and Jaques 1948, Gollub and Ulin 1962, Natelson et al. 1969, Babcock et al. 1976, Bell 1976, Rhodes et al. 1977, Kapsch et al. 1979). No correlation between the heparin dose and the degree of thrombocytopenia has been established (Rhodes et al. 1977).

There is some evidence of an immunologic etiology, with heparin-dependent platelet antibodies belonging to the IgG or IgM class (Babcock et al. 1976, Rhodes et al. 1977, Nelson et al. 1978, Trowbridge et al. 1978, Wahl et al. 1978, Kapsch et al. 1979). It has been suggested that the antibody reacts with a heparin-platelet complex located on the platelet membranes, whereupon a release reaction and aggregation occur (Green et al. 1978).

Recently, a double-blind study was performed on the incidence of thrombocytopenia with administration of various heparin preparations (Bell and Royall 1980). Thrombocytopenia was defined as a decrease in the number of platelets to less than $100\,000/mm^3$, and was significantly more common after administration of bovine lung heparin (26%) than after heparin derived from intestinal mucosa (9%). No corresponding difference in the effect of various heparin preparations could be shown in a prospective but open study by Eika et al. (1980). However, bovine lung heparin appears to induce thrombocytopenia more often (Godal 1980).

It has also recently been reported that heparin injection may give rise to complement-mediated platelet damage with subsequent thrombocytopenia (Cines et al. 1980).

Some case reports on thrombocytopenia in connection with low-dose heparin have recently been published (Galle et al. 1978, Hrushesky 1978, Chu Cheng 1981).

On the basis of these case reports, studies were performed in order to establish prospectively the incidence of heparin-induced thrombocytopenia. They are compiled in Table 32. The incidence varies, but the conclusion must be that, although rare, this is a complication to be taken into account in clinical situations. In none of the thromboembolism prophylactic studies previously discussed were the hemorrhagic complications related to a possible thrombocytopenia.

Table 32. Prospective studies on the incidence of heparin-induced thrombocytopenia

Author	Heparin administration	Number of patients	Number of patients with thrombocytopenia	Number of platelets
Ansell et al. (1980)	Continuous i.v.	43	16	< 150 000
Ayars and Tikoff (1980)	Low-dose s.c.	50	3	30% decrease
Bell et al. (1976)	Continuous i.v.	52	16	< 100 000
Eika et al. (1980)	Continuous i.v.	129	2	< 100 000
Powers et al. (1979)	Continuous i.v.	117	4	< 150 000
Malcolm et al. (1979)[a]	Continuous i.v.	13	5	< 150 000
	Intermittent i.v.	36	4	< 150 000
	S.c.	38	4	< 150 000
	Mixed	17	0	< 150 000

[a]Only one patient had less than 100 000 platelets, and it was not possible to show that the decrease in the other cases was due to heparin.

Thrombocytopenia occurs after administration of heparin for 2 or 3 days to 3 weeks (Godal 1980). A few fatal cases have been described, but these patients are often seriously ill. In the majority of cases, the reaction is reversible when the heparin supply is stopped. It is important that all patients receiving heparin are at risk for the development of thrombocytopenia. The route of administration, heparin dosage, or heparin source do not seem to modify the risk. The incidence of this complication has been found to be approximately 0.6% of patients who have received heparin (Kapsch and Silver 1981).

Other Complications

Other complications are rare. Allergic reactions occur sometimes (Chernoff 1950, Gotz 1951, Bernstein 1956, Curry et al. 1973). In Törngren's study (1979b), two patients out of 259 (0.8%) exhibited this complication.

Necrosis of the skin has been observed (O'Toole 1973, Hill et al. 1976, White et al. 1979, Jackson and Pollock 1981). White et al. (1979) reported several cases of necrosis of the skin at the site of the heparin injection, in all cases occurring in patients who had received the injections for more than 6 days before the complications developed. Most patients exhibited a heparin-induced platelet aggregation in vitro.

Progress of a thrombus or the development of fresh ones may occur in rare cases during ongoing heparin administration (Weissmann and Tobin 1958, Roberts et al. 1964, Rhodes et al. 1973, 1977, Hussey et al. 1979). These patients have an abnormal heparin-induced platelet aggregation in vitro (Hussey et al. 1979). When such a reaction occurs, the heparin administration should be stopped immediately. Platelet antiaggregating substances such as dextran 40 or dipyridamole have been reported to have a favorable effect (Hussey et al. 1979).

Osteoporosis is rare and develops only after heparin treatment for long periods of time (Stinchfield et al. 1956, Griffith et al. 1965, Jaffe and Willis 1965, Miller and De Wolfe 1966, Schuster et al. 1969). This complication is possibly due to the fact that heparin binds collagenase by forming a complex, and that this complex binds to collagen, resulting in a local increase in enzyme activity (Sakamoto et al. 1975).

Summary

Low-dose heparin can be defined as heparin administered subcutaneously for thromboprophylactic purposes and in such a low dose that the usual coagulation parameters are not influenced. The primary effect is considered to be an inhibition of activated factor X. Heparin should therefore be administered to the organism before the coagulation activity has started, i.e., preoperatively.

In general surgery, gynecology, neurosurgery, and possibly urology, a thromboprophylactic effect is undeniable. In orthopedic surgery the effect is more dubious, and much less pronounced in any case. The prophylactic effect on pulmonary embolism must be considered as certain. There are some differences in the resorption between sodium and calcium heparin, but these are probably of little practical importance both with regard to efficacy and adverse effects.

Low-dose heparin prophylaxis should be introduced 2 h preoperatively and then be administered every 8 or 12 h according to the different studies. The effect appears to be equal for these two dosage intervals, but hemorrhagic complications are more often observed on administration every 8 h. Injection three times a day is therefore not indicated at present. Epidural analgesia and low-dose heparin prophylaxis can thus be combined without any inconvenience. Dextran and low-dose heparin should not be combined, since there are some indications of a hemorrhage-potentiating effect.

Hemorrhagic complications are a fact to be taken into account in low-dose heparin prophylaxis, but they do not occur very frequently and are seldom of clinical importance. Other adverse effects (thrombocytopenia, allergic reactions, necrosis of the skin) are exceedingly rare.

Heparin Analogues

In the past few years, part of the thromboprophylactic research has been aimed at developing heparin-like substances, sulfated polysaccharides (glucosaminoglycans). Jaques (1976) suggested a classification into heparins, heparinoids, heparitins, chondroitins, and hyaluronic acids. There is a large number of glucosaminoglycans, and in interstitial tissue there are several of physiologic importance (see Comper and Laurent 1978, Lindahl and Höök 1978).

For thrompoprophylactic purposes, analogues with a more specific action as Xa-inhibitors, and also more homogenous than heparin, are of interest (Teien et al. 1976a, Yin and Tangen 1976). A series of such substances are known (Jaques 1967, 1978a), and new ones are continuously being developed, but they have as yet not been properly standardized (Jaques 1978b, Thomas 1978a).

A semisynthetic heparin analogue (SSHA-A 73025) has been compared with heparin in vitro and in vivo (Lane et al. 1977, Michalski et al. 1977, Thomas et al. 1977). The substance is a galactosaminoglycan polysulfate from the respiratory tract of horned cattle. It is composed of disaccharide units with almost equimolar amounts of hexuronic acid and hexosamine and has a mean molecular weight of 7000 (range 6000–10 000). There are no sulfamine groups and it contains an insignificant amount of heparin.

In vitro, this analogue has only a slight influence on the coagulation time of koalin and cephalin as well as the heparin level according to Yin et al. (1973). In vivo, antithrombin III was potentiated in the same way as by heparin, whereas the coagulation time was not affected. Thomas et al. (1979, 1980) reported data indicating an SSHA-induced release of a component with a Xa-inhibitor effect in vivo. It could possibly be heparan sulfate, a natural glucosaminoglycan present in vascular endothelium. SSHA prolongs the prothrombin time in doses where heparin has no effect (Kakkar et al. 1981a).

In a prospective randomized study, this heparin analogue was compared with low-dose heparin (Kakkar et al. 1978). Two hundred patients undergoing various abdominal surgical operations were studied, employing the ^{125}I-fibrinogen test confirmed by phlebography to establish the diagnosis. The heparin analogue group exhibited 6.3% thrombi compared with 12.5% in the low-dose heparin group, a difference which is not significant. No differences in intraoperative blood loss and hemorrhagic complications could be shown.

Sodium pentosan polysulfate (SP 54, average molecular weight 2000) is another sulfated polysaccharide. According to Jaques' classification it is a heparinoid. Oral and rectal administration in doses up to 150 mg does not influence the thrombin time or partial thromboplastin time according to Greten et al. (1978). However, other authors previously showed a prolongation of the thrombin time and fibrinolysis stimulation (Schneider et al. 1967, Coccheri et al. 1978). Inhibition of activated factor X has been demonstrated by several authors (Yin et al. 1980, Soria et al. 1978, Coccheri et al. 1979, Czapek et al. 1980). Like heparin, this heparin analogue causes platelet aggregation (Kindness et al. 1979). There are, however, experimental data indicating a decrease in aggregation of erythrocytes and platelets by SP 54 (Bicher 1970). Release of platelet factor 4 is diminished by SP 54 (Vinazzer et al. 1980).

In a thromboprophylactic study by Joffe (1976), this sulfated polysaccharide was compared with low-dose heparin and no treatment. The incidence of thrombosis was 15%, 9%, and 51%, respectively, as assessed by the ^{125}I-fibrinogen test. Thus the incidence of thrombosis for this sulfated polysaccharide was the same size as for low-dose heparin prophylaxis. A similar study was performed in elective hip surgery patients by Morin et al. (1978), who found that sodium pentosan polysulfate administered intramuscularly reduced the incidence of thrombosis from 43% to 4% (total of 46 patients; P < 0.01). Immelman et al. (1981) found that SP 54 and low-dose heparin gave the same thromboprophylactic effect. PZ 68 is also a sodium pentosan polysulfate with an average molecular weight of about 4000 and a rather narrow molecular weight range (1500–5000). It is produced semisynthetically from raw plant material and is constructed of pentose units, contrary to the hexose units of heparin. After subcutaneous injection, the substance has a stronger influence on the APT time and about the same influence on the Xa-inhibitor test as heparin in low doses (Bergqvist and Nilsson 1981). In vitro, it is equal to heparin per weight unit in an APT time test system, but is considerably less effective than heparin in a thrombin test system. Ryde et al. (1981) showed that PZ 68 markedly inhibits factor Xa, but not thrombin et all, and that the individual variation in effect is much less pronounced than for heparin. The results agree well with those of Czapek et al. (1980) mentioned previously.

The substance is equivalent to the dihydroergotamine — heparin combination with respects to thromboprophylaxis, but in a dose of 100 mg × 2 subcutaneously it results in a significantly increased need of transfusion in elective surgery (Bergqvist et al. 1980). With a dose of 75 mg every 12 h, this increased need of transfusion is not observed, but the thromboprophylactic effect is still good, in abdominal surgery significantly superior to dextran 70 (Bergqvist and Ljungnér 1981), and in hip fracture surgery equally as good as dextran 70 (Fredin et al. 1982). Also, in hip fracture surgery, no tendency toward hemorrhage could be shown for the higher dose.

Summary

Heparin is a heterogeneous substance with a wide molecular weight range which can be responsible for the variable effect. For this reason, part of the thromboprophylactic research has been aimed at developing heparin analogues with a more specific inhibition of activated factor X. At present, there are a few such substances with a good thromboprophylactic effect, at least as good as low-dose heparin. This research ist still in a preliminary phase, however, but a rapid expansion of new synthetic or semisynthetic heparin analogues is likely.

Dihydroergotamine and a Combination of Dihydroergotamine and Low-Dose Heparin

Mode of Action

Dihydroergotamine (DHE) is an α-adrenergic receptor stimulant as well as an α-adrenergic receptor blocker (see Salzman and Bucher 1978). In addition, it directly increases the tone of the venous walls by stimulation of the smooth muscle cells (Lange and Echt 1972a, Müller-Schweinitzer 1974, Müller-Schweinitzer and Brundell 1975a, Aellig 1976, Chu et al. 1976, Stürmer 1976). The effect on the resistance vessels is much less pronounced (Berde and Stürmer 1978) and is largely due to the preexisting sympathetic tone (Aellig 1967). The increased vein tonus can be seen phlebographically as a diminished vein diameter (Felix and Louven 1972) and plethysmographically as a decreased calf volume (Laube et al. 1977). The resting arterial blood flow is not influenced (Ulrich et al. 1973). Zimpfer et al. (1981), however, found a decreased femoral arterial flow and increased femoral resistance in dogs.

The constrictive effect on the veins is stronger for dihydroergotamine than for noradrenaline (Mellander and Nordenfelt 1970). As a consequence, the venous flow rate in the lower extremities increases, but for 2 min following administration a transient increase in the venous volume flow can also be observed (Rieckert 1971). The flow rate is also accelerated in the pelvic region (Mühe et al. 1975). The effect appears to be optimal at a dose of 0.5 mg and lasts for about 8 h (Lange and Echt 1972b, Mühe et al. 1975). The blood flow through the calf muscle as measured by [133]Xenon increases significantly 2 h after subcutaneous injection, but returns to normal in 5 h (Stamatakis et al. 1977a). After administration of DHE the blood volume is redistributed, decreasing in the arms and legs and increasing in the thorax and liver (Mostbeck and Partsch 1978). Intraoperative administration of DHE decreases the intravascular volume in the legs (Walser et al. 1980).

During extracorporeal circulation about ½ liter blood is mobilized from extrathoracic capacitance vessels (Reichelt et al. 1980).

In humans submitted to a centrifugal force the blood volume in the lungs is redistributed so that there is less perfusion of the apices. This redistribution can be prevented by pretreatment with dihydroergotamine (Koppenhagen et al. 1979). Tissue blood flow measured with radioactive microspheres in dogs decreases to the pancreas and the thyroid gland and increases to the central nervous system, other organs being uninfluenced by DHE (Lindblad and Bergqvist 1982b).

The central hemodynamics are influenced in different ways depending on the experimental situation (Clark et al. 1978). However, systolic systemic blood pressure and pressure in the pulmonary artery seem to increase as well as stroke volume and central venous pressure. In dogs total peripheral resistance increases whereas the pulmonary vascular resistance remains unchanged (Lindblad and Bergqvist 1982a).

Very little is known about other mechanisms which may contribute to the thromboprophylactic effect. Adrenalin-induced platelet aggregation is competitively inhibited (Barthel and Markwardt 1974), but this effect is only of short duration (Markwardt et al. 1978). There seems to be an inhibition of the platelet release of β-thromboglobulin and platelet factor 4 (Kakkar 1981). A prostaglandin-like substance is released from the endothelium of the vein walls under the influence of DHE (Müller-Schweinitzer and Brundell 1975a, b). Cyclic AMP phosphodiesterase is inhibited, which may be of potential importance for the function of the platelets (Meier-Ruge and Iwangoff 1976).

Since DHE causes increased venous tone, factors which may be of importance in association with thrombosis could be released from the vein wall endothelium. It is known that for instance venous stasis, vasopressin, and adrenalin induce the release of fibrinolytic activators and factor VIII-related antigen. Svanberg et al. (1980) studied certain coagulation and fibrinolytic factors and a possible influence of DHE in gynecologic surgery. The patients received DHE preoperatively and twice daily for 7 days. Blood samples were drawn preoperatively and on day 7. There was no control group, which makes it difficult to draw any conclusions from the slight changes occurring in fibrinogen, factor VIII, plasminogen, antithrombin III, and α_2-macroglobulin. Some of the changes can be ascribed to the surgical trauma.

Clinical results will be discussed in more detail later. On the basis of the study by Buttermann et al. (1977) it could be expected that a combination of DHE and low-dose heparin would result in a better prophylactic effect than each agent separately. This study was not randomized, but contained different consecutive groups of patients. Objections can thus be raised against it, but it has initiated several studies on the combination effect. The effect has also been documented experimentally (Schlag et al. 1981).

Sagar et al. (1976) measured the plasma heparin concentration after administration of low-dose heparin and DHE. They were able to demonstrate significantly higher heparin levels when heparin was combined with DHE, and put forward the hypothesis that by preventing venous stasis, the local thrombin generation will also be reduced, consequently reducing heparin neutralization. It was not possible to confirm this effect in other studies, however (Beermann and Lahnborg 1979, Briel et al. 1979, Kunz et al. 1979).

The combination of DHE and low-dose heparin is significantly better than placebo in preventing deep vein thrombosis in patients with recent cerebrovascular accident (Czechanowski and Heinrich 1981).

Clinical Documentation

In Germany four large studies on the thromboprophylactic effect of DHE have been performed. These studies suffer from substantial methodologic defects, particularly through the lack of randomization, and can hardly be used for the assessment of the method (Höör et al. 1976, Buttermann et al. 1977, Koppenhagen et al. 1977, Tscherne et al. 1978). The gynecologic patient population in Buttermann's study has also been reported separately (Adolf et al. 1978). In still another nonrandomized study, DHE was compared with dextran in gynecologic surgery (Bernstein et al. 1980).

In Table 33 a compilation of the studies is presented, using DHE as well as a combination of dihydroergotamine and low-dose heparin (DHE-LDH), and employing objective methods to establish the diagnosis. These studies are acceptable from a

Table 33. Thromboprophylactic effect of dihydroergotamine (DHE) alone as prophylactic method, or in combination with low-dose heparin (LDH)
Diagnosis of thrombosis by the ^{125}I-fibrinogen test

Author	Patient population	Number of patients	Incidence of thrombosis (%)				Significance
			Control	DHE	LDH	DHE-LDH	
Buttermann et al. (1975)	General surgery	106	35	9[x]	–	–	[x]S
Fey et al. (1975)	General surgery	148	57	33[x]	–	–	[x]S
Kakkar et al. (1979)	Abdominal surgery	197	–	20	4[x]	6[x]	[x]S
	Elective hip surgery	100	–	–	52	20[x]	[x]S
Koppenhagen et al. (1979)	General surgery gynecologic surgery	253	–	–	14	6.5[x]	[x]S
Kunz et al. (1977)	Gynecologic surgery	178	–	–	15	7[x]	[x]S
Lahnborg (1980)	Hip fracture	210	39	–	20[x]	16[x]	[x]S
Morris and Hardy (1981)	Elective hip surgery	81	56	22	–	4[x]	S
Mühe et al. (1975)	General surgery	150	44	24[x]			[x]S
Sagar et al. (1976a)	Elective hip surgery	82	69	–	32	16[x]	[x]S
Schöndorf and Weber (1980)	Elective hip surgery	108	–	–	15	4	$P = 0.05$
Sechas et al. (1978)	General surgery, urologic	80	12	2[x]	–	–	[x]S
Stamatakis et al. (1977d)	General surgery	100	–	16	4[x]	4[x]	[x]S

statistical viewpoint. DHE per se has a certain reducing effect on the incidence of thrombosis.

More studies are still required to establish to what extent the LDH-DHE combination is superior to either substance separately. Still, this seems to be the case, and combination appears to be effective also in hip surgery patients, which is otherwise a difficult group where effective thromboprophylaxis is concerned.

In a Swedish study, DHE-LDH was compared with a new sulfated polysaccharide in general surgery and was shown to have an equal and good prophylactic effect (Lindblad et al. 1979, Bergqvist et al. 1980b). The same prophylactic methods in comparison with dextran 70 in elective and post-traumatic hip surgery were shown to have an equal or superior effect to dextran 70 (Lindblad et al. 1979).

In the previously mentioned nonrandomized studies the results indicate a prophylactic effect on pulmonary embolism. This observation requires confirmation in controlled studies, however.

It has also been suggested that when using the combination, it would be possible to lower the heparin dose to 2500 IU instead of 5000 IU, thereby reducing the risk of hemorrhage (Stamatakis et al. 1977d, Hohl et al. 1980a). In three recent studies it has been clearly shown that a combination of 2500 units of heparin with 0.5 mg DHE gives the same thromboprophylactic effect as 5000 units of heparin, but causes significantly less bleeding complications (Hohl et al. 1980a, Koppenhagen and Häring 1981, Butterman et al. 1981).

In a Swiss multicenter study the LDH-DHE combination was compared with dextran to determine the prophylaxis of pulmonary embolism in patients undergoing orthopedic surgery. Of the 8001 patients included, 7413 fulfilled the criteria of the study. The two methods are equally effective (Gruber et al. 1981, 1982). Also the total mortality was identical in the two groups.

No adverse effects were noted, and in the publications studied there was no indication of an increased tendency toward hemorrhage. In one study there was even a decreased bleeding in the DHE group, and the authors considered this to be due to the venoconstrictor effect of DHE (Morris and Hardy 1981). Sagar et al. (1976a) found that the intra- and postoperative blood loss in elective hip surgery was equally large in the controls and in a DHE group (1159 ± 106 ml versus 1127 ± 110 ml). In the gynecologic patients studied by Kunz et al. (1977) this intra- and postoperative blood loss amounted to more than 500 ml in 6.8% of the heparin patients, in 3.3% of the DHE patients, and in 3.7% of the patients receiving oral anticoagulants. As the latter prophylaxis was not introduced until 36 h postoperatively, this group can be regarded as a control series.

As most ergot alkaloids, DHE has an oxytocin-like effect (see Saameli 1978). The contraction amplitude and frequency as well as the tone at rest increase in the pregnant human uterus on administration of DHE (Jeffcoate and Wilson 1955, Kremer and Narik 1955, Alvarez 1961). For this reason pregnant women should not be treated with this substance.

DHE can be administered intravenously, intramuscularly, and subcutaneously, but since it will mainly be used together with low-dose heparin, the subcutaneous route should be chosen. The dosage is 0.5 mg for each injection. Peroral administration of DHE is less suitable. Around 30% of an oral dose is resorbed (Aellig and Nuesch 1977), but some patients have an extremely low biovailability (Jennings et al. 1979, Olver et al. 1980).

A side effect, which in the postoperative period can be beneficial, is a shortening of the bowel transit time (Schütze et al. 1979, 1980).

It has been proposed that DHE should be contraindicated in patients with angina pectoris because of the finding of an increased resistance in coronary arteries (Raberger et al. 1981). The tissue blood flow to the different parts of the heart muscle does not, however, decrease after the administration of DHE but remains constant (Lindbland and Bergqvist 1982b). In the prophylactic studies performed so far there are no clinical data indicating an increased complication risk in patients with angina or hypertension.

In rare cases DHE can increase the tonus also in resistance vessels. Seven patients have been reported with a vascular spasm similar to that seen in ergotism (Echterhoff et al. 1981, van den Berg et al. 1982a, b). However, in most of the cases there were complicated and severe illnesses, and several possible factors could contribute to the vasospasm. The cases must also be considered in relation to the millions of doses of DHE, which have been administered.

Summary

Dihydroergotamine (DHE) is both an α-adrenergic receptor stimulant and blocker, also having a direct tonus-increasing effect on the smooth muscles of the vein walls. This is particularly true for the veins of the extremities. The substance produces an increase in the venous flow rate in the lower extremities. For this reason DHE was tried as a thromboprophylactic agent. It seems to have a certain effect, but the most important finding was that a combination of DHE and low-dose heparin results in an improved effect compared with either substance separately. The combination is also effective in hip surgery. When DHE is used, the heparin dose can possibly be reduced, and consequently also the risk of hemorrhage, without any accompanying reduction of the prophylactic effect.

Platelet-Influencing Agents

A number of substances have been shown to inhibit platelet function in vitro (see e.g., Wautier and Caen 1979), but the effect on both experimental and clinical venous thrombi in vivo has been more dubious. This may partly be due to a discrepancy between the in vivo and in vitro effects, and partly to the fact that the initial role of the platelets in the thrombotic process is not as important as first assumed (see above, p. 49). In in vitro and ex vivo studies, the blood has been anticoagulated in most cases, and Baumgartner (1979) has shown that both acetylsalicylic acid and sulfinpyrazone have a much stronger platelet-inhibiting effect in citrated blood than in native blood, where the effect is quite modest.

In this context six substances will be analyzed in more detail: acetylsalicylic acid (ASA), sulfinpyrazone, dipyridamole, hydroxychloroquine, flurbiprofen, and ticlopidine. All of them have been discussed as possible thromboprophylactic substances and have also, to some degree, been studied as such.

Acetylsalicylic Acid (ASA)

Mode of Action

ASA inhibits the platelet release of a number of substances, e.g., adenosine diphosphate, platelet factor 4, serotonin, and adenosine triphosphate, which is induced for instance by adrenalin and collagen, while thrombin-induced release is only slightly inhibited (Weiss and Aledort 1967, Evans et al. 1968, O'Brien 1968, Packham et al. 1968, Weiss et al. 1968, Zucker and Peterson 1968, Doery et al. 1969, Mustard and Packham 1970, Clagett et al. 1974, Vinazzer et al. 1975). The ability of ASA to inhibit platelet adherence to collagen and subendothelium has been shown experimentally to be hematocrit-dependent and effective especially at hematocrit below normal physiologic levels (Cazenave et al. 1978).

Since the release of ADP is prevented, interplatelet aggregation is inhibited also. This inhibition persists up to about 1 week after a single dose of ASA (Harker and Schlichter 1972a, Hirsh et al. 1973, Kocsis et al. 1973, Mielke et al. 1973, Baele et al. 1975, MacIntyre and Gordon 1975). The aforementioned influence on the platelets manifests itself as an ASA-induced prolongation of the bleeding time by influencing the primary hemostasis (Quick 1966, Mielke et al. 1969, Mielke and Britten 1970, Sahud and Cohen 1971, Harker and Schlichter 1972a, Hirsh et al. 1973, Mielke et al. 1973, Bick et al. 1976).

The distribution of the bleeding time following ASA intake indicates that people do not normally respond as one single population (Mielke et al. 1969). Some people have a prolonged bleeding time, whereas others are not affected at all. However, some experimental animals such as rabbits and rats seem to react differently and respond by a shortened bleeding time (Arfors et al. 1972, Stella et al. 1975). Certain results also indicate that the apparently contradictory results may be due to different doses, with inhibition only of thromboxane A_2 formation at low doses, and also prostacyclin (PGI_2) inhibition at high doses (see below: O'Grady and Moncada 1978).

The biochemical rationale for the mode of action of ASA is being focused more and more on an influence on prostaglandin synthesis (Fig. 3, p. 39). Activated platelets synthesize and release prostaglandin E_2, $F_2\alpha$, the cyclic endoperoxides PGG_2 and PGH_2, thromboxane A_2 and B_2, and malondialdehyde (Kocsis et al. 1973, Silver et al. 1973, Smith et al. 1973, 1974, 1976a, b). Different platelet-activating substances induce prostaglandin synthesis, and its release is closely associated with the release of ADP and serotonin (Kocsis et al. 1973, Silver et al. 1973, Smith et al. 1973, 1974, 1976a, b).

This prostaglandin synthesis is inhibited by ASA both in vitro and in vivo (Smith and Willis 1971, Kocsis et al. 1973, Willis 1974). More specifically, ASA irreversibly inhibits the prostaglandin synthetase enzyme (a cyclo-oxygenase); therefore the cyclic endoperoxides PGG_2 and PGH_2 are not formed from arachidonic acid (Flower 1974, Willis 1974, Hamberg et al. 1975, Needleman et al. 1976). The platelet-aggregating thromboxane A_2 is not formed. ASA inhibits cyclo-oxygenase by acetylating amino-terminal serine, the active part of the platelet membrane (Roth et al. 1975, 1978, Roth and Siok 1978). This is an irreversible process, and the effect lasts throughout the life of the platelet, explaining the long duration of the effect of an ASA dose.

The effect is obtained at low ASA concentrations (Patrano et al. 1980, Ellis et al. 1980, Hanley et al. 1981). At higher concentrations, the cyclo-oxygenase of the endothelial cells is also acetylated. This is 60–250 times less sensitive to ASA than platelet cyclo-oxygenase (Burch et al. 1978). Thereby the synthesis of PGI_2 in the vessel wall is inhibited (Baenzinger et al. 1977). Another possibility is a parallel inhibition of both endothelial cell and platelet cyclo-oxygenase, but with a shorter effect on endothelial cells, which would indicate a fairly long administration interval (Preston et al. 1981). PGI_2 is a potent platelet aggregation inhibitor, and recent experiments have shown that high ASA doses can in fact have a thrombogenic effect (Kelton et al. 1978b). This is also supported by the observation that low doses of ASA prolong the bleeding time more than high doses (O'Grady and Moncada 1978, Rajah et al. 1978).

Clinical Documentation

Some relatively early studies demonstrated the efficacy of ASA as a prophylactic agent against postoperative venous thrombosis (Salzman et al. 1971, Weber et al. 1971, Loew et al. 1974), but these studies can rightly be criticized. The diagnosis of thrombosis was based on clinical findings, which must be considered unfortunate in this situation, since it is possible that the anti-inflammatory and analgesic effect of ASA may conceal thrombotic symptoms. In a sequential study a prophylactic effect on pulmonary embolism was suggested (Hellgren and Scheibe 1975).

Salzman's group in Boston was later able to show that ASA, dextran, and warfarin were of equal thromboprophylactic value in patients undergoing elective hip surgery, who underwent phlebograms (Harris et al. 1974). However, this study did not include an untreated control group.

Table 34 shows the effect of ASA according to controlled studies employing objective diagnosis of thrombosis. An effect was shown only in two studies (Harris

Table 34. Thromboprophylactic effect of acetylsalicylic acid (ASA)
Diagnosis by the ^{125}I-fibrinogen test except for Clagett et al., Harris et al., and Soreff et al. (phlebography)

Author	Patient population	Dose (mg)	Number of patients	Incidence of thrombosis (%)		Significance
				Control	ASA	
Clagett et al. (1975)[a]	General surgery	650 × 2	105	20	13	NS
Encke et al. (1976)[b]	Abdominal surgery	330 × 3	66	38	28	NS
Harris et al. (1977)[b]	Elective hip surgery	600 × 2	95	45	25	$P < 0.03$
McKenna et al. (1980)[b]	Knee surgery	325 × 3	33	75	78	NS
		1300 × 3			8	S
Med. Res. Council (1972)[b]	General surgery	600 × 1	303	22	27	NS
O'Brien et al. (1971)[b]	General surgery		58	65	74[c]	NS
Schöndorf and Hey (1976)[a]	Elective hip surgery	900 every 2nd day	45	60	53	NS
Soreff et al. (1975)[a]	Elective hip surgery	500 × 4	51	36	47	NS

[a]Prophylaxis introduced postoperatively.
[b]Prophylaxis introduced intraoperatively.
[c]The ASA group was divided into one low (0.6 g daily) and one high (0.6 × 4) dose, but the incidence of thrombosis was identical.

et al. 1977, McKenna et al. 1980), in one of them only males (Harris et al. 1977). The results are difficult to evaluate, however, and the incidence of thrombosis in the control group was higher in males than in females, a sex difference which has not been reported by other authors. Channon and Wiley (1979) administered ASA to all hip fracture patients during a certain period of time. Thrombosis was diagnosed by a combination of ultrasound impedance plethysmography and phlebography, and the incidence was the same in males and females.

Still, in patients with cerebral transitory ischemic attacks, a positive response to ASA therapy favored males (The Canadian Cooperative Study Group 1978, Gent 1979). Such a sex difference was also noted experimentally (Kelton et al. 1978a). In a thrombosis model in rabbits, the weight of the thrombus was significantly reduced by aspirin in male animals, whereas no effect was obtained in females. The platelet prostaglandin synthesis was assessed by measurement of malondialdehyde, which was significantly decreased after aspirin ingestion, but no sex difference was noted.

McKenna et al. (1980) studied patients undergoing knee joint arthroplasty, finding that ASA in high doses was as equally effective for prophylactic purposes as intermittent calf muscle compression.

Stamatakis et al. (1978) reported a very high incidence of thrombosis — 80% — in patients undergoing elective hip surgery who had received ASA prophylaxis. In the study by Zekerts et al. a prophylactic effect on fatal pulmonary embolism in hip fracture surgery was observed, but the incidence of thrombosis was not studied in detail. It was not possible to confirm the results in later studies, even though a similar tendency was noted in a Austrian multicenter study (Loew et al. 1974).

The other studies do not contain sufficient data for an adequate analysis of the effect on fatal pulmonary embolism. As appears in Table 35, different doses and administration intervals were tried with no effect on the result. From a theoretical viewpoint, the doses so far used were too high to have an optimal platelet-inhibiting effect. Thromboprophylactic studies using lower doses are therefore anticipated with great interest. Harris et al. (1982) compared 3.6 g daily with 1.2 g in patients undergoing total hip replacement, the thromboprophylactic effect being equal.

Adverse Effects

The adverse effects that may occur are dyspepsia, an increased tendency toward hemorrhage, particularly from the intestinal tract, and, in rare cases, anaphylactoid reactions or allergic skin manifestations.

In the studies previously discussed, no increased tendency toward hemorrhage was observed either from the gastrointestinal tract or as a complication of the surgical operation. In two of the studies no hemorrhagic complications occurred (Soreff et al. 1975, Encke et al. 1976); however, in three hemorrhagic complications were not mentioned at all (O'Brien et al. 1971, Medical Research Council 1972, Clagett et al. 1975). Harris et al. (1977) and Zekert et al. (1974) reported the number of hemorrhagic complications, finding no difference between the groups. Schöndorf and Hey (1976) measured the blood loss in drainage during 2 days following hip surgery. The loss was equally large in the patients receiving ASA and the controls.

Comments

The studies performed so far lend very little support to a prophylactic effect on thromboembolism of acetylsalicylic acid. The substance cannot at present be recommended as a prophylactic against venous thromboembolism in trauma or surgery.

Dipyridamole

Dipyridamole was originally used as a vasodilator. Emmons et al. (1965a, b) were able to show that this substance has an inhibiting effect on ADP-induced platelet aggregation. Moreover, collagen-induced aggregation and release reaction are inhibited (Best et al. 1979).

Dipyridamole induces a reversible inhibition of the phosphoesterase activity in platelets, thereby increasing the concentration of cyclic AMP, which is involved in the inhibition of the platelet function (Mills and Smith 1971, Mills 1972). This is possible, since platelet adenylcyclase is activated by circulating prostacyclin (PGI_2), which is potentiated by dipyridamole (Moncada and Korbut 1978). In dipyridamole-inhibited aggregation, the thromboxane A_2 production of the platelets is reduced (Best et al. 1979). Platelet adhesiveness is not affected.

An inhibiting effect both on arterial and venous experimental thrombi has been demonstrated (Emmons et al. 1965b, Didisheim 1968, Polterauer et al. 1975). Different analogues to dipyridamole have also been synthesized, several of which are capable of a much more effective inhibition of the platelet function (Hampton et al. 1972, Holmes et al. 1977).

Clinically, a reduction of the incidence of emboli emanating from artificial cardiac valves (Sullivan et al. 1968) and of small-vessel occlusion in transplanted kidneys (Kincaid-Smith 1969) has been observed. On the basis of studies employing clinical diagnosis of thrombosis, Browse and Hall (1969) and Salzman et al. (1971) arrived at the conclusion that dipyridamole has no prophylactic effect.

There is only one study using objective diagnosis of venous thromboembolism (Morris and Mitchell 1977b). No effect could be shown in patients undergoing hip fracture surgery.

Thus, thromboprophylaxis using dipyridamole is still an open question, even if a very large effect is not to be expected.

RA 233 is a dipyridamole analogue, which in a small study on hip fracture patients was shown to have no effect whatsoever (Wood et al. 1973).

Combination of ASA and Dipyridamole

A few studies have been performed using a combination of the these substances, which have an effect on the platelet function, although they act in different ways. Some results indicate a synergistic effect (Genton et al. 1977), and at least in cases of arterial thrombosis after reconstructive surgery, the effect seems established, both experimentally (Josa et al. 1981) and clinically (Harjola et al. 1981). The synergistic effect may, however, be dependent on the dosage of ASA (Moncada and Korbut 1978). While low ASA doses inhibit the formation of the platelet-aggregating thromboxane A_2, high doses also inhibit prostacyclin formation, leading to a reduced dipyridamole effect. Nevertheless, it is too early to venture an opinion as to the clinical relevance of this hypothesis. Moreover, ASA administration appears to produce an increased plasma concentration of dipyridamole. This could possibly happen by blocking the excretory route of dipyridamole, and is valid at least experimentally (Buchanan et al. 1979). The combination gives a prolonged platelet survival (^{51}Cr-labeled platelets) compared with placebo (Steele 1980).

The results of prophylaxis by means of a combination of ASA and dipyridamole are presented in Table 35. A prophylactic effect appears to be achieved by the combination, but this does not apply to the studies performed in hip surgery patients (McBride et al. 1975, Encke et al. 1976, Morris and Mitchell 1977b, Silvergleid et al. 1977). Nor did the combination of RA 233 (see above) and ASA have any prophylactic effect on hip fracture patients (Wood et al. 1973). In patients with recurrent deep vein thrombosis, the combination of ASA and dipyridamole is as effective as prophylaxis against recurrence (Steele 1980).

Table 35. Thromboprophylactic effect of a combination of acetylsalicylic acid (ASA) and dipyridamole
Diagnosis of thrombosis using the ^{125}I-fibrinogen test, except in the case of Silvergleid et al., who used phlebography

Author	Patient population	Number of patients	Incidence of thrombosis (%)		Significance
			Control	ASA dipyridamole	
Encke et al. (1976)	General surgery	64	38	10	$P > 0.05$
	Hip surgery	18	44	67	NS
McBride et al. (1975)	Elective hip surgery	43	37	38	NS
Morris and Mitchell (1977b)	Hip fracture	64	66	63	NS
O'Sullivan et al. (1972)	General surgery	200	47	18	$P < 0.01$
Plante et al. (1979)	General surgery	104	21	8	$P < 0.05$
Renney et al. (1976)	General surgery	160	32	14	$P < 0.02$
Silvergleid et al. (1977)	Elective hip surgery	67	33	24	NS
Weiss et al. (1977)	Gynocologic surgery	66	31	3	$P < 0.05$

Sulfinpyrazone

Sulfinpyrazone, a nonsteroidal anti-inflammatory agent, is chemically closely related to phenylbutazone. It lowers the uric acid level in serum (Burns et al. 1958), but has a relatively low anti-inflammatory activity.

In 1965 it was reported that long-term treatment with sulfinpyrazone results in a prolonged platelet survival time and a reduced platelet turnover, while the coagulation mechanism is not influenced (Smythe et al. 1965). Moreover, the serotonin uptake of the platelets is higher after treatment (Mustard et al. 1967). The same group of investigators were able to show that the compound blocks the platelet-aggregating effect of collagen and inhibits the release reaction of the platelets, but not the platelet-aggregating effect of ADP or thrombin (Packham et al. 1967).

The explanation of the inhibitory effect on the platelets is not known. Certain experiments indicate that sulfinpyrazone inhibits the platelet prostaglandin synthesis (Ali and McDonald 1977), probably through cyclo-oxygenase inhibition (Cerskus et al. 1978). The effect lasts only as long as sulfinpyrazone remains in the serum — contrary to ASA — and the effect can also be neutralized on washing the platelets (Gallus and Hirsh 1976a). The platelet-inhibitory effect is maximal when sulfinpyrazone in plasma has begun to decrease (Buchanan et al. 1978), and it seems probable that a thio ether metabolite is responsible for the effect and ten times more potent than sulfinpyrazone itself (Pedersen and Jakobsen 1979, Pay et al. 1981). An inhibiting effect on platelet aggregation in the microcirculation in vivo was shown in several different species (Lewis and Westwick 1977, Adams and Mitchell

1979, Wiedeman 1980). Sulfinpyrazone also seems to have a protective effect against substances capable of damaging the endothelium (Harker et al. 1978). Some studies have raised hopes of an antithrombotic effect on the arterial side (Kaegi et al. 1975, Sherry 1979, Margulies et al. 1980). Experimental venous thrombosis could not be prevented by administration of sulfinpyrazone (Arfors et al. 1975).

There are only two studies on the prophylactic effect of sulfinpyrazone on postoperative venous thrombosis (Gruber et al. 1977a, Arapakis et al. 1981). In the first study 119 patients undergoing elective general and urologic surgery were randomized to one of three treatment groups, i.e., low-dose heparin, dextran 70, and sulfinpyranzone. The incidence of thrombosis assessed by the ^{125}I-fibrinogen test was 9%, 31%, and 43%, respectively. In the second study on 96 patients, the frequency of thrombosis was 8.3% in the control group and 14.5% in the sulfinpyrazone group.

Thus, there is no indication that sulfinpyrazone might have a prophylactic effect on postoperative venous thromboembolic complications.

Hydroxychloroquine

Hydroxychloroquine is an antimalarial agent also used in rheumatology. Its effect on the hemostatic system has not been thoroughly investigated.

Carter et al. (1971) were able to show that the substance has a significant inhibiting effect on ADP-induced platelet aggregation. The effect in vitro is established, but it is more difficult to reach concentrations with an inhibitory effect also in vivo (Johansson et al. 1981). Phospholipase A_2 is inhibited in vitro by hydroxychloroquine (Flower and Blackwell 1976). This enzyme is necessary for the release of arachidonic acid from fatty acids bound to the membrane, and of phospholipids. Arachidonic acid is the precursor to prostaglandin synthesis.

Carter et al. (1971) also showed that the substance has a significant reducing effect on the incidence of thrombosis assessed by phlebography following general surgery (from 23% to 0% in 52 patients; $P < 0.05$). They then repeated the investigation in surgical patients employing the ^{125}I-fibrinogen test, and also found a significant reduction (Carter and Eban 1974; from 16% to 2% in 204 patients; $P < 0.05$).

A significantly lower incidence of thrombosis in general surgery patients treated with hydroxychloroquine than in those untreated was noted by Wu et al. (1977), and the effect was as effective as for low-dose heparin. A similar and good effect was shown also by Sechas et al. (1977) in a study where the postoperative incidence was lowered from 23% to 5%.

No prophylactic effect of hydroxychloroquine could be shown in patients who underwent hip arthroplasty (Johansson and Forsberg 1976, Cooke et al. 1977b, Hume et al. 1977, Johansson et al. 1981).

Flurbiprofen

Flurbiprofen, dl-2-(2-fluoro-4-biphenylyl)-propionic acid, is a nonsteroidal anti-inflammatory agent. It is capable of inhibiting collagen-induced platelet aggregation in vitro and has been shown experimentally to have a prophylactic effect on pulmonary embolism also after oral administration. The mode of action is essentially unknown, but differs from that of aspirin and dipyridamole (Nishizawa et al. 1973). It has been shown to inhibit the prostaglandin synthesis in tumor tissue (Bennett et al. 1979). In a study on hip fracture patients no decreased incidence of thrombosis could be shown (Morris and Mitchell 1977b).

Ticlopidine

Ticlopidine, 5-(2-chlorobenzyl)-4, 5, 6, 7-tetra hydrothieno-(3,2-*C*)-pyridine hydrochloride, is a new antiplatelet agent. It inhibits collagen-induced platelet aggregation (Thebault et al. 1975, Ashida and Abiko 1978, 1979, Kirstein et al. 1980, Nunn and Lindsay 1980, Brommer 1981), ADP-induced aggregation (Kirstein et al. 1980, Brommer 1981), but not prostaglandin G_2-induced aggregation (Kirstein et al. 1980). Aggregation induced by arachidonic acid or ristocetin is partially inhibited but not abolished (Kirstein et al. 1980, Brommer 1981). Ticlopidine probably interferes with platelet membrane function (O'Brien et al. 1978), inhibiting the binding of ADP to membrane receptors (Lips et al. 1980) and increasing the activity of adenyl cyclase (Ashida and Abiko 1978). Aggregation-associated release of serotonin is inhibited (Nunn and Lindsay 1980). Bleeding time is prolonged (Brommer 1981). There is disagreement about the influence upon platelet adhesiveness (David et al. 1979, Paleirac et al. 1979, Brommer 1981). Antithrombotic effects have been shown in experimental animal models (Ashida et al. 1980, Kumada et al. 1980). Coagulation and fibrinolysis are not influenced (Tomikawa et al. 1978).

In one randomized study with 46 patients undergoing transvesical prostatectomy the thromboprophylactic effect of preoperative ticlopidine was compared with that of acenocoumarol from the day of surgery (Brommer 1981). By means of the ^{125}I-fibrinogen test the frequency of postoperative thrombosis was 13% in the ticlopidine group and 29% in the acenocoumarol group, the difference being insignificant.

Summary

Six substances with differing effects on the platelet function are of interest in thromboprophylaxis: acetylsalicylic acid (ASA), dipyridamole, sulfinpyrazone, hydroxychloroquine, flurbiprofen, and ticlopidine. There is little indication that ASA, dipyridamole, sulfinpyrazone, flurbiprofen, or ticlopidine have any effect. However, there are now theoretical grounds for assuming that the ASA dose was generally too high, and studies using a lower dose can be expected in the near future. Hydroxychloroquine and a combination of ASA and dipyridamole seem to have a prophylactic effect in general surgery, but not in hip surgery. Whether or not there is any prophylactic effect on pulmonary embolism is unknown.

Several of these substances influence the complex prostaglandin system. This system contains natural platelet inhibitors which are of theoretical interest. Prostacyclin or prostaglandin I_2 (PGI$_2$) is the most potent inhibitor of platelet aggregation known so far. It is very unstable and cannot for this reason be used clinically. Intensive work is in progress to synthesize stable PGI$_2$ analogues with the same effect, which hopefully may be used clinically. Such an analogue is 13—14-deydroprostacyclin methyl ester, which inhibits platelet aggregation induced by arachidonic acid, ADP, collagen, and prostaglandin G_2 (Fried and Barton 1977). Still more substances have been tested (Nicalaon et al. 1977, Scholkens et al. 1979).

Another approach is to stimulate the release of PGI_2 from the vessel wall, and substances with such an action are being developed (Vermylen et al. 1979).

One more method is a selective inhibition of the thromboxane synthetase to decrease the aggregatory function of the platelets. Clinical trials with a derivate of imidazole with such an effect have started (Tyler et al. 1981, Vermylen et al. 1981).

Dextran

Dextran was introduced in the 1940s as a plasma-substituting agent (Grönwall and Ingelman 1944). When studying high molecular weight substances in sugar beets, a polysaccharide of uncommonly high molecular weight was discovered, yielding only glucose on hydrolysis. This polysaccharide was described as early as the 1870s with the name of dextran. It is formed when the *Leuconostoc mesenteroides* B512 streptococcus acts on saccharose mediated by the enzyme dextran sucrase.

It was thought possible by partial hydrolysis and fractionation to develop a molecule of the same size as albumin in plasma. This ought to be an inert and atoxic substance, and therefore possible to use in humans. With World War II, the need for a good blood substituting agent and volume expander became evident. With about 450 glucose molecules, dextran forms a unit of approximately the same molecular weight as albumin (Grönwall 1966).

The first clinical studies on dextran as a volume expander were performed by Bohmansson et al. (1946). In 1947 the first dextran preparation was launched. Today, dextran is available in Sweden in two forms, i.e., dextran 70 with an average molecular weight of 70 000 (Macrodex), and dextran 40 with an average molecular weight of 40 000 (Rheomacrodex). Dextran 40 has been used clinically since 1961 (Gelin and Ingelman 1961).

Around 1953 dextran production was changed so that the average molecular weight became lower and the molecular weight distribution narrower (Ebert 1958, Gruber 1968). The glucose molecules in dextran are bound to each other by α-1-6 glucose bonds, forming a main chain, side chains being formed through 1–3 glucose bonds (Fig. 7). The number of side chains depends on which bacterial strain is used in the manufacture. For the B512 strain of *Leuconostoc mesenteroides*, the side chain frequency is about 1 per 20 glucose units. The chains are very flexible (Ingelman and Siegbahn 1944). Dextran, with a higher degree of branching, has been shown to induce more adverse effects (Kabat et al. 1957).

Molecules with molecular weights below 40 000–50 000 are quickly excreted via the kidneys (Ricketts et al. 1950, Wallenius 1954, Howard et al. 1956, Arturson and Wallenius 1964). This means that dextran 40 and dextran 70 have different excretion rates. After 6 h about 60% of dextran 40 and 30% of dextran 70 has been excreted, after 40 h 75% and 55%, respectively (Arturson et al. 1964). Dextran is temporarily taken up by various organs, and what is not excreted via the kidneys is degraded to carbon dioxide and water. The degradation is achieved by means of dextranase, dextran-1-6-glucosidase, which is present in various animal tissues, e.g., the reticuloendothelial system (Terry et al. 1953, Rosenfeld and Lukomskaja 1957, Ammon 1963). Dextran does not pass the placental barrier (Falk et al. 1967, Kivikoski et al. 1966, Ricketts et al. 1966). A certain part of the smaller dextran molecules pass the capillary membranes and are able to recirculate via the lymphatic system (Grotte 1956, Areskog et al. 1964, Schwartzkopff 1965).

In the 1950s several reports appeared on hemorrhage associated with dextran infusion (see also p. 140), and later experimental (Borgström et al. 1959) and clinical

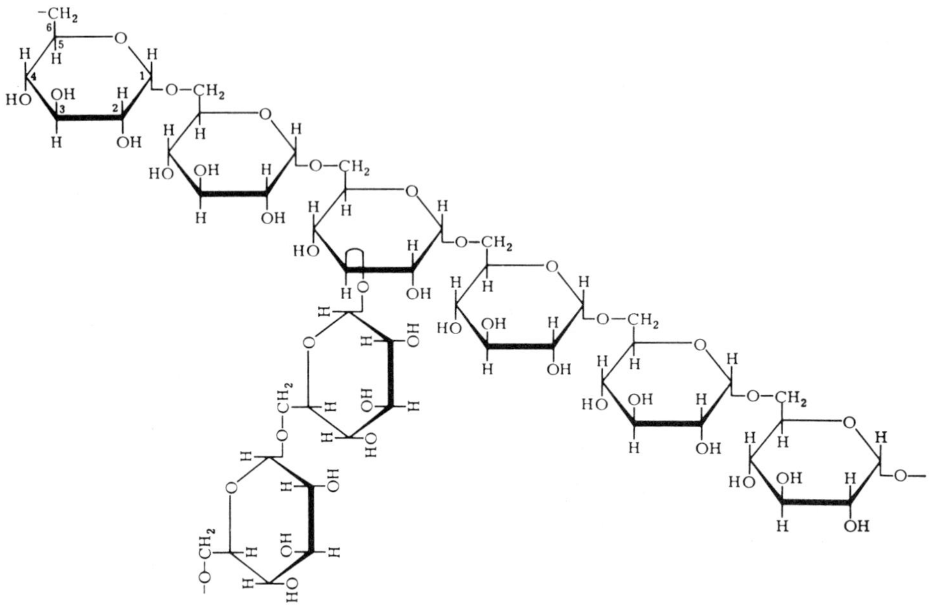

Fig. 7. Structure of dextran

(Koekenberg 1961) evidence was also presented that dextran might have antithrombotic properties. These two "side effects" of the plasma volume expanding effect — hemorrhage and thromboprophylaxis — showed that dextran was not the inert substance so far assumed. This led to intensive researche in to the mode of action of dextran.

Mode of Action

Dextran exerts a number of effects on various physiologic systems (Grönwall et al. 1968, Thorén 1978).

1. Colloid osmotic (oncotic) effect (Hint 1965, 1968). This property is vital for the water-binding capacity and thus for plasma volume expansion. In clinical molecular weight areas the water-binding capacity is 20–25 ml water/g dextran; this can be compared with albumin, which binds 18 ml/g (Hammarsten and Heller 1952, Eckert et al. 1954, Köster et al. 1957). The water that is not available in the circulatory system is absorbed from the extracellular volume. In this way, dextran achieves a very effective volume expansion (Gruber and Messmer 1977, Lamke and Liljedahl 1977). The higher the molecular weight of dextran, the higher the concentration must be to maintain a constant colloid osmotic pressure (Hint 1964). An approximately 2.5% solution of dextran 40 and an approximately 3.5% solution of dextran 70 are nearly iso-oncotic with blood (Gruber 1968). In hypovolemic individuals and persons with a lowered colloid osmotic pressure, the vol-

ume expanding effect lasts longer than in normovolemic individuals (Hammarsten et al. 1953, Semple 1954).

2. Penetration of semipermeable membranes. The permeability of the glomerular membranes for different dextrans has been studied in investigations in the dog and in humans (Wallenius 1954, Arturson and Wallenius 1964). Dextran with a molecular weight of 10 000 proved to pass freely, and molecular weights of 50 000 were the largest molecules capable of passing. By using a spectrum of different molecular weights (2300–145 000) the macromolecular transport and macromolecular leakage in the microcirculation can be studied (Svensjö 1978, Arfors et al. 1979).

3. Erythrocyte aggregation. In the presence of high molecular weight proteins, the aggregation of the erythrocytes tends to increase, and the same applies to the presence of high molecular weight dextran. The erythrocyte aggregation increases with the molecular weight of the dextran molecules (Thorsén and Hint 1950, Rφ et al. 1974). As a consequence of the erythrocyte aggregation, peripheral resistance and nutritive flow are impaired (Gelin 1956, Zederfeldt 1957, Gelin and Zederfeldt 1961, Groth and Löfström 1966). When the average molecular weight exceeds 150 000, the aggregation may cause an impaired microcirculatory flow and hypoxic organic manifestations (Swank 1958, Gelin and Schoemaker 1961, Stalker 1964).

4. Erythrocyte disaggregation. With low molecular weights a disaggregating effect is obtained (Thorsén and Hint 1950, Gelin and Zederfeldt 1960, Gelin and Ingelman 1961, Engeset et al. 1966, Richter 1966, Litwin 1972). The intravascular cellular aggregation increases in association with trauma, and thus also the viscosity. Infusion of dextran 40 results in a reduced viscosity on account of the cell-disaggregating effect (Gelin and Thorén 1961, Bergentz et al. 1963, Hoyt et al. 1964, Schoemaker et al. 1965, Ehrly 1966, Dawidson et al. 1975, Litwin 1976, Heidrich and Wachta 1978). It was this property of low molecular weight dextran that formed the basis of the development of Rheomacrodex (Gelin and Ingelman 1961, Gelin and Thorén 1961).

5. Flow-improving effect (Schwartz et al. 1964). The improved blood flow is believed to be due to: (a) an effect on erythrocyte aggregation, (b) hemodilution, and (c) passive capillary dilation as a result of the colloid osmotic effect.

6. Influence on the hemostatic system (see below).

7. Histamine and 5-hydroxytryptamine release, at least in animal experiments (Haining 1955, Westerholm 1966).

8. Antilipemic effect (Wallenius 1950, Mollison and Rennie 1954, Flotte and Buxton 1963, 1965).

9. So-called coating, i.e., vessel wall endothelium and blood corpuscles are coated with a thin dextran film (Rothman et al. 1957, Florey et al. 1959, Ponder and Ponder 1961, Bloom et al. 1964, Zingg and Linday 1964). This phenomenon has been discussed as a possible thromboprophylactic mechanism (Gruber 1968). The possibility has also been suggested that this is achieved via electropotential changes (Ross and Ebert 1959, Corley and Joseph 1966).

10. Alteration in the electrical charge of erythrocytes (Bernstein et al. 1963). Increased electronegativity is supposed to diminish the aggregability of erythrocytes.

The dextran effects currently considered to contribute to the explanation of a thromboprophylactic effect are hemodilution and flow improvement, but also the influence on the hemostatic system. The latter will therefore be dealt with in more detail.

Influence on the Hemostatic System

Infusion of dextran in doses up to 1.5 g/kg body wt. does not affect the number of platelets (Bergentz et al. 1961, Gelin et al. 1961, Nilsson and Eiken 1964, Bennett et al. 1966, Cronberg et al. 1966, Dhall et al. 1967, Weiss 1967, Rø et al. 1974). However, in a few studies a decreased number of platelets after dextran 70 infusion has been reported (Gelin et al. 1961, Abildgaard and Skjörten 1968, Langsjoen and Murray 1971).

After dextran infusion, the platelet adhesiveness to foreign surfaces decreases, the decrease reaching a maximum 2–6 h after the infusion, i.e., when the dextran concentration in serum is decreasing (Bennett et al. 1966, Bygdeman et al. 1966, Cronberg et al. 1966, Dhall et al. 1967, Weiss 1967, Jacobsson 1969, Atik et al. 1970, Åberg 1978). In these studies various adhesiveness tests were used (Borchgrevink 1960, Hellem et al. 1963, Salzman 1963, Weiss 1967).

No reduced adhesiveness could be shown after dextran administration in vitro (Bygdeman and Eliasson 1966, Cronberg et al. 1966), which excludes a direct effect of dextran on the platelets. In certain studies, dextran in vitro even induced platelet aggregation (Dhall and Matheson 1968), a phenomenon explained by a transient platelet ADP release (Paterson and Dhall 1971). Other authors were unable to demonstrate such an aggregation (Weiss 1967, Bygdeman and Tangen 1973). Also platelet aggregation induced by ADP (Bennett et al. 1966, Bygdeman and Eliasson 1967, Dhall et al. 1967, Kidess et al. 1978), collagen (Weiss 1967, Kidess et al. 1978), or ristocetin (Åberg et al. 1979) is inhibited by dextran. Dextran infusion also prevents platelet adherence to artificial surfaces during extracorporeal circulation (Watson and Chang 1975).

Using a laser ray, ADP-induced platelet aggregation can be achieved in the microcirculation in vivo, e.g., in a rabbit ear chamber (Arfors et al. 1970, Hovig et al. 1974, McKenzie et al. 1974). This reaction is also counteracted by dextran, with a maximum effect 4–6 h after the infusion (Arfors et al. 1968, 1971, 1973). In addition, the effect is dependent on the quantity injected. In an experimental dog model, performing transluminal angioplasty in normal coronary arteries, the platelet adhesion was almost totally inhibited by dextran 40 (Pasternack et al. 1980).

In experimental intestinal vascular obstruction, the pulmonary uptake of labeled platelets is diminished if the animals are treated with dextran 70 (Haglind 1981). This can at least in part explain the reduced mortality after dextran administration in this experimental situation.

Dextran is adsorbed to the platelet surface (Rothman et al. 1957, Bloom et al. 1964, Barnhardt and Quintana 1967, Rampling 1976), and the negative charge of the platelets may increase (Sawyer et al. 1973). Both these properties are believed capable of reducing platelet adhesiveness to the endothelium of the vessel wall.

With the exception of factor VIII, the various coagulation factors, including factor XIII, are not influenced more than can be explained by the dextran hemodilution effect (Jacobaeus 1957, Bergentz et al. 1961, Gelin et al. 1961, Nilsson and Eiken 1964, Ewald et al. 1965, Cronberg et al. 1966, Alexander 1971, Berliner and Lackner 1972, Fedderson et al. 1975, Åberg et al. 1975, Popov-Cenić et al. 1977). A similar effect that can be ascribed to hemodilution is also observed after infusion of hydroxyethyl starch (HES) — another plasma volume expander (Vinazzer and Bergmann 1975). HES lacks the more specific effect of dextran on the hemostasis, however.

Following dextran infusion, factor VIII, on the contrary, falls considerably more than can be explained by hemodilution (Bergentz et al. 1961, Cronberg et al. 1966), and it was later shown that it is the antigen-related activity of factor VIII (VIII R:Ag) that falls significantly, whereas the coagulation activity of factor VIII (VIII:C) remains at the initial level (Kladetzky et al. 1977, Åberg et al. 1979). This effect also appears a few hours after dextran infusion (Åberg et al. 1979).

In vitro, dextran accelerates fibrinogen coagulation on addition of thrombin — the so-called fibrinoplastic effect (Laurell 1951, Ricketts 1952, Jacobaeus 1957, Bergentz et al. 1961, Abildgaard 1966, Dugdale et al. 1966, Carlin et al. 1976a). The effect is considered to be due to steric exclusion, reducing the amount of effective water (Laurent 1963, Abildgaard 1966). In high concentrations (more than 3%), dextran induces precipitation of fibrinogen (Laurent 1963, Iverius and Laurent 1967, Naleczynska et al. 1970, Rampling 1974, 1976). In pure in vitro systems the fibrin structure is also changed into a coarser network. This has been shown turbidimetrically (Muzaffar et al. 1972a, b), by measuring the elasticity and tensile strength (Dugdale et al. 1966, Dhall et al. 1976), by thromboelastography (Bryant et al. 1961), and morphologically (Gollub and Schaefer 1968, Tangen et al. 1972, Carlin et al. 1976b). Whether or not this is reflected in alterations in the fibrin structure in vivo remains to be shown.

The fibrinolytic system per se is not influenced by dextran (Nilsson and Eiken 1964, Cronberg et al. 1966), but some authors have reported a certain increase in plasminogen activators following dextran infusion or addition of dextran in vitro (Deutsch 1964, Fischer and Wimmer 1965, Vinazzer and Bergmann 1968, Wallenbeck and Tangen 1975, Popov-Cenić et al. 1977). The plasminogen level in plasma is not influenced by dextran (Fischer and Wimmer 1965, Cronberg et al. 1966, Popov-Cenic et al. 1977, Carlin et al. 1979).

Dextran does not influence the concentrations of plasminogen activation inhibitors (with urokinase) (Cronberg et al. 1966) or α_2-macroglobulin, an unspecific protease inhibitor (Åberg et al. 1979). However, other authors were able to show that dextran is capable of reducing the fibrinolysis-inhibitive activity (α_2-antiplasmin) in serum both in the rabbit and in man (Saldeen 1977, Carlin and Saldeen 1978, Carlin et al. 1980). Dextran is not supposed to interact specifically with the various protease inhibitors (paricularly α_2-antiplasmin and α_2-macroglobulin), but the coarser fibrin network provides better protection for plasmin against the inhibitors (Carlin 1980). Clots formed in vitro in the presence of dextran are more easily lysed by plasmin than control clots (Tangen et al. 1972, Wallenbeck and Tangen 1975).

If blood is allowed to rotate at a constant velocity in a plastic coil, ex vivo thrombi are formed which have a close histologic resemblance to thrombi formed in vivo (Chandler 1958, Jacobsen and Chandler 1965). By incubating these thrombi with plasmin, and either measuring the release of fibrinogen degradation products or using radioactively labeled fibrinogen, a measure of the lysability of the thrombus can be obtained (Åberg et al. 1975). If blood for such an ex vivo thrombus is drawn from dextran-treated patients, the lysability increases, reaching a maximum 2–4 h after the dextran infusion, while dextran added in vitro does not induce any increase in lysability (Åberg et al. 1975). An addition of streptokinase results in a reduction of the size of the thrombus, if dextran has been administered to the blood in vitro (Metcalf et al. 1974, Metcalf 1980). Thrombocytopenia induces an increased lysability as well, but the mechanism is different than that of dextran (Åberg et al. 1977b). The dextran effect on platelet adhesiveness as well as lysability appears to be mediated by its influences on factor VIII R:Ag (Åberg 1978). Concurrently with the increased lysability, the structure of the Chandler thrombi is altered. The platelets are thus more evenly distributed throughout the thrombus instead of being localized to its head (Åberg and Rausing 1978, Åberg and Bergentz 1979). The weight of the thrombi is also significantly less (Esquivel et al. 1982b), this effect being dose dependent and true both for dextran 70 and dextran 40. A corresponding plasma volume expansion with albumin does not effect the thrombi.

Clinical Documentation

Dextran is capable of preventing experimental venous thrombi (Borgström et al. 1959, Bryant et al. 1961, 1966, Ernst et al. 1964, Merck et al. 1964, Flemma et al. 1965, Gruber and Bergentz 1966, Hobson et al. 1973, Brais et al. 1973, Ah-see et al. 1974, Ricotta et al. 1979).

The first clinical study was reported in 1961 by Koekenberg. He substituted intra-operative blood loos with either bank blood or dextran in a randomized way, finding that the incidence of clinically diagnosed thrombi decreased from 21% to 4% when dextran was used. In a double-blind study including 901 patients, Jansen (1972) also observed a reduction of clinically diagnosed thrombi.

In studies employing objective diagnosis, the results are partly contradictory. Table 36 presents the results of the controlled studies published so far. In the studies on general surgery, gynecology, and urology patients, the ^{125}I-fibrinogen test was used to establish the diagnosis. Dextran was effective in only three of these investigations (Bonnar and Walsh 1972, Carter and Eban 1973, Sechas et al. 1977). In the two former studies the controls had an uncommonly low incidence of thrombosis.

The effect seems to be better in patients with hip fracture. In three of these studies, phlebography was used as the method of diagnosis. In five of the seven orthopedic studies, dextran had a beneficial effect. In their study, Johnson et al. (1968) employed Armitage's sequential method for statistical analysis, which is a dubious method in this context (see p. 80). This could possibly explain the dramatic reduction of the incidence of thrombosis, which is unique in hip fracture patients. A large dose of dextran and late phlebography are other factors of importance. McManus (1976) administered dextran intraoperatively and postoperatively on days 3 and 5 (in total 1500 ml), finding a phlebographically confirmed incidence of thrombosis of 6.6%

Table 36. Thromboprophylactic effect of dextran 70
Phlebography was used in four orthopedic studies: Ahlberg (2–10 months postoperatively), Harper et al. (5–10 days postoperatively), Johnson et al. (within 3 months postoperatively), and Myhre and Holen (2–3 weeks postoperatively). Hurson et al. used isotope venography. In the other studies the ^{125}I-fibrinogen test was the method of diagnosis employed

Author	Patient population	Number of patients	Incidence of thrombosis (%)		Significance
			Control	Dextran	
Ahlberg et al. (1968)	Hip fracture	84	36	13	$P < 0.05$
Becker and Schampi (1973)	General surgery	77	31	31	NS
Bergqvist and Hallböök (1980)	General surgery	103	27	29	NS
Bergqvist et al. (1979)	Hip fracture	49	91	48	$P < 0.01$
	Elective hip surgery	141	63	57	NS
Bonnar and Walsh (1972)	Gynecology	260	11	0.8	$P < 0.01$
Carter and Eban (1973)	General surgery	207	10	0.4	$P < 0.02$
Daniel et al. (1972)	Hip fracture	66	61	60	NS
Harper et al. (1973)	Amputation	27	67	8	$P < 0.05$
Hedlund (1975)	Urology	77	45	27	NS
Hurson et al. (1979)	Elective hip surgery	106	18	27	NS
Huttunen et al. (1977)	General surgery	150	33	27	NS
Johnson et al. (1968)	Hip fracture	52	52	4	$P < 0.05$
Kline et al. (1975)	General surgery	214	26	21	NS
Multi-unit-Contr. Trial (1974)	General surgery	258	37	25	NS
Myhre and Holen (1969)	Hip fracture	110	40	20	$P < 0.025$
Renney et al. (1970)	General surgery	190	24	29	NS
Sechas et al. (1977)	General surgery	85	23	2	$P < 0.05$
Stephenson et al. (1973)	General surgery	80	35	29	NS

following elective hip surgery. The study included no control series, yet the incidence reported is so low in association with hip surgery that it deserves to be mentioned.

It has sometimes been discussed whether or not the reduction in the incidence of thrombosis observed after dextran administration is dependent on the diagnostic method employed. According to this line of thought, thrombi are formed also in dextran-treated patients, and are thus detected by the ^{125}I-fibrinogen test. The thrombi formed should then be more easily lysed — which is theoretically supported by e.g., Åberg's (1978) studies — and should not be detected to the same extent by phlebography relatively late in the postoperative phase. Becker and Schampi (1973) and Bergqvist et al. (1973) observed a discrepancy in the incidence of thrombosis between these two diagnostic methods. They suggested as a possible explanation that thrombi formed in the presence of dextran are more easily lysed. However, in two prospective studies, which admittedly included a comparatively small number of patients followed both by the ^{125}I-fibrinogen test and by phlebography, this hypothesis could not be verified (Bergqvist et al. 1976a, Hongler et al. 1976).

"Big" thromboembolic complications classified arbitrarily (bilateral thrombi, thrombi above the knee, and/or pulmonary emboli in patients undergoing hip surgery) are significantly reduced by dextran as compared with oral anticoagulants (Bergqvist and Dahlgren 1973) and no treatment or low-dose heparin (Bergqvist et al. 1979). An analysis of thrombi diagnosed by the ^{125}I-fibrinogen test in general surgery patients revealed no differences in size or extension between patients given placebo, low-dose heparin, and dextran (Stutz and Gruber 1978).

Dextran 40 as a thromboprophylactic agent has been much less studied than dextran 70 (Table 37). As appears from the table, the results can be ambiguous. Bergman et al. (1975) studied relatively young patients undergoing gallbladder operations, finding an overall very low incidence of thrombosis. In the study by Evarts and Feil (1971) in patients who underwent elective hip surgery, very large doses of dextran 40 were given: 500 or 1000 ml daily for 10 days.

In some studies dextran and oral anticoagulants were compared. In all studies except one (Myhre and Holen 1969) it was considered unethical to include an untreated control series (Table 38). The incidence varies according to different patient populations and diagnostic principles, but the two prophylactic methods are equal in all studies except one (Lambie et al. 1970a). The anticoagulant treatment was not introduced in this study until 36 h postoperatively. The risk of hemorrhage is greater in prophylaxis using anticoagulants than in dextran prophylaxis.

In a comprehensive randomized prospective study from Tübingen (Lüders et al. 1973) dextran 60 (2945 patients) was compared with heparin and oral anticoagulants (3014 patients). The incidence of fatal pulmonary embolism was 0.36% in the anticoagulant group, and 0.30% in the dextran group. Hemorrhagic complications were noted in 1.12% of the anticoagulant group and in 0.61% of the subjects treated with dextran ($P < 0.05$).

Table 37. Thromboprophylactic effect of dextran 40
Phlebography was used by Evarts and Feil (days 10–12) and Harris et al. (days 7–10). In the other studies the ^{125}I-fibrinogen test was the method of diagnosis employed

Author	Patient population	Number of patients	Incidence of thrombosis (%)		Significance
			Control	Dextran	
Bergman et al. (1975)	Cholecystectomy	60	0	3.3	NS
Evarts and Feil (1971)	Elective hip surgery	106	54	26[a]	$P < 0.05$
				6[a]	$P < 0.001$
Harris et al. (1974)	Elective hip surgery	106	36[b]	25	NS
Hutter et al. (1976)	General surgery, urology	192	36	22	$P < 0.05$
Huttunen et al. (1977)	General surgery	150	33	43	NS
Lindström (1982)	General surgery	75	30	20	NS

[a]The patients with a 26% incidence had received 500 ml dextran 40 daily; those with a 6% incidence had received 1000 ml. Both groups were treated for 10 days.
[b]Acetylsalicylic acid.

Table 38. Thromboprophylactic studies comparing dextran and oral anticoagulants

Author	Patient population	Number of patients	Incidence of thrombosis (%)		Incidence of hemorrhage (%)	
			Dextran	Anti-coagulant	Dextran	Anti-coagulant
Barber et al. (1977)[a]	Elective hip surgery	109	51	58	?	
Bergqvist et al. (1972)[b]	Hip fracture	138	30	33	0	7.9
Bergqvist and Dahlgren (1973)[a]	Hip fracture	75	44	50	0	6.2
Bronge et al. (1971)[b]	Hip fracture	135	42	34	0	1.0
Davidson et al. (1972)[a]	Gynecologic surgery	60	10	13	?	
Harris et al. (1974)[b]	Elective hip surgery	107	25	20	11	20
Lambie et al. (1970a)[a]	Gynecologic surgery	80	10	30	?	
Myhre and Holen (1969)[b]	Hip fracture	105	20	18	2	5

[a] ^{125}I-fibrinogen test.
[b] Phlebography.

The incidence of scintigraphically detected pulmonary emboli was not reduced by dextran in a study in patients who underwent elective hip surgery (Bergqvist et al. 1979), whereas Browse et al. (1976) reported a reduction if dextran was combined with intermittent calf muscle compression in general surgery patients.

Kline et al. (1975) noted a significant reduction of the number of fatal pulmonary emboli following administration of 1 liter dextran 70 at the operation. The study was double-blind, including 831 patients. In the control series 14 fatal pulmonary emboli occurred among 435 patients, and in the dextran group four in 396 patients ($P < 0.05$). The incidence of venous thrombi as measured by the ^{125}I-fibrinogen test was not reduced. As a consequence of these results, all adult patients in Cardiff undergoing surgery are treated with dextran 70 (Davies 1979). However, this study has been criticized on epidemiologic, diagnostic, and statistical grounds (Kakkar 1979a, Salzman 1979, Vessey 1979).

In Table 31, the available low-dose heparin studies were compiled to give an idea of the incidence of fatal pulmonary embolism, although this is a rare complication. Table 39 presents a corresponding compilation concerning dextran 70. The incidence of fatal pulmonary embolism is significantly lower in the dextran group, which reduces the total mortality.

There are also three time-sequential studies, providing a certain indication of the prophylactic effect of dextran on pulmonary embolism. King and Daly (1975) compared control patients from 1971–1972 with dextran 40 treated patients from

Table 39. Prophylactic effect of dextran 70 on fatal pulmonary embolism (FPE) and total mortality

Author	Controls			Dextran 70		
	Number of patients	Number of deaths	Number of FPE	Number of patients	Number of deaths	Number of FPE
Ahlberg (1969)	114	19	4	84	14	1
Atik et al. (1970)	77	14	5	49	7	1
Becker and Schampi (1973)	35	1	0	42	1	0
Bergman et al. (1975)	30	0	0	30	0	0
Bergqvist et al. (1979)	93	5	2	97	2	0
Bergqvist and Hallböök (1980)	51	7	0	52	2	0
Bonnar and Walsh (1972)	140	0	0	120	0	0
Brisman et al. (1971)	90	5	3	89	8	3
Carter and Eban (1973)	101	0	0	106	0	0
Edwards et al. (1975)	31	7	6	31	3	2
Elsner-Mackey et al. (1969)	427	0	0	391	0	0
Hartshorn et al. (1969)	104	2	2	99	0	0
Hedlund (1975)	40	0	0	37	0	0
Huttunen et al. (1971)	100	6	4	100	1	1
Huttunen et al. (1977)	75	0	0	75	1	0
Jansen (1972)	301	19	4	304	13	1
Johnson et al. (1968)	25	0	0	27	0	0
Kline et al. (1975)	435	35	7	396	27	1
Koekenberg (1962)	105	1	1	94	0	0
Multi-unit-Contr. Trial (1974)	128	1	1	130	0	0
Myhre and Holen (1969)	55	6	2	55	3	0
Stadil (1970)	397	22	5	424	21	1
Stephenson et al. (1973)	46	0	0	34	0	0
Total	*3000*	*150*	*46*	*2866*	*104*	*11*
Mean incidence		*5.0%*	*1.5%*		*3.6%*	*0.4%*

1972–1974 and found a significantly reduced incidence of fatal pulmonary embolism
during the latter period. Ljungström (1975, 1977) investigated the number of fatal
pulmonary emboli during an 8-year period in Danderyd, Sweden, where general
dextran prophylaxis was practiced during the second and fourth 2-years periods. During these years all patients of more than 50 years of age undergoing surgery of the
bone, abdomen, and urinary tract received dextran 70. The number of operations
was equally large throughout the investigation period. The numbers of fatal pulmonary emboli during the four 2-year periods were 15, 6, 15, and 3. During the
last 2-year period the incidence was significantly reduced. Atik and Broghamer (1979)
analyzed the 1960–1974 period in a Veterans Administration Hospital in Louis-

ville. During the first 6-year period, when no prophylaxis was offered, 41 patients died of pulmonary embolism, and during the last 9-year period, when dextran prophylaxis had been introduced, the number of deaths was 24. Out of these 24 patients, 21 had not received the prophylaxis recommended, however. During the period 1968–1979 dextran prophylaxis was regularly used at the Orthopedic Clinic in Malmö, Sweden. During this period 1498 patients underwent elective hip arthroplasty, nine of whom died of pulmonary embolism (0.6%) (Fredin and Nillius 1982).

Nevertheless, no strictly controlled study has been performed with the purpose of comparing the incidence of postoperative fatal pulmonary embolism in untreated controls and in a series of patients treated with dextran.

Dosage

There is considerable variation in dosage and dose interval in the various studies (Edwards et al. 1975, Steinmann et al. 1975). The optimal dose remains to be established.

There seems to be no certain correlation between dose and effect, even though this is indicated in a few studies. Evarts and Feil (1971) noted a superior effect of 1000 ml dextran 40 to 500 ml, but Wilhelm et al. (1978), on the other hand, reported a much better prophylactic effect using "low-dose dextran." A series of general surgery patients received 500 ml intraoperatively, followed by 100 ml daily for 5 days. The incidence of thrombosis as measured by the ^{125}I-fibrinogen test was 30% versus 4%. A moderate hemodilution using dextran 70 to a hematocrit of 25–30 results in a lower incidence of pulmonary embolism, as assessed by perfusion scintigraphy, than intraoperative dextran administration without concurrent hemodilution (Nillius 1978, Nillius et al. 1979b). The phlebographically assessed incidence of thrombosis was not influenced in this study. In a small study plasma volume expansion with hydrolyzed gelatin (Haemaccel) had no effect on postoperative frequency of thrombosis (Fuglsang et al. 1980).

On the basis of the studies performed so far, it is reasonable to recommend infusion of dextran with 500 ml intraoperatively and 500 ml after the operation, i.e., 1000 ml during the day of operation. An additional 500 ml should then be administered at least on the first postoperative day. In hip surgery, it has been suggested that additional infusions, for instance on days 3 and 5, would be of prophylactic value (Evarts and Feil 1971, McManus 1976). Provided that it could be confirmed that dextran has a reducing effect on the inhibition of fibrinolysis (Bagge and Saldeen 1978, Carlin and Saldeen 1978, Carlin et al. 1980), which reaches its maximum 3–6 days postoperatively, there would be support for such a hypothesis.

As mentioned previously, a number of aspects remain to be studied with regard to dextran administration, such as optimal dose, dose interval, duration, and time of the first infusion.

Adverse Effects

Cardiac Overloading

Owing to the volume expanding effect, there is some risk of cardiac overloading especially in elderly patients with latent cardiac failure. However, this side effect is unusual and can be avoided by slow infusion. The effect on factor VIII has been reported to be independent of variations in the duration of the infusion from 15 min to 2 h (Åberg et al. 1977a).

Hemorrhagic Complications

In the first few dextran studies, no effect on the bleeding time was observed (Bohmanson 1947, Thorsén 1947, Nittis et al. 1953). Later, several observations were reported, especially from the United States, of a prolonged bleeding time in association with dextran infusion.

Carbone et al. (1954) found that the bleeding time increased on administration of 1000 ml, and that the increase reached a maximum 3–9 h after the infusion, i.e., at the time when the influence on the platelets was at its highest (see p. 132). Bronwell et al. (1954) found that the prolongation of the bleeding time was molecular weight dependent, and were able to show an increased blood loss when skin was removed from burn patients after dextran infusion. The bleeding time in thrombocytopenic patients was still more prolonged by dextran (Adelson 1958).

Several authors were later able to confirm this dextran-induced prolongation of the bleeding time (Adelson et al. 1955, Jaenike and Waterhouse 1955, Jacobaeus 1957, Langdell et al. 1958, Ewald et al. 1965, Cronberg et al. 1966).

The time it takes for an effective hemostatic plug to form depends on the molecular weight as well as the quantity of dextran supplied (Bergqvist D, to be published). It has been shown both clinically (Cronberg et al. 1966) and experimentally (Arfors and Bergqvist 1975) that dextran doses of 1 g/kg body w. or less do not lead to a defect in hemostasis.

In the studies on thrombosis previously referred to, no increased blood loss was reported in association with dextran prophylaxis, even if the exact quantity of the hemorrhage was *not* stated (Koekenberg 1962, Ahlberg et al. 1968, Johnson et al. 1968, Elsner-Mackey et al. 1969, Myhre and Holen 1969, Huttunen et al. 1971, Bonnar and Walsh 1972, Harris et al. 1974, Hedlund 1975, Kline et al. 1975).

In Jansen's (1972) double-blind study including 901 patients, no difference in intraoperative blood loss was noted between patients receiving glucose, dextran 40, or dextran 70. Reoperation because of postoperative hemorrhage was required in five, none, and three patients, respectively. Two, three, and four patients, respectively, were reoperated due to postoperative rupture of the wound. Zederfeldt (1957) had previously shown that dextran did not affect the wound healing process.

In a few studies (Table 40) the blood loss was stated. No significant increased blood loss occurred after dextran administration in thromboprophylactic doses in any of these studies. In one study, an increase in the number of hemorrhagic complications occurred (Smith et al. 1978b). Under certain circumstances an increased diffuse oozing

Table 40. Hemorrhage in association with prophylactic use of dextran

Author	Patient popula-tion	Number of patients	Intraoperative hemorrhage (ml)		Postoperative need of transfusion (units)		Hemorrhagic com-plications (number of patients)	
			Controls	Dextran	Controls	Dextran	Controls	Dextran
Bergqvist et al. (1979)[a]	Hip fracture	49	240 ± 170	171 ± 139	0.5 ± 0.8	1.1 ± 1.5	0	0
	Elective hip surgery	141	552 ± 404	734 ± 390	0.7 ± 0.9	1.0 ± 1.0	0	1
Bergqvist and Hallböök (1980)[a]	General surgery	103	240 (0–1000)	344 (0–2200)	0.2 (0–5)	0.5 (0–3)	0	0
Ruckley (1976)[b] Smith et al. (1978)[c, d]	General surgery	258	530 (38–3800)	485 (10–6197)				
Smith et al. (1978)[c,d]	General surgery	293	175 (5–1300)	245 (10–7500)			2	17

[a]Measured in all patients.
[b]Measured in 63% of patients.
[c]Measured in 75% of patients.
[d]The controls were treated with calf muscle compression intermittently.

was reported in association with dextran administration, but this is difficult to assess in objective terms, and is probably related to the improved capillary perfusion. This could possibly cause difficulties, e.g., in neurosurgery. In patients with hemostatic defects, dextran should be administered with caution.

Anaphylactoid Reactions

The fact that dextran infusion may induce hypersensitive reactions has been known since dextran became clinically available (Pulaski 1951, Maurer 1953, Heistø and Lund 1953). Several cases have been described in the literature (Henley et al. 1957, Meissner 1961, Getzen and Speiggle 1963, Bailey et al. 1967, Brisman et al. 1968, Michelson 1968, Maddi et al. 1969, Kohen et al. 1970, Carlsson et al. 1972, Misgeld and Mende 1974, Fanous et al. 1977). The reactions are induced both by dextran 40 and dextran 70.

During the past decade, a number of comprehensive case reports have been published (Bauer and Östling 1970, Hedin et al. 1976, Furhoff 1977, Hedin 1977, Ring 1978). Furhoff's (1977) material is based on adverse effects reported to the Swedish National Board of Health and Social Welfare during the years 1966–1975, with an incidence figure per infused unit of dextran 70 (1975) of 1:2500 (0.04%).

In a prospective multicenter study Ring and Messmer (1977) compared different plasma volume expanders (200 906 infusions), finding serious reactions in 0.003% of the plasma infusions, the corresponding figure being 0.006% for hydroxyethyl starch, 0.008% for dextran, and 0.038% for gelatin. As is the case with Furhoff's (1977) investigation, this study has a fundamental defect in that it does not relate the incidence of reactions to the numer of patients, but to the number of infusions, the latter ranging from one to ten per patient. This study shows that all volume expanders may give rise to anaphylactoid reactions, but it can hardly be used for assessing the incidence of such reactions.

A randomized adverse effect study was performed by Schöning and Koch (1975) in 750 patients who underwent orthopedic surgery. The patients received infusion of Haemaccel, Gelifundol-S, Neo-plasmagel, plasma-sterile, or dextran. Of the 150 dextran patients, seven exhibited limited skin reactions and one a serious asthma attack (this patient was an asthmatic). As the group is small, the figures can hardly be used for an estimation of the incidence, but the results suggest that the incidence is probably higher for other plasma volume expanders than for dextran.

In a recent prospective multicenter study, where 2159 patients underwent treatment with dextran as a thromboprophylactic, 22 allergic reactions were observed, five of which were serious, i.e., 0.23%, which is a considerably higher figure than stated in the aformentioned compilations, and also in the prospective study from Bavaria by Ring and Messmer (1977) (Gruber et al. 1980).

Reactions of this type are usually divided into (Ring and Messmer 1976):

I   Skin symptoms and/or slight fever
II Measurable, but not life-threatening, cardiovascular reaction (tachycardia, hypotension). Respiratory disturbance
III Shock, life-threatening smooth muscle spasm (e.g., in the bronchi)
IV Cardiac and/or respiratory arrest

III–IV are considered to be serious reactions. Deaths of such causes occur particularly in elderly patients (over 70 years of age).

The reactions always occur initially during dextran infusion, and after administration of a very small quantity. As a rule, the earlier the reaction, the more serious the symptoms. No differences as to sex and age or any relation to other diseases could be demonstrated (Hedin 1977, Ring 1978). Fanous et al. (1977) reported that asthmatics are particularly prone to anaphylactic reactions, however. Whether the infusion of dextran is introduced pre- or intraoperatively does not seem to influence the incidence of reactions.

Kabat and Bezer (1958) and Grönwall (1959) showed that the ability of dextran to induce antibody formation can be ascribed to molecules with a molecular weight exceeding 70 000–80 000.

High titers of hemagglutinating dextran-reactive antibodies (of the IgG, IgA, and IgM types) can be observed in 14%–15% of the population, but most of these people tolerate dextran infusions (Hedin et al. 1976). IgE is within the normal range (Hedin et al. 1976). Cross-reaction occurs for instance between dextran and certain bacterial polysaccharides, especially from pneumococci, streptococci, and *Salmonella* typhi (Zozoya 1932, Hehre et al. 1952). Other potential sources of cross-immunization are dental plaques and food additives (Hedin et al. 1976).

It is probable that specific immune complexes are involved in the serious dextran reactions, and the reaction pattern (the symptoms as well as the complement and antibody response) closely resembles experimental aggregate anaphylaxis in the monkey (Hedin and Smedegård 1979). There is a correlation between the titer of hemagglutinating dextran-reactive antibodies and the severity of the dextran reaction (Richter et al. 1980). Pathoanatomic examination revealed similarities between the microembolism syndrome in the monkey lung, and patients who had died of dextran anaphylaxis (Saldeen et al. 1979, Revenäs et al. 1980). The pulmonary vessels contained platelet and leukocyte aggregates as well as hyaline globules, mainly composed of fibrin. With aggregate anaphylaxis, serious pulmonary vasoconstriction develops, resulting in an increased resistance in the pulmonary artery circulation, and right heart failure (Smedegård 1980). Prostaglandin-like vasoactive substances are possibly released from the platelets (Revenäs 1979).

On this basis it would be theoretically possible to counteract this dextran complication by interfering with the immune complex formation, which can be achieved by the hapten inhibition principle (Richter 1971, 1973a, b). Using low molecular weight dextran, the binding sites on the antibody are blocked, and aggregate formation is prevented. Richter (1971) was able to show that preinjection of low molecular weight dextran could provide complete protection against dextran anaphylaxis in guinea pigs, which otherwise led to a 100% mortality. The principle was shown to provide significant protection also in a dog model (Seemann et al. 1978, Richter et al. 1980).

Preliminary results from the study of about 30 000 patients given a preinjection of hapten dextran (dextran 1, mean mol · wt. = 1000) showed that the number of serious reactions can probably be substantially reduced (Messmer et al. 1980). This study is based on a historical control population, however, which is a great disadvantage, but the immunologic theory as well as experimental data indicate that the principle works. A randominzed prospective study would be of great value.

A dextran solution with a sufficient amount of small molecules, which function according to the hapten inhibition principle, protects guinea pigs from dying from anaphylactoid reactions (Richter 1973a). Thus, there are experimental indications that an excess of low molecular weight dextran in the infusion solution should be effective, which has in fact been shown in a dog model (Richter et al. 1980). Studies are in progress to test whether or not this hypothesis is also valid under clinical conditions.

When a serious dextran reaction occurs, the infusion should be stopped immediately, oxygen should be administered as well as fluid and volume in the form of salt solutions, and perhaps albumin. Moreover, large doses of corticosteroids are supplied (e.g., 0.3–1 g prednisolone i.v.) and adrenalin (0.05–0.1 mg i.v.). In the case of pronounced respiratory symptoms, theophylline may be useful (Schöning and Koch 1975). However, our experience of such ractions is still very limited, and no therapeutic recommendations can as yet be made.

Kidney Damage

Since the dextran solution is hyperoncotic, concurrent fluid administration is required, which is of course particularly important in dehydrated patients (Gelin 1966, Bergentz 1978).

Kidney damage may ensue if large quantities of dextran are administered to dehydrated patients (Fournier et al. 1968, Matheson and Diomi 1970). This applies primarily to dextran 40, which in the form of Rheomacrodex is a 10% solution. Large quantities of dextran 40 induce a pronounced but reversible morphologic vacuolization (osmotic nephrosis) of the cytoplasm of the proximal tubular cells, but their function is not influenced (Engberg 1969). The vacuoles consist of enlarged endocytic vacuoles and enlarged lysozymes, while other cell organelles are morphologically intact (Engberg and Ericsson 1969).

Summary

Dextran is a plasma volume expander with a structure of glucose units. It has a good water-binding capacity and improves hemodilution and perfusion. It also has a complex way of influencing the hemostatic system. The platelet adhesiveness is reduced, while the lysability of thrombi is increased, and both these effects can probably be explained by an influence on the structure and function of factor VIII.

Dextran has a thromboprophylactic effect, especially in connection with hip surgery, where the effect appears to be equal to that of oral anticoagulants. It has been more difficult to demonstrate an effect when the ^{125}I-fibrinogen test was used to establish the diagnosis than when phlebography was employed. The prophylactic effect on pulmonary embolism has been proved and is equal to that of low-dose heparin.

The dextrans used for clinical purposes have average molecular weights of 40 000 and 70 000. The optimal thromboprophylactic dose is unknown, but 500 ml should be administered intraoperatively, followed by an additional 500 ml during the first 24 h postoperatively, and 500 ml at least the 1st day after the operation.

Cardiac overloading may occur in elderly individuals with threatening heart failure. Using modern dextrans in doses not exceeding 1.5 g/kg body wt., no hemorrhagic complications need be feared. Anaphylactoid reactions occur with an incidence of 0.01%–0.25%, which is of the same magnitude as for other plasma volume expanders. The number of serious reactions can probably be reduced by using the hapten inhibition principle, i.e., by injection of a low molecular weight dextran.

Comparative Studies of Low-Dose Heparin and Dextran

Low-dose heparin and dextran are at present the two therapeutic alternatives for thromboprophylaxis with the most comprehensive scientific documentation. Yet, there are relatively few studies comparing the two methods. Table 41 summarizes the available investigations with respect to the incidence of venous thrombosis. Control series are lacking in five of these studies, making it somewhat difficult to obtain a complete picture.

Largely, the results are the same as for the separate studies of either method of prophylaxis. Dextran seems to have a better effect in hip surgery, a fact which is further stressed by the marked reduction of large thrombi (Bergqvist and Dahlgren 1973,

Table 41. Thromboprophylactic studies comparing dextran and low-dose heparin
Harris et al. and Myrvold et al. used phlebography to establish the diagnosis. In the other studies, the ^{125}I-fibrinogen test was used

Author	Patient population	Number of patients	Incidence of thrombosis (%)		
			Controls	Heparin	Dextran
Barber et al. (1977)	Elective hip surgery	70	–	52	51
Bergqvist et al. (1979)	Elective hip surgery	213	63	48	57
	Hip fracture	77	91	63[a]	48[b]
Bergqvist and Hallböök (1980)	General surgery	149	27	13[a]	29
Gruber et al. (1975b)[c]	General surgery, urology	261	36	13[b]	21[a]
Harris et al. (1974)[d]	Elective hip surgery	71	–	73	25[a]
Hohl et al. (1980b)	Gynecologic surgery	232	–	2[b]	15
McCarthy et al. (1974)	Gynecologic surgery	132	–	11	16
Multi-unit Contr. Trial (1974)	General surgery	245	43	15[b]	25[a]
	Gynecologic surgery	82	14	0[b]	22
	Thoracic surgery	54	44	15[a]	31
Myrvold et al. (1973)[e]	Hip fracture	94	–	41	36

[a] $P < 0.05$
[b] $P < 0.01$
[c] Dextran 40
[d] Change of dose interval during the study from heparin 5000 IU every 12 h to every 8 h.
[e] Heparin dosage: 5000 IU × 2 until operation, then 10 000 IU × 2 on postoperative days 1–4, and finally, 5000 IU × 2 on days 5–7.

Bergqvist et al. 1979). In other types of surgery, i.e., when the trauma is not so extensive, the incidence of thrombosis is clearly more reduced using low-dose heparin.

To judge from previous studies, both forms of prophylaxis should be effective against fatal pulmonary embolism, but it is difficult on the basis of these studies to assess their mutual relationship. In 1975 an opinion was expressed in leading articles in *Lancet* (Editorial 1975b) and *British Medical Journal* (Editorial 1975a) that there were no data available that made it possible to give one prophylactic method priority over the other, and also that a comprehensive multicenter study comparing the two methods was clearly needed.

In January 1977 the design of such a study was presented (Svensjö 1977), which was mainly based on the International Multicenter Trial (1975) on the effect of low-dose heparin. This study has now been completed (Gruber et al. 1980). Eight hospitals in Norway, Switzerland, and Sweden participated, and the primary purpose was to establish the incidence of fatal pulmonary embolism within 30 days following surgery, and also to compare the adverse effects involved in the two methods. The Swiss part of the study has also been published separately (Gruber et al. 1979, Hohl et al. 1980).

Five hundred milliliters of dextran 70 was administered intraoperatively, immediately postoperatively, and postoperatively on day 1; 1500 ml in total. Low-dose heparin was administered as sodium heparin at a dose of 5000 IU every 8 h for 6 days. After exclusion of 368 patients for various reasons, 1993 patients remained in the dextran group and 1991 in the low-dose heparin group. Seventy-five patients died, 38 in the dextran series, and 37 in the low-dose heparin group. The autopsy frequency was 87%.

Six patients in each series exhibited pulmonary embolism at autopsy; in the dextran group pulmonary embolism was the sole cause of death in five cases, in the heparin group in three. Only two of the patients with pulmonary embolism in the heparin series had received adequate prophylaxis compared with five of the dextran

Table 42. Total mortality, and the pulmonary embolism mortality (FPE, fatal pulmonary embolism) in studies of the prophylactic effect of low-dose heparin and dextran on embolism

Authors	Total number of patients	Control		Low-dose heparin		Dextran	
		Deaths (%)	FPE (%)	Deaths (%)	FPE (%)	Deaths (%)	FPE (%)
Gruber et al. (1980)[a]	3984	–	–	1.9	0.10	1.9	0.25
Int. Multicentre Trial (1975)[b]	4121	4.8	0.77	3.9	0.10	–	–
Kiil et al. (1978)[c]	1296	?	1.1	?	0.16	–	–
Kline et al. (1975)[d]	831	8.0	1.6	–	–	6.8	0.25
Sagar et al. (1975)[c]	488	16.1	3.4	11.1	0	–	–

Follow-up time:
[a] 1 month.
[b] Until discharge or death at the hospital.
[c] Not stated.
[d] 3 months.

Table 43. Adverse effects of dextran and low-dose heparin in the multicenter study. (Gruber et al. 1980)

	Dextran 70	Low-dose heparin	Significance
Excluded because of hemorrhage	6 patients	94 patients	$P < 0.01$
Reoperation because of hemorrhage	47 patients	31 patients	NS
Wound hematoma	68 patients	135 patients	$P < 0.01$
Intraop. hemorrhage of > 800 ml	15%	12%	NS
Intraop. transfusion > 2 units	24%	21%	$P < 0.01$
Postop. transfusion	equal	equal	NS
Allergic reaction	22 patients	3 patients	$P < 0.01$

patients. This difference is not statistically significant, however. It is not quite clear why patients who had not received adequate prophylaxis had not been excluded from the final compilation. As appears from Table 42, the figures are difficult to compare with other studies.

When the multicenter study on dextran and low-dose heparin was started, it was considered unethical to study an untreated control series, but it would certainly have been of great value if such a series had been included. Nevertheless, the conclusion in Gruber's study that both methods are equally useful for the prophylaxis of fatal pulmonary embolism appears to be justified.

Table 43 shows the adverse effects in this multicenter study. As could be expected, low-dose heparin dominates where hemorrhages are concerned, and dextran with respect to allergic reactions. Also, the number of patients excluded from the heparin series because the protocol had not been followed properly was significantly higher than in the dextran series (331 patients excluded versus 118). Apart from the hemorrhagic complications, this was also due to the technical problem involved in injecting heparin subcutaneously on 21 occasions compared to three infusions of dextran.

As mentioned previously, the design of this study was mainly based on Kakkar's multicenter study, but it has at least partly succeeded in avoiding the factors that gave rise to the criticism of Kakkar's work, e.g., by Sherry (1975). The autopsy frequency was thus considerably higher, and the pathologic assessment of the autopsy protocol more homogeneous.

In Table 44 the various facts are presented which must be taken into account when assessing the two prophylactic methods, i.e., dextran and low-dose heparin. An evaluation was performed by Verstraete (1976a, b), who suggested low-dose heparin in extensive abdominal and thoracic surgery operations as well as in gynecologic surgery, and dextran in orthopedic surgery.

Summary

There are few studies which directly compare low-dose heparin and dextran from a thromboprophylactic viewpoint, while both methods separately have been thoroughly documented.

Table 44. Schematic comparison between low-dose heparin and dextran

	Low-dose heparin	Dextran
Effect on thrombosis (fibrinogen test)	+++	+ ?
Effect on thrombosis (phlebography)	+	+
Effect on fatal pulmonary embolism	+	+
Effect on post-thrombotic syndrome	?	?
Effect in hip surgery	+	+++
Effect on trauma patients	−	+
Duration of prophylaxis	About 1 week	A day or two
Introduction of prophylaxis	Preop.	Intraop.
Administration	15–21 5000-IU s. c. injections	1–5 500-ml i.v. infusions
Allergy	+	++
Cardiac overloading	−	+
Hemorrhage	++	+
Concomitant volume expansion	−	+

In general surgery, the incidence of thrombosis is clearly more effectively reduced by low-dose heparin. In hip-surgery dextran is superior. Judging from previous studies, the two methods appear to be equally effective in the prophylaxis of pulmonary embolism.

In a recently performed multicenter study, dextran was compared with low-dose heparin with respect to fatal pulmonary embolism as well as administration reliability. This study did not contain any control series. The prophylactic effect on pulmonary embolism was equal. Low-dose heparin induced more hemorrhagic complications, dextran more allergic side effects. The protocol was followed less often in the low-dose heparin series, indicating the technical problem involved in administering 21 subcutaneous injections of heparin as compared to three infusions of dextran.

Other Prophylactic Methods

Vitamin C (Ascorbic Acid)

Since vitamin C is necessary for an intact supporting tissue, and a deficiency of this vitamin causes vascular fragility, it has been suggested that it could be used for thromboprophylactic purposes (Spittle 1973). However, other authors have not been able to confirm such a hypothesis (Andrews and Wilson 1973).

Taylor et al. (1979) performed a double-blind study on preoperative administration for 1 week of vitamin C to general surgery patients. The incidence of thrombosis assessed by the ^{125}I-fibrinogen test was not reduced, but the ascorbate concentration in the leukocytes was significantly increased.

Stimulation of Fibrinolysis

A large group of patients with recurrent idiopathic venous thrombosis have an abnormally low level of plasminogen activator in the vein walls (Pandolfi et al. 1969, Isacson and Nilsson 1972b, Nilsson et al. 1981) and a decreased fibrinolytic activity in plasma (Menon et al. 1971a). A combination of phenformin and ethylestrenol stimulates the spontaneous fibrinolytic activity in the blood (Fearnley et al. 1967). Such treatment has also been shown to normalize the plasminogen activator in the vein walls of patients with a low concentration of this substance, but the treatment must be continued for at least 6 months to obtain such an effect (Nilsson et al. 1975). Preoperative treatment for 6 weeks will increase the postoperative fibrinolytic activity (Brown et al. 1971).

This combination has been used in a few studies as possible prophylaxis against postoperative venous thrombosis, but without any evident effect (Fossard et al. 1974a, Atkins et al. 1978). It is also a cumbersome prophylactic method in association with surgery, since medication must be introduced several weeks preoperatively. Fossard et al. (1974a) treated their patients for 3 weeks preoperatively, Atkins et al. (1978) for 6 weeks. This is a short time compared to what is considered necessary for normalization of the fibrinolytic activator concentration in the vein walls of patients with spontaneous thrombosis. The fibrinolytic activation obtained is obviously not sufficient for a thromboprophylactic action in the postoperative situation.

L7035 is a fibrinolysis-activating substance (Jardon 1976). The effect is optimal after 2 weeks' treatment with 50 mg/kg body wt. It is neutralized by epsilon-aminocaproic acid. This substance has also been shown to induce total thrombolysis of occluding experimental arterial thrombi in the dog. It also reduces platelet adhesiveness and aggregation with adenosine diphosphate without influencing the number of platelets. It does not affect the coagulation system. The substance has no central hemodynamic effects.

This substance was studied as a possible thromboprophylactic agent in a double-blind controlled study including 34 patients who underwent elective hip surgery

(Jardon 1976). The patients were treated with 400 mg L 7035 $\times$ 3 for 15 days pre-operatively, and during the first postoperative week. Eight out of 14 patients treated with placebo (57%) and seven of 20 patients receiving L 7035 (35%) exhibited thrombi, diagnosed by the ^{125}I-fibrinogen test ($P > 0.3$).

Xantinol Nicotinate

Xantinol nicotinate is the nicotinate of 7-[2-hydroxy-3-((2-hydroxyethyl) methyl-amino) propyl] theophylline. It induces peripheral vasodilatation and an increase of the stroke volume and minute volume of the heart. Xantinol nicotinate had no effect as a thromboprophylactic agent in a study in which thrombi diagnosed by the ^{125}I-fibrinogen test and fatal pulmonary emboli were recorded (Gruber et al. 1977b). The incidence of thrombosis was 36% in the control series and 41% in the treatment group.

O-(β-Hydroxyethyl)-rutoside (HR)

HR is a flavonoid which is semisynthetically produced from a plant material. It affects the microrheological conditions of the blood in two ways: by reducing the aggregating tendency of the erythrocytes, and by decreasing their rigidity in an acid milieu (van Haeringen et al. 1973, Schmid-Schönbein et al. 1975). There are also indications of an inhibition of the platelet-aggregating capacity (Kahlé et al. 1975). Furthermore, the blood viscosity is somewhat decreased (Thulesius and Gjöres 1972). The formation of the hemostatic plug in a rabbit mesenterium model is delayed, which is an indirect measure of a defect in platelet function (Bergqvist et al. 1978). At the same time the leakage of macromolecules in postcapillary venules decreases, and the prostaglandin content in the tissues falls (Bergqvist et al. 1978). The capillary filtration rate in the lower extremities decreases (Roztocil et al. 1977, Bergqvist et al. 1981), and the venous tone increases (Forconi et al. 1977), for which reason the substance is some-times used in venous insufficiency (Rose 1970, Prerovsky et al. 1972, Rish and Rod-riguez 1972). Clinical effects have been summarized by Golden (1978).

Experimental models of thrombosis have yielded contradictory results (Mirko-vitch et al. 1972, Hladovec 1977, Bergqvist et al. 1978). However, the theoretical background has made HR interesting in connection with thromboprophylaxis, but only a few investigations have been published so far. In 120 patients undergoing various hip joint operations, HR was compared with low-dose heparin or no prophy-laxis at all (Protoulis et al. 1976). The incidence of thrombosis assessed by the ^{125}I fibrinogen test was 52% in the control series, 63% in the HR series, and 25% in the heparin group ($P < 0.01$ in favor of heparin). Calnan (1972) compared HR with placebo in 30 cancer patients undergoing surgery, finding no difference in the inci-dence of thrombosis.

Lidocaine

The possible role of leukocytes in the pathogenesis of thrombosis has previously been discussed (p. 37). Lidocaine — a local anesthetic — prevents leukocyte adhesion to and invasion of the vein wall (Giddon and Lindhe 1972, Stewart et al. 1974). The effect can be ascribed to the influence on the leukocytes rather than on the vein wall per se. The coagulation and fibrinolytic activities are not affected (Cooke et al. 1977a). Being membrane-active substances (Seeman 1972), local analgesics also change the platelet reaction pattern, at least in vitro (O'Brien 1977).

Intravenous administration of 1 mg/kg body wt. preoperatively, followed by 2 mg/min for 6 days, was studied as thromboprophylaxis (Cooke et al. 1977a). Twenty-eight patients were randomized to a control or treatment group, after which the study was discontinued because of the significantly higher incidence of thrombi in the control series — 11 out of 14 (78%), eight of which were in the femoral veins. The lidocaine group exhibited only two thrombi (14%), none of which occurred in the femoral veins. No complications were observed. The blood loss through suction drainage and need of transfusion were identical in the two groups.

Intramuscular administration does not have the same thromboprophylactic effect (Cooke and Bowcock 1979a), but work is in progress to evaluate a preparation with a similar mechanism of action, which can be administered orally — tocainide (Cooke and Bowcock 1979b). In a recent study the effect of oral tocainide had no effect on the frequency of phlebographic thrombi or scintigraphic emboli in patients undergoing elective hip surgery (Modig et al. 1981).

Saponin-β aescin

Aescin is a substance with an antiphlogistic and antiexudative effect (Vogel and Ströcker 1966, Vogel et al. 1970). It has been investigated as a prophylactic agent against thromboembolism in a study including 200 female patients undergoing various general surgery operations (Prexl et al. 1976). The incidence of thrombosis assessed by the ^{125}I-fibrinogen test was 16% in the aescin series versus 27% in the control group, a difference which is not statistically significant ($\chi^2 = 3.58, P = 0.07$).

Antithrombin III

A low antithrombin III level is a factor predisposing to thrombus formation, and several studies have demonstrated a lowered level after surgery (see p. 47). Purified antithrombin III (Andersson et al. 1974) has been shown to raise the antithrombin III level in experiments (Medén-Britth et al. 1976) and in patients undergoing hip fracture surgery (Medén-Britth and Teien 1979). Whether or not antithrombin III can function as a prophylactic against thrombosis remains to be studied. Because of manufacturing difficulties and consequent high prices, it can certainly be used only in very special situations, mainly operations in patients with a congenital antithrombin III deficiency.

Summary

Apart from the more firmly established prophylactic methods against thromboembolism, an additional number of medicinal methods have been studied. For each separate substance, however, only one or two reports concerning projects still being investigated have been published.

Antithrombin III deficiency predisposes to thrombosis. Administration of antithrombin III raises the serum level, but the thromboprophylactic effect has so far not been studied in detail.

Vitamin C, fibrinolytic stimulation, xantinol nicotinate, O-(β-hydroxyethyl)-rutoside, and aescin all seem to be without effect.

Lidocaine — a local anesthetic — on the other hand, appears to be of interest. It prevents leukocyte adhesion to the vein wall and, in a few studies, has been shown to have a thromboprophylactic effect in elective hip surgery.

Combination Prophylaxis

The most interesting combination of prophylactic agents is dihydroergotamine – low-dose heparin (see p. 115). A combination of acetylsalicylic acid and dipyridamole has also been discussed (p. 124). Both combinations appear to have a prophylactic effect. Using dihydroergotamine, it also seems possible to reduce the heparin dose without interfering with the effect, thereby reducing the incidence of hemorrhagic complications (Hohl et al. 1979).

Only a few reports have been published on other combinations of prophylactic methods. Since thrombosis is a multifactorial disease, it is logical to assume that the assessment of various combination alternatives will be an important feature of future thromboprophylactic research.

A combination of low-dose heparin and aspirin was shown to have a potentiating effect in a study in general surgery patients (Loew et al. 1977) and in another study concerning patients undergoing hip surgery (Schöndorf and Hey 1976), while a third investigation in patients undergoing elective hip surgery did not show such an effect (Flicoteaux et al. 1977). In a small hip fracture study, the hemorrhagic complications increased markedly using a combination of heparin 5000 IU every 12 h and 0.6 g ASA every 12 h (Yett et al. 1978).

Rogers et al. (1978) found that a combination of sulfinpyrazone and low-dose heparin was effective in hip fracture patients. As this study contained only one control series apart from the combination group, the results are difficult to assess. Also, the population was small (30 patients in all).

A combination of aspirin and hydroxychloroquine was not shown to be effective in elective hip surgery (Hume et al. 1976). Aspirin combined with RA 223 (a dipyridamole analogue) had no effect in hip fracture surgery either (Wood et al. 1973).

In one study, an elastic bandage was combined with the platelet-inhibiting agent oxyphenbutazone in patients who underwent elective hip surgery (Tillberg 1974). The incidence of thrombosis was 57% in the control series, and 19% in the treatment group ($P < 0.01$, 50 patients in all).

Browse et al. (1976) combined dextran 70 and intermittent calf muscle compression, resulting in a significant reduction of the incidence of pulmonary embolism (from 24% to 8%; $P < 0.02$) as assessed by scintigraphy. Since there was only one control series, the effect of each prophylactic method cannot be analyzed separately. However, Smith et al. (1978b) did not find a lower incidence of thrombosis in a combination series of dextran 70 and intermittent calf muscle compression than in either group separately. By administration of low-dose heparin, Roberts and Cotton (1975) did not succeed in reducing the incidence of thrombosis observed when employing intermittent calf muscle compression.

Korvald et al. (1973) combined warfarin with dextran 70, comparing this combination with dextran only. The incidence of thrombosis confirmed by phlebography in hip fracture patients was reduced from 35% in the dextran series to 10% in the combination group ($P < 0.05$). A total of six hematomas developed, the majority in the combination series. No other serious hemorrhagic complications were observed.

Nevertheless, this combination can hardly be recommended for routine use because of the risk of hemorrhage.

Dextran 40 combined with low-dose heparin is not superior to low-dose heparin alone in association with elective hip surgery (Schöndorf and Weber 1980).

Intraoperative administration of dextran 40 combined with anticoagulants introduced postoperatively was tried by van Geloven et al. (1977). They found that the combination was significantly superior to anticoagulants only in a study comprising patients undergoing thoracotomy, laparotomy, or hip joint surgery. The ^{125}I-fibrinogen test was employed to establish the diagnosis, and the incidence of thrombosis was 11% in the combination series versus 25% in the anticoagulants series ($P < 0.05$). No difference was observed in the same study between a group treated with low-dose heparin and another group receiving a combination of low-dose heparin and oral anticoagulants (19% vs 18%). Nevertheless, the heparin dose was changed during the investigation, since during the first part of the study heparin had been administered in very low doses (see p. 106). The incidence of pulmonary perfusion defects, as assessed by scintigraphy, was not reduced by any of the four prophylactic methods.

Törngren (1980) studied a combination of low-dose heparin and graded elastic compression (TED stocking, see p. 67). All patients undergoing abdominal surgery in the study were treated with low-dose heparin (5000 IU × 2), and an elastic stocking was applied to one leg and allowed to remain for 6 days. In the leg treated with the stocking, a significantly lower incidence of thrombosis was observed than in the untreated leg.

To sum up, there are relatively few studies on different prophylactic combinations, the most interesting being a combination of low-dose heparin and dihydroergotamine, allowing a lower heparin dose, which leads to fewer hemorrhagic complications. It is also effective in elective hip surgery.

Summary

A number of combinations have been tried in the hope of increasing the thromboprophylactic effect. In the majority of studies, no potentiation could be shown. However, combinations of ASA and dipyridamole as well as low-dose heparin and dihydroergotamine seem to have a clear effect, the latter combination also in hip surgery. In hip fracture surgery, a combination of oral anticoagulants and dextran has also been shown to be of value, although involving a risk of hemorrhage.

Since thrombosis is a multifactorial disease, future thromboprophylaxis will probably be directed toward finding effective combinations of prophylactic methods. On the other hand, any form of combination is often complex and more demanding from a technical viewpoint in the care of the patient.

Use of Prophylaxis

In spite of the intensive scientific production in the field of thromboprophylaxis, comparatively little is known about its use in clinical practice. An American (Simon and Stengle 1974) and an English (Morris and Mitchell 1976a) survey among orthopedic surgeons, and an American survey among general surgeons (Conti 1980), revealed that only approximately half of the surgeons interviewed used any kind of thromboprophylaxis. The reply rate in these investigations was low, however, about 63%.

Morris (1980) later performed another survey in England, involving orthopedic surgeons as well as general surgeons. This time the reply rate was somewhat higher, about 75%. This study also shows that the use of prophylaxis is not very common. Surprisingly, prophylaxis seems to be less commonly employed the greater the risk of thrombosis.

To obtain an idea of the practice in Sweden, an inquiry was made among all inpatient clinics within general surgery, urology, orthopedics, and gynecology (Bergqvist 1980c). Ninety-four percent of the clinics replied, 76% stating that they used some kind of prophylaxis (general surgery clinics 81%, urologic clinics 65%, orthopedic clinics 96%, and gynecologic clinics 57%). The estimated percentage of patients in these clinics receiving prophylaxis is low, however, being about 19%, with no difference between specialities. Among the clinics using no prophylaxis, the general opinion was that the risk of thromboembolism is slight (67%), while 28% considered the risk of complications with the available prophylactic methods too great to justify any prophylaxis.

Table 45. The use of thromboprophylactic methods in Swedish clinics

Prophylactic method	Percentage of clinics				
	Surgery ($n = 76$)	Urology ($n = 13$)	Orthopedics ($n = 44$)	Gynecology ($n = 35$)	All ($n = 168$)
Oral anticoagulants	42	–	27	9	28
Low-dose heparin (LDH)	78	54	39	69	64
Dextran 40	22	8	11	17	17
Dextran 70	76	69	75	66	73
Acetylsalicylic acid	12	–	2	3	7
Dihydroergotamine (DHE)	–	–	2	3	1
LDH + DHE	1	–	–	–	0.6
Elastic bandage	29	23	46	3	27
Electric calf muscle stimulation	1	8	–	–	1
Intermittent calf muscle compression	7	8	9	3	7

Table 46. Thromboprophylactic practice in orthopedic surgery in the United States, Great Britain, and Sweden. Results of surveys

Method of prophylaxis	Percentage of clinics					
	United States, hip surgery[a]		Great Britain[b]	Great Britain, hip surgery[c]		Sweden[d,e]
	Elective	Fracture	Hip fracture	Elective	Fracture	Orthopedic surgery
Oral anticoagulant	17	11	3	3	2	27
Dextran	17	7	8	6	2	86
Acetylsalicylic acid	11	9	1	1	1	2
Low-dose heparin	2	2	1	7	3	39
Other methods, incl. mechanical ones	7	5	36	31	20	11
No prophylaxis	47	66	51	52	72	4

[a]Simon and Stengle 1974 (637 surgeons, reply frequency 63%).
[b]Morris and Mitchell 1976a (643 surgeons, reply frequency 64%).
[c]Morris 1980 (752 surgeons, reply frequency 74%).
[d]Bergqvist 1980c (46 clinics, reply frequency 100%).
[e]Since several clinics use more than one prophylactic method, the sum exceeds 100%.

Among the risk factors stated as indicating need of prophylaxis, the major ones are the extent of the operation and previous thromboembolic disease. Only 45% of the clinics considered age to be an essential factor. The median age for the introduction of prophylaxis is 40 years in the orthopedic clinics and 50 years in the others.

Among the drug therapy methods, dextran and low-dose heparin are the agents most commonly used (Table 45). Oral anticoagulants are used in several general surgery clinics, but almost exclusively where fracture surgery is practiced. The relatively common use of elastic bandages is probably due to the comparative simplicity of the method. Fifty-eight percent of the clinics practice two or more prophylactic methods concurrently. About half of the clinics using prophylaxis have noted some kind of adverse effect of the method concerned, but only two clinics have abandoned a certain method because of its adverse effect.

Table 46 presents a comparison between the four surveys from three different countries in which orthopedic surgeons were interviewed as to their principles of prophylaxis. It is apparent that the attitude toward prophylaxis is considerably more radical in Sweden than in England and the United States. Recently, a similar survey concerning general and gynecologic surgery was made in Finland (Kettunen 1981). The reply rate was 88% and the general attitude toward prophylaxis is in agreement with that in Sweden: 83% use drug therapy methods, predominantly oral anticoagulants, dextran, and low-dose heparin. But just as in Sweden only 13% of operated patients receive prophylaxis.

To sum up, the number of surgical clinics in Sweden using prophylaxis is great, but the percentage of patients receiving prophylaxis is low. Taking 50 years as the age limit for introduction of prophylaxis, at least three times as many patients ought to receive some kind of prophylaxis. Low-dose heparin and dextran are the most commonly employed prophylactic methods. Adverse effects appear to be of minor importance.

Summary

On inquiry, 81% of the general surgery, 65% of the urologic, 96% of the orthopedic, and 57% of the gynecologic inpatient clinics in Sweden today stated that they use some kind of thromboprophylaxis. The estimated percentage of patients receiving prophylaxis is low, about 19%. Clearly the most common methods of prophylaxis are low-dose heparin and dextran. Adverse effects appear to be a minor problem. The prophylactic attitude seems to be more aggressive than in the United States and England.

Prophylaxis Against Thromboembolism in Various Clinical Situations

Summarizing Comments

Pulmonary embolism as well as post-thrombotic venous insufficiency are relatively common conditions, the former often having a fatal outcome, the latter leading to prolonged suffering.

The course of fatal pulmonary embolism is so rapid that the diagnosis is often inadequate. Within 15 min of the onset of the symptoms 39% of the patients have died, 57% within 1 h (MacIntyre and Ruckley 1974). Studies with a still higher 1 h mortality have been published (Hermann et al. 1961, Donaldson et al. 1963, Morrison 1963). For untreated pulmonary embolism, the mortality is about 30% (Zilliacus 1946, Barritt and Jordan 1960, Hermann et al. 1961, Morell et al. 1963, Coon et al. 1969, Dalen and Alpert 1975), and may be still higher in surgical patients (Inberg et al. 1974).

These circumstances underline the importance of prophylaxis since the time to establish the diagnosis is so short. Moreover, many pulmonary emboli are silent, i.e., there are no warning symptoms before the acute embolization.

A more advanced surgical and anesthesiologic technique makes it possible to operate on older patients. It is important to reduce the risk of fatal pulmonary embolism in these patients, since age is one of the major risk factors predisposing to this complication.

The course of post-thrombotic venous insufficiency, on the other hand, is so slow that the pathogenetic development is only partly known.

Today, the possibility of foreseeing the risk of these two complications in the individual case, e.g., through some form of prognostic index, is small. Provided that the prophylactic methods are relatively effective and the frequency of adverse effects low, and that they are easy to apply, it is reasonable to offer such prophylaxis to a large part of the patients undergoing surgery.

The risk factors of major importance, which should influence the decision whether prophylaxis should be provided or not, are the age of the patient, the extent of the operation, previous thromboembolic disease, and malignancy. The lower age limit for a more general prophylaxis should be 45–50 years.

The ideal prophylactic method, as presented in Table 47, does not exist. It will be the aim of future research to come as close to this ideal as possible. Since thrombosis is a multifactorial disease, we will probably have to accept a few different solutions or perhaps combination prophylaxis in one form or another.

Different methods can, in a certain situation, be of equal thromboprophylactic value. The important points are to use a method which is already effective intraoperatively, and that patients at risk are not left without any prophylaxis. On the other hand, it is reasonable to assume that a reduced incidence of thrombosis also reduces the risk of pulmonary embolism.

With the present public health economy, it is important to analyze the costs of different prophylactic methods in relation to their efficacy. These calculations are

Table 47. Conditions for a satisfactory thromboprophylactic method

Effective against venous thrombosis
Effective against pulmonary embolism
Effective against post-thrombotic venous insufficiency
Few adverse effects
Few contraindications
Effective intraoperatively
Effective during the whole risk period
Simple mode of administration requiring little time
Exact dosage
Acceptable for the patient
No laboratory controls
Suitable to all patients and types of surgery
Low costs

Table 48. Use of various thromboprophylactic methods in different surgical specialties

Type of operation	Oral anti- coagulants	ASA- dipyri- damole	LDH	LDH-DHE	Dextran	ICF
General surgery	+	+	+	+	+ ?	+
Urology	?	?	+ ?	?	+ ?	+ ?
Gynecology	+	+ ?	+	+	+	?
Orthopedics						
Elective	+ ?	–	–	+	+	–
Fracture	+	–	–	+	+	–
Neurosurgery	?	?	+	?	?	+

ASA, acetylsalicylic acid; LDH, low-dose heparin; DHE, dihydroergotamine; ICC, intermittent calf muscle compression; +, effect certain; –, no effect; ?, effect uncertain or unknown

very complex, but attempts in that direction have been made concerning American (Salzman and Davies 1980) and Swedish conditions (Bergqvist and Ousbäck 1982). It can be concluded that prophylaxis is reasonable also from the economic point of view.

Table 48 is a compilation of different prophylactic methods in different clinical situations. In the assessment of a suitable prophylactic method it is also important to take the patient's bleeding tendency into account, both with respect to the nature of the operation and to possible defects in the hemostatic system of the individual patient. It is of vital importance to obtain a preoperative bleeding history from all patients (Bergqvist 1980a).

In *general surgery, thoracic surgery,* and *gynecologic surgery* most types of prophylaxis can be employed. If only the thromboprophylactic effect is taken into account, the effect of dextran is somewhat dubious, but this agent reduces the incidence of fatal pulmonary embolism. Low-dose heparin is useful in most studies, and the addition of dihydroergotamine appears to improve the effect.

In *urologic surgery* comparatively few prophylactic studies have been performed. Patients undergoing transvesical prostatectomy run a special risk of hemorrhage, with the raw wound surface of an enucleated prostatic lobe. None of the methods is altogether satisfactory. One can choose between low-dose heparin, dextran, or calf muscle compression. With thrombosis in mind, transurethral surgery is preferable to transvesical prostatectomy.

Orthopedic patients form a special high-risk group with respect to thrombo-embolic complications. Oral anticoagulants, dextran, and low-dose heparin combined with dihydroergotamine can be used. Low-dose heparin and intermittent calf muscle compression do not reduce the incidence of thrombosis satisfactorily. In fracture surgery, low-dose heparin is clearly unsuitable, since it cannot be introduced prior to the activation of factor X by the trauma.

Neurosurgical patients also form a special group. The incidence of thrombosis is higher than previously believed, and patients are in danger even with small local hemorrhagic complications. Low-dose heparin has been shown to have a thrombo-prophylactic effect, but should be administered with caution due to the risk of hemor-rhage, although this is slight. Intermittent calf muscle compression is an ideal alternative in this special situation, and the thromboprophylactic effect has been established.

References

Åberg M (1978) On effect of dextran on lysability and structure of ex vivo thrombi, platelet function and factor VIII.Thesis. Malmö University

Åberg M, Bergentz S-E (1979) The effect of dextran on the platelet distribution and lysability of ex vivo thrombi in dogs. Eur Surg Res 11:282

Åberg M, Nilsson IM (1968) Fibrinolytic activity of the vein wall after surgery. Br J Surg 65:259

Åberg M, Rausing A (1978) The effect of dextran 70 on the structure of ex vivo thrombi. Thromb Res 12:1113

Åberg M, Nilsson IM, Hedner U (1973) Antithrombin III after operation. Lancet II:1337

Åberg M, Isacson S, Nilsson IM (1974) The fibrinolytic system and postoperative thrombosis following operation of rectal carcinoma. A preliminary report. Acta Chir Scand 140:352

Åberg M, Bergentz S-E, Hedner U (1975) The effect of dextran on the lysability of ex vivo thrombi. Ann Surg 181:342

Åberg M, Arfors K-E, Bergentz S-E (1977a) Effect of dextran on factor VIII and thrombus stability in humans. Significance of varying infusion rates. Acta Chir Scand 143:417

Åberg M, Bergentz S-E, Hedner U (1977b) Effect of dextran and induced thrombocytopenia on the lysability of ex vivo thrombi in dogs. Acta Chir Scand 143:91

Åberg M, Hedner U, Bergentz S-E (1979) Effect of dextran on factor VIII (antihemophilic factor) and platelet function. Ann Surg 189:243

Abbott W (1980) Renal failure complicating vascular surgery. In: Bernhard V, Towne J (eds) Complications in vascular surgery. Grune & Stratton, New York London Toronto Sidney San Francisco

Abernathy E, Hartsuck J (1974) Postoperative pulmonary embolism. A prospective study utilising low dose heparin. Am J Surg 128:739

Abildgaard U (1966) Acceleration of fibrin polymerization by dextran and ficoll. Interaction with calcium and plasma proteins. Scand J Clin Lab Invest 18:518

Abildgaard U (1968) Highly purified antithrombin III with heparin cofactor activity prepared by disc electrophoresis. Scand J Clin Lab Invest 21:89

Abildgaard U, Skjörten F (1968) Influence of low molecular weight dextran and thrombin infusions on blood platelets and fibrinogen. J Atheroscler Res 8:69

Abou-Abdallah E, Rausis C, Loup P, Mosimann E (1975) Etude cooperative héparinate de sodium et de calcium dans la prophylaxie des maladies thromboemboliques en chirurgie. Helv Chir Acta 42:691

Abraham-Inpijn L, Vreeken J (1975) Effect of low-dose heparin on incidence of postoperative thrombosis in orthopaedic patients. Arch Chir Neerl 27:63

Adams J, DeWeese J (1966) Partial interruption of the inferior vena cava with a new plastic clip. Surg Gynecol Obstet 123:1087

Adams JH, Mitchell JRA (1979) The effect of agents which modify platelet behaviour and of Mg ions on thrombus formation in vivo. Thromb Haemost 42:603

Adelson E (1958) Bleeding time prolongation after dextran influsion. Bibl Haematol 7:275

Adelson E, Crosby WH, Roeder WH (1955) Further studies of a haemostatic defect by intravenous dextran. J Lab Clin Med 45:441

Adelson J, Steer M, Glotzer D, Skillman J, Simon M, Salzman E (1980) Thromboembolism after insertion of the Mobin-Uddin caval filter. Surgery 87:184

Adelsten-Jensen RA (1952) Postoperative thrombo-embolism. Acta Chir Scand 103:263

Adiseshiah M (1979) Preventing thromboembolic complications in high-risk surgical patients. Br Med J 1:1707

Adolf J, Buttermann G, Weidenbach A, Gmeineder F (1978) Optimierung der postoperativen Thromboseprophylaxe in der Gynäkologie. Ein Vergleich von Heparin, Dihydroergotamin, ihrer Kombination und Azetylsalizylsäure. Geburtshilfe Frauenheilkd 38:98

Aellig WH (1967) Periphere Kreislaufwirkungen von Ergotamin, Dihydroergotamin und l-Methylergotamin an der innervierten, perfundierten Hinterextremität des Hundes. Helv Physiol Pharmacol Acta 25:374

Aellig WH (1976) Influence of ergot compounds on compliance of superficial hand veins in man. Postgrad Med J 52:[Suppl 1]21

Aellig WH, Nuesch E (1977) Comparative pharmakokinetic investigations with tritium-labelled ergot alkaloids after oral and intravenous administration in man. Int J Clin Pharmacol 15:106

Ahlberg Å (1969) Thromboprophylaxis with dextran in hip fracture surgery (In Swedish) Studentlitteratur, Lund

Ahlberg Å, Nylander G, Robertson B, Cronberg S, Nilsson IM (1968) Dextran in prophylaxis of thrombosis in fractures of the hip. Acta Chir Scand [Suppl] 387:83

Ah-see A-K, Arfors K-E, Bergqvist D, Tangen O (1974) Effect of dextran on experimental venous thrombosis in rabbits. Thromb Diath Haemorrh 32:284

Ah-see AK, Arfors K-E, Bergqvist D, Dahlgren S (1976) The haemodynamic and antithrombotic effects of intermittent pneumatic calf compression on femoral vein blood flow. A comparison between different pump types. Acta Chir Scand 142:381

Albrechtsson U, Olsson C-G (1976) Thrombotic side-effects of lower-limb phlebography. Lancet I: 723

Aldrete J, Halperin N, Ward S, Wright J (1979) Factors determining the mortality and morbidity in hepatic injuries. Analysis of 108 cases. Ann Surg 189:466

Alexander B (1971) Effect of dextran and other macromolecules on coagulation and hemostasis. In: Derrick JR, Guest MM (eds) Dextrans. Current concepts of basic actions and clinical applications. Thomas, Springfield, Ill

Alho A, Rokkanen P (1973) Recovery of patients after intensive care for blunt injuries. Ann Chir Gynecol Fenn 62:64

Ali M, McDonald JW (1977) Effects of sulfinpyrazone on platelet prostaglandin synthesis and platelet release of serotonin. J Lab Clin Med 89:868

Allen AW (1947) Interruption of the deep veins of the lower extremities in the prevention and treatment of thrombosis and embolism. Surg Gynecol Obstet 84:519

Allen A, Linton R, Donaldson G (1945) Venous thrombosis and pulmonary embolism. JAMA 128: 397

Allen EV, Barker NW, Waugh JM (1942) A preparation from spoiled sweet clover [3,3′-methylene-bis-(4-hydroxycoumarin)] which prolongs coagulation and prothrombin time of the blood: A clinical study. JAMA 120:1009

Allen EV, Hines E, Kvale W, Barker N (1947) The use of dicumarol as an anticoagulant: experience in 2307 cases. Ann Intern Med 27:371

Allen JG, Arendrup H, Toftgaard C, Lindegaard P, Madsen EM, Sørensen SS (1979) Calcium-heparin or sodium-heparin in low-dose heparin prophylaxis? Thromb Haemost 42:1064

Allen NH, Jenkins JD, Smart CJ (1978) Surgical haemorrhage in patients given subcutaneous heparin as prophylaxis against thromboembolism. Br Med J 1:1326

Allenby F, Boardman L, Pflug JJ, Calnan JS (1973) Effects of external pneumatic intermittent compression on fibrinolysis in man. Lancet II:1412

Allgood R, Cook J, Weedn R, Speed HK, Whitcomb W, Greenfield L (1970) Prospective analysis of pulmonary embolism in the postoperative patient. Surgery 68:116

Almén T, Nylander G (1962) Serial phlebography of the normal lower leg during muscular contraction and relaxation. Acta Radiol 57:264

Alvarez H (1961) Discussion: motility of parts of human uterus. In: Caldeyro-Barcia R, Heller H (eds) Oxytocin. Pergamon, Oxford

Amados E (1965) Adrenal hemorrhage during anticoagulant therapy. Ann Intern Med 63:559

Ammon R (1963) Das Vorkommen von Dextranase im menschlichen Gewebe. Enzymologia 25: 245

Andersson J, Eklöf B, Neglén P, Thomson D (1979) Metabolic changes in blood and skeletal muscle in reconstructive aortic surgery. Ann Surg 189:283

Andersson L (1964) Anti-fibrinolytic treatment with ε-amino-caproic acid in connection with prostatectomy. Acta Chir Scand 127:552

Andersson L (1965) Combined prophylaxis of haemorrhage and thrombosis after prostatectomy. Acta Chir Scand 130:393

Andersson L, Nilsson IM, Olow B (1962) Fibrinolytic activity in man during surgery. Thromb Diath Haemorrh 7:391

Andersson L-O, Borg H, Miller-Andersson M (1974) Purification of antithrombin III by affinity chromatography. Thromb Res 5:439

Andersson L-O, Barrowcliffe TW, Holmer E, Johnson EA, Sims GEC (1976) Anticoagulant properties of heparin fractionated by affinity chromatography on matrix-bound antithrombin III and by gel filtration. Thromb Res 9:575

Andersson L-O, Barrowcliffe TW, Holmer E, Johnson EA, Söderström G (1979) Molecular weight dependency of the heparin potentiated inhibition of thrombin and activated factor X. Effect of heparin neutralization in plasma. Thromb Res 15:531

Andrassy K, Salzmann W, Saggan W, Storch H, Ritz E (1981) Is more heparin necessary for low-dose heparin prophylaxis in uremic patients? Thromb Haemost 46:740

Andreasen C, Krieger Lassen H (1965) Fatal pulmonary embolism in a surgical department during a period of 15 years. Acta Chir Scand [Suppl] 343:42

Andrews CT, Wilson TS (1973) Vitamin C and thrombotic episodes. Lancet II:39

Angelides NS, Nicolaides AN, Fernandes J, Gordon-Smith I, Bowers R, Lewis JD (1977) Deep venous thrombosis in patients having aorto-iliac reconstruction. Br J Surg 64:517

Ansay J, Fastres R, Kutnowski M, Kraytman M (1977) Prevention des thromboses veineuses profondes post-opératoires par l'héparine sous-cutanée à faible doses. Ann Chir 31:263

Ansell J, Slepchuk N, Kumar R, Lopez A, Southard L, Deykin D (1980) Heparin induced thrombocytopenia: a prospective study. Thromb Haemost 43:61

Antila LE, Markkula H, Iisalo E (1966) Ten years' experience of geriatric aspects in surgery of patients with benign prostatic hyperplasia. Acta Chir Scand [Suppl] 357:95

Arapakis G, Trovas A, Orphanoudakis G, Vassilikos P (1981) Sulfinpyrazone and prevention of postoperative deep venous thrombosis (DVT). Thromb Haemost 46:401

Arbeit J, Lowny S, Line B, Jones D, Brennan M (1981) Deep venous thromboembolism in patients undergoing inguinal lymph node dissection for melanoma. Ann Surg 194:648

Ardlie NG, Kirlough RL, Schwartz CJ (1967) In-vitro thrombosis and platelet behaviour after operation. Australas Ann Med 16:269

Arenander E (1957) Varicosity and ulceration of the lower limb. A clinical follow-up study of 247 patients examined phlebographically. Acta Chir Scand 112:135

Arendrup H, Toftgaard C (1979) Low-dose heparin treatment. An investigation of local reactions with 5000 IU sodium and calcium heparin (In Danish). Ugeskr Laeg 141:1203

Areskog NG, Arturson G, Grotte G, Wallenius G (1964) Studies on heart lymph. Arch Dis Child 39:182

Arfors K-E, Bergqvist D (1975) Microvascular haemostatic plug formation in the rabbit mesentery. Effect of blood flow velocity, thrombocytopenia and dextran treatment. Bibl Haematol 41:84

Arfors K-E, Hint HC, Dhall DP, Matheson NA (1968) Counteraction of platelet activity at sites of laser-induced endothelial trauma. Br Med J 4:430

Arfors K-E, Jonsson J, McKenzie FN (1970) A titanium rabbit ear chamber: assembly, insertion and results. Microvasc Res 2:516

Arfors K-E, Hint HC, McKenzie FN, Matheson NA, Svensjö E (1971) The effect of dextran and heparin on platelet reactivity in vivo. In: Ditzel I, Lewis DH (eds) 6th Eur Conf Microcirc, Aalborg 1970. Karger, Basel, p 348

Arfors K-E, Bergqvist D, Bygdeman S, McKenzie FN, Svensjö E (1972) The effect of inhibition of the platelet release reaction on platelet behaviour in vitro and in vivo. Scand J Hameatol 9:322

Arfors K-E, Bergqvist D, McKenzie FN, Nilsson G (1973) Platelet response to laser-induced microvascular injury in the rabbit mesentery and the rabbit ear chamber. A statistical comparison. Thromb Res 3:75

Arfors K-E, Bergqvist D, Tangen O (1975) The effect of platelet function inhibitors on experimental venous thrombosis formation in rabbits. Acta Chir Scand 141:40

Arfors K-E, Rutili G, Svensjö E (1979) Microvascular transport of macromolecules in normal and inflammatory conditions. Acta Physiol Scand [Suppl] 463:93

Arnadottir M, Konrad P, Bergqvist D, Lindholm T, Husberg B (1982) Venous thromboembolism after renal transplantation. Transplant Proceed 14:79

Arnesen H, Bjerkedal I, Skjaeggestad Ø, Godal HC (1979a) Plasma free-fatty-acids and small doses of subcutaneous heparin in acute myocardial infarction. Thromb Res 14:541

Arnesen H, Kristiansen L, Godal HC (1979b) The local reaction of subcutaneous heparin (In Norwegian). 35:13

Arnesen H, Skjaeggestad Ø, Wik B (1980) Plasma free fatty acids and the incidence of arrhytmias in acute myocardial infarction during treatment with small doses of subcutaneous heparin or warfarin. Acta Med Scand 207:21

Arnoldi C (1976) The effect of elastic compression on the flow velocity of the deep veins in the leg (In Danish). Ugeskr Laeger 138:274

Aronsen K-F, Ekelund G, Kindmark C-O, Laurell C-B (1972) Sequential changes of plasma proteins after surgical trauma. Scand J Clin Lab Invest [Suppl] 124:127

Aronson DL (1976) Comparison of the actions of thrombin and the thrombin-like venom enzymes ancrod and batroxibin. Thromb Haemost 36:9

Arturson G, Wallenius G (1964) The renal clearance of dextran of different molecular sizes in normal humans. Scand J Clin Lab Invest 16:81

Arturson G, Granath K, Thorén L, Wallenius G (1964) The renal excretion of low molecular weight dextran. Acta Chir Scand 127:543

Aschoff L (1912) Thrombose und Sandbankbildung. Beitr Pathol Anat 52:207

Ashford A, Ross J, Southgate P (1968) Pharmacology and toxicology of a defibrinating substance from Malayan pit viper venom. Lancet I:486

Ashford T, Freiman D (1967) The role of the endothelium in the initial phases of thrombosis. Am J Pathol 50:257

Ashida SI, Abiko Y (1978) Inhibition of platelet aggregation by a new agent, Ticlopidine. Thromb Haemost 40:542

Ashida S, Abiko Y (1979) Mode of action of ticlopidine in inhibition of platelet aggregation in the rats. Thromb Haemost 41:436

Ashida SI, Ishihara M, Ogawa H, Abiko Y (1980) Protective effect of Ticlopidine on experimentally induced peripheral arterial occlusive disease in rats. Thromb Res 18:55

Ashton H (1966) Effect of inflatable plastic splints on blood flow. Br Med J 2:1427

Ask-Upmark E (1963) Bedside medicine. Selected topics. Almqvist & Wiksell, Uppsala

Åstedt B (1971) Low fibrinolytic activity of veins during treatment with ethinyloestradiol. Acta Obstet Gynecol Scand 50:279

Åstedt B, Pandolfi M, Nilsson IM (1971) Quantitation of fibrinolytic agents released in tissue culture. Experientia 27:358

Åstedt B, Liedholm P, Wingerup L (1978) The effect of tranexamic acid on the fibrinolytic activity of vein walls. Ann Chir Gynecol 67:203

Åstedt B, Bernstein K, Casslén B, Ulmsten U (1980) Estrogens and postoperative thrombosis evaluated by the radioactive iodine method. Surg Gynecol Obstet 151:372

Astrup T (1966) Tissue activators of plasminogen. Fed Proc 25:42

Astrup T, Glas-Greenwalt P, Dalton BC, Caulfield JB, Munth ED (1971) Localization of fibrinolytic activity at the lining of valves from heart and veins. Am Heart Assoc Meeting, November 1971

Atik M, Broghamer W (1979) The impact of prophylactic measures in fatal pulmonary embolism. Arch Surg 114:366

Atik M, Harkness JW, Wichman H (1970) Prevention of fatal pulmonary embolism. Surg Gynecol Obstet 130:403

Atkins P, Brown IK, Downie RJ, Haggart BG, Littler J, Robb PM, Santer GJ, Jones I (1978) The value of phenformin and ethyloestrenol in the prevention of deep venous thrombosis in patients undergoing surgery. Thromb Haemost 39:89

Awbrey BJ, Hoak JC, Owren WG (1979) Binding of human thrombin to cultured human endothelial cells. J Biol Chem 254:4092

Ayars G, Tikoff G (1980) Incidence of thrombocytopenia in medical patients on "mini-dose" heparin prophylaxis. Am Heart J 99:816

Azam (1864) De la morte subite par embolie pulmonaire dans les contusions et les fractures. Gazette Hebdomad Med Chir 1:611

Babcock RB, Dumper CW, Scharfman WB (1976) Heparin-induced immune thrombocytopenia. N Engl J MEd 295:237

Backer-Gröndahl N (1944) The influence of "early rising" on the postoperative complications. Acta Chir Scand 91:193

Baele G, Verdonck L, Vermeulen A, Barbier F (1975) Duration of the inhibition effect of acetylsalicylic acid on human platelet function. Thromb Diath Haemorrh 34:576

Baenzinger NL, Dillender MJ, Majerus PW (1977) Cultured human fibroblasts and arterial cells produce a labile platelet-inhibitory prostaglandin. Biochem Biophys Res Commun 78:294

Baertschi U, Schaer A, Bader P, Huber L, Morf P (1975) Thromboseprophylaxe nach gynäkologischen Operationen: Eine Vergleichstudie von Low-Dose-Heparin und oralen Antikoagulantien. Geburtshilfe Frauenheilkd 35:754

Bagge L, Saldeen T (1978) The primary fibrinolysis inhibitor and trauma. Thromb Res 13:1131

Bagge L, Carlin G, Hjelmstedt Å, Högstorp H, Jacobsson H, Modig J, Saldeen T (1979) Fibrinolysis inhibition after a standardized trauma, total hip replacement surgery. Thromb Haemost 42:278

Bailey G, Strub RL, Klein RC, Salvaggio J (1967) Dextran-induced anaphylaxis. JAMA 200:889

Baker LW, Houlder A (1973) Deep vein thrombosis in Bantu and Indian patients. S Afr Med J 47: 1689

Baker LW, Prajapat DK (1976) Deep vein thrombosis in African and Indian patients. S Afr J Surg 12:127

Ballard RM, Bradley-Watson PJ, Johnstone FD, Kenney A, McCarthy TG, Campbell S, Weston J (1973) Low doses of subcutaneous heparin in the prevention of deep vein thrombosis after gynaecological surgery. J Obstet Gynaecol Br Commonw 80:469

Bangham DR, Woodward P (1970) A collaborative study of heparins from different sources. Bull World Health Org 42:120

Barber HM, Feil EJ, Galasko CSB, Edwards DH, Sutton RA, Haynes DW, Bentley GA (1977) A comparative study of dextran-70, warfarin and low-dose heparin for the prophylaxis of thromboembolism following total hip replacement. Postgrad Med J 53:130

Barker NW, Nygaard KK, Walters W, Priestley JT (1941) A statistical study of postoperative venous thrombosis and pulmonary embolism. III. Time of occurrence during the postoperative period. Proc Staff Meet Mayo Clin 16:17

Barlow GH, Holleman WH, Lorand L (1970) The action of arvin on fibrin stabilizing factor (Factor XIII). Res Commun Chem Pathol Pharmacol 1:39

Barner HB, Willman VL, Kaiser GC, Hanlon CR (1969) Thrombectomy for iliofemoral venous thrombosis. JAMA 208:2442

Barnes R, Slaymaker E (1976) Postoperative deep vein thrombosis in the lower extremity amputee: a prospective study with Doppler ultrasound. Ann Surg 183:429

Barnes R, Brand R, Clarke W, Hartley N, Hoak J (1978) Efficacy of graded-compression anti-embolism stockings in patients undergoing total hip arthroplasty. Clin Orthop Rel Res 132:61

Barnett H, Clifford J, Llewellyn R (1977) Safety of mini-dose heparin administration for neurosurgical patients. J Neurosurg 47:27

Barnhardt MI, Chen ST (1978) Vessel wall models for studying interaction capabilities with blood platelets. Semin Thromb Haemost 5:112

Barnhardt MI, Quintana C (1967) Platelet alterations with dextran. Blood 30:541

Barr M, Burdi AR (1976) Warfarin-associated embryopathy in a 17 week old abortus. Teratology 14:129

Barrie W, Wood EH, Crumlish P, Forbes CD, Prentice CRM (1974) Low-dosage ancrod for prevention of thrombotic complications after surgery for fractured neck of femur. Br Med J 4:130

Barritt DW, Jordan SC (1960) Anticoagulant drugs in treatment of pulmonary embolism: controlled trial. Lancet I:1309

Barrowcliffe TW (1978) Antithrombin III and heparin. Br Med Bull 34:143

Barrowcliffe TW, Johnson EA, Eggleton CA, Thomas DP (1977) Anticoagulant activities of lung and mucous heparins. Thromb Res 12:27

Barthel W, Markwardt F (1974) Aggregation of blood platelets by biogenic amines and its inhibition by antiadrenergic and antiserotoninergic agents. Biochem Pharmacol 23:37

Bauer GA (1942) A roentgenological and clinical study of the sequels of thrombosis. Acta Chir Scand [Suppl] 74
Bauer G (1944) Thrombosis following leg injuries. Acta Chir Scand 90:229
Bauer G, Boström H, Jorpes E, Kallner S (1950) Intramuscular administration of heparin. Acta Med Scand 136:188
Bauer Å, Östling G (1970) Dextran-induced anaphylactoid reactions in connection with surgery. Acta Anaesth Scand [Suppl] 37:182
Baumgartner H (1979) Effects of acetylsalicylic acid, sulfinpyrazone and dipyridamole on platelet adhesion and aggregation in flowing native and anticoagulated blood. Haemostasis 8:340
Baumgartner HR, Haudenschild C (1972) Adhesion of platelets to subendothelium. Ann NY Acad Sci 201:22
Bechthol CO, Crickenberger DP, O'Rourke FM (1976) Pneumatic venous pump and thromboembolism in total hip replacement surgery: a retrospective study. In: Madden J, Hume M (eds) Venous thromboembolism. Prevention and treatment. Appleton-Century-Crofts, New York
Becker HM (1965) Die Lungenembolie. Münch Med Wochenschr 107:66
Becker J (1972a) Fibrinolytic activity of the blood and its relation to postoperative venous thrombosis of the lower limbs. A clinical study. Acta Chir Scand 138:787
Becker J (1972b) Postoperative venous thrombosis. A clinical and experimental study with special reference to early diagnosis, prophylaxis, course and some haematological findings. Acta Chir Scand [Suppl] 431
Becker J (1972c) The relation of platelet adhesiveness to postoperative venous thrombosis in the legs. Acta Chir Scand 138:781
Becker J, Borgström S (1968) Incidence of thrombosis associated with epsilonaminocaproic acid administration and with combined epsilonaminocaproic acid and subcutaneous heparin therapy. Acta Chir Scand 134:343
Becker J, Schampi B (1973) The incidence of postoperative venous thrombosis of the legs. A comparative study on the prophylactic effect of dextran 70 and electrical calf-muscle stimulation. Acta Chir Scand 139:357
Becker J, Borgström S, Saltzman C-F (1970) Incidence of thrombosis associated with epsilon-aminocaproic acid administration and with combined epsilon-aminocaproic acid and subcutaneous heparin therapy. II. A clinical study with the aid of intravenous phlebography. Acta Chir Scand 136:167
Becker M, Genieser N, Finegold M, Miranda D, Sparkman T (1975) Chondrodysplasia punctata. Is maternal warfarin therapy a factor? Am J Dis Child 129:356
Beermann B, Lahnborg G (1979) Pharmacokinetics of heparin administered with and without dihydroergotamine. Thromb Haemostas 42:380
Beermann B, Lahnborg G (1981) Pharmakokinetics of heparin in healthy and obese subjects and in combination with dihydroergotamine. Thromb Haemost 45:24
Behrens M, Taubert M (1952) Der Nachweis von Heparin in den basophilen Leukocyten. Klin Wochenschr 30:76
Belch JJF, Lowe GDO, Pollock JG, Forbes CD, Prentice CRM (1979) Subcutaneous heparin in the prevention of venous thrombosis after selective aortic bifurcation graft surgery. Thromb Haemost 42:303
Belch JJF, Meek D, Lowe GDO, Drummond MM, Campbell AF, Forbes CD, Prentice CRM (1981) An assessment of subcutaneous ancrod in prevention of deep vein thrombosis after surgery for hip replacement. Thromb Haemost 46:93
Bell W (1971) Current status of therapy with arvin. Thromb Diath Haemorrh [Suppl] 47:371
Bell W (1974) Defibrinogenation with arvin in thrombotic disorders. In: Sherry S, Scriabine A (eds) Platelets and thrombosis. Urban & Schwartzenberg, Munic Berlin Vienna
Bell W (1976) Thrombocytopenia occurring during heparin therapy. N Engl J Med 295:276
Bell W, Royall R (1980) Heparin-associated thrombocytopenia: a comparison of three heparin preparations. N Engl J Med 303:902
Bell W, Zuidema G (1979) Low-dose heparin — concern and perspectives. Surgery 85:469
Bell W, Bolton G, Pitney WR (1968a) The effect of arvin on blood coagulation factors. Br J Haematol 15:589

Bell W, Pitney WR, Goodwin JF (1968b) Therapeutic defibrination in the treatment of thrombotic disease. Lancet I:490

Bell W, Tamasulo P, Alving B, Duffy T (1976) Thrombocytopenia occurring during the administration of heparin. A prospective study in 52 patients. Ann Intern Med 85:155

Bell W, Shapiro S, Martinez J, Nossel H (1978) The effects of ancrod, the coagulating enzyme from the venom of Malayan pit viper (A. rhodostoma) on prothrombin and fibrinogen metabolism and fibrinopeptide. A release in man. J Lab Clin Med 91:592

Bender F, Aronson L, Hougle C, Moser K (1980) Bioequivalence of subcutaneous calcium and sodium heparins. Clin Pharmacol Ther 27:224

Bennett A, Houghton J, Leaper DJ (1979) Cancer growth, response to treatment and survival time in mice: beneficial effect of the prostaglandin synthesis inhibitor flurbiprofen. Prostaglandins 17:179

Bennett PN (1967) Postoperative changes in platelet adhesiveness. J Clin Pathol 20:708

Bennett PN, Dhall DP, McKenzie FN, Matheson NA (1966) Effects of dextran infusion on the adhesiveness of human blood-platelets. Lancet II:1001

Benson EA (1970) Prevention of fatal postoperative thromboembolism by heparin prophylaxis. Lancet II:1135

Berde B, Stürmer E (1978) Introduction to the pharmacology of ergot alkaloids and related compounds as a basis of their therapeutic application. In: Berde B, Schild HO (eds) Ergot alkaloids and related compounds. Springer, Berlin Heidelberg New York

Berge T, Bergqvist D, Efsing HO, Hallböök T (1978) Local complications to ascending phlebography. Clin Radiol 29:691

Berge T, Bergqvist F, Efsing HO, Hallböök T, Lindblad B, Lindhagen A (1981) Complications of phlebography: A randomized comparison between an ionic and a non-ionic contrast medium. Clin Radiol 32:595

Bergentz S-E (1978) Dextran in the prophylaxis of pulmonary embolism. World J Surg 2:19

Bergentz S-E, Nilsson IM (1961) Effect of trauma on coagulation and fibrinolysis in dogs. Acta Chir Scand 122:21

Bergentz S-E, Eiken O, Nilsson IM (1961) The effect of dextran of various molecular weight on the coagulation in dogs. Thromb Diath Haemorrh 6:15

Bergentz S-E, Gelin L-E, Rudenstam C-M, Zederfeldt B (1963) The viscosity of whole blood in trauma. Acta Chir Scand 126:289

Bergman B, Bergqvist D, Dahlgren S (1975) The incidence of venous thrombosis in the lower limbs following elective gall-bladder surgery. A study with the ^{125}I-fibrinogen test. Ups J Med Sci 80:41

Bergquist E, Bergqvist D, Bronge A, Dahlgren S, Lindquist B (1972) An evaluation of early thrombosis prophylaxis following fracture of the femoral neck. A comparison between dextran and dicoumarol. Acta Chir Scand 138:689

Bergquist E, Bergqvist D, Bronge A, Dahlgren S, Hallböök T (1973) Diagnosis of venous thrombosis in the lower limbs. A comparative study between ^{125}I-fibrinogen test, strain gauge plethysmography and phlebography. Ups J Med Sci 78:191

Bergqvist A, Bergqvist D, Hallböök T (1979) Acute deep vein thrombosis (DVT) after Caesarean section. Acta Obstet Gyneacol Scand 58:473

Bergqvist A, Bergqvist D, Hallböök T (1983) Diagnosis and treatment of patients with deep vein thrombosis during pregnancy. Acta Obstet Gynecol Scand

Bergqvist A, Bergqvist D, Tangen O (to be published b) The influence of oral contraceptives on XaI-activity. A prospective study

Bergqvist A, Bergqvist D, Hedner U (1982a) Oral contraceptives and venous thromboembolism. Brit J Obstet Gynecol 89:381

Bergqvist A, Bergqvist D, Hedner U (1982) Clinical manifestations of thrombosis during pregnancy (In Swedish). Läkartidningen 79:901

Bergqvist B (1938) Über die Häufigkeit der Thromboembolie nach Bruchoperationen. Acta Chir Scand 81:555

Bergqvist D (1977) Critical evaluation of some methods used in the diagnosis of deep vein thrombosis. In: Lewis D (ed) Dextran – 30 years. Uppsala

Bergqvist D (1978) Venous thrombosis and embolism. Prophylaxis with dextran (In Swedish). In: Thoren L (ed) Anticoagulants and coagulants. Symposium. The Swedish Health Authorities Committee on Drug Information, No 3, p 67

Bergqvist D (1979) Prophylaxis of postoperative thromboembolic complications with low-dose heparin. An analysis of different administration intervals. Acta Chir Scand 145:7

Bergqvist D (1980a) Investigations and treatment of patients with haemorrhagic diatheses (In Swedish). Läkartidningen 77:3639

Bergqvist D (1980b) Prophylaxis against postoperative venous thrombosis — a survey of the practice in Sweden (In Swedish). Läkartidningen 77:3251

Bergqvist D (1980c) Prevention of postoperative deep vein thrombosis in Sweden. Results of a survey. World J Surg 4:489

Bergqvist D, Arfors K-E (1974) Influence of fibrinolysis and coagulation on haemostatic plug formation. An experimental study in rabbits. Thromb Res 4:345

Bergqvist D, Arfors K-E (1980) Haemostatic platelet plug formation in the isolated rabbit mesenteric preparation — an analysis of red blood cell participation. Thromb Haemost 44:6

Bergqvist D, Dahlgren S (1973) Leg vein thrombosis diagnosed by ^{125}I-fibrinogen test in patients with fracture of the hip: a study of the effect of early prophylaxis with dicoumarol or dextran 70. Vasa 2:121

Bergqvist D, Hallböök T (1978a) The frequency and significance of postoperative plantar vein thrombosis judged by the ^{125}I-fibrinogen test. Acta Chir Scand 144:343

Bergqvist D, Hallböök T (1978b) The use of thermography in screening postoperative deep vein thrombosis (DVT); a comparison with the ^{125}I-fibrinogen test. Br J Surg 65:993

Bergqvist D, Hallböök T (1978c) A comparison between subcutaneous low-dose sodium and calcium heparin. Prophylaxis of postoperative deep vein thrombosis and side effects of treatment. Acta Chir Scand 144:339

Bergqvist D, Hallböök T (1979a) Biphasic venous emptying from the calves in venous occlusion plethysmography. Scand J Clin Lab Invest 39:271

Bergqvist D, Hallböök T (1979b) Venous function after thigh vein thrombosis diagnosed by the ^{125}I-fibrinogen test — a study with occlusion plethysmography. J Cardiovasc Surg 20:561

Bergqvist D, Hallböök T (1980) Prophylaxis of postoperative venous thrombosis in a controlled trial comparing dextran 70 and low-dose heparin. A study with the ^{125}I-fibrinogen test. World J Surg 4:239

Bergqvist D, Hedner U (1983) Pregnancy and venous thromboembolism. Acta Obstet Gynecol Scand

Bergqvist D, Ljungnér H (1981) A comparative study of dextran 70 and a sulphated poly-saccharide in the prevention of postoperative thromboembolic complications in patients undergoing abdominal surgery. Br J Surg 68:449

Bergqvist D, Nilsson IM (1981) A sulphated polysaccharide — the effects in vivo and in vitro on the haemostatic system in healthy volunteers. Thromb Res 23:309

Bergqvist D, Ousbäck L (1982) Prophylaxis or routine screening of postoperative thromboembolism. An economic analysis (In Swedish). Läkartidningen 79:3302

Bergqvist D, Elvelin R, Eriksson U, Hjelmstedt A (1976a) Thrombosis following hip arthroplasty. A study using phlebography and ^{125}I-fibrinogen test. Acta Orthop Scand 47:549

Bergqvist D, Hallböök T, Hessman Y (1976b) Anticoagulation and retroperitoneal haematoma. Vasa 5:329

Bergqvist D, Hallböök T, Lindblad B, Lindhagen A (1981) A double-blind trial of O-(β-hydroxy-etyl)-rutoside in patients with chronic venous insufficiency. Vasa 10:253

Bergqvist D, Hedelin H, Karlsson G, Lindblad B, Lindhagen A, Mätzsch T (to be published) Abdominal trauma in elderly persons. Acta Chir Scand

Bergqvist D, Ljungnér H, Nilsson M (to be published) Venous emptying from the calves. A methodological report and the effect of intermittent pneumatic compression. Acta Chir Scand

Bergqvist D, Svensjö E, Arfors K-E (1978) The effect of O-(beta-hydroxyethyl)-rutoside (HR) on macromolecular leakage, thrombosis and haemostasis in experimental animals. Ups J Med Sci 83:123

Bergqvist D, Efsing HO, Hallböök T, Hedlund T (1979) Thromboembolism after elective and post-traumatic hip surgery — a controlled prophylactic trial with dextran and low-dose heparin. Acta Chir Scand 145:213

Bergqvist D, Efsing HO, Hallböök T, Lindhagen A (1980a) Analysis of preoperative and postoperative lung scintigraphy in patients undergoing elective hip surgery. Vasa 9:311

Bergqvist D, Efsing HO, Hallböök T, Lindblad B (1980b) Prevention of postoperative thromboembolic complications. A prospective comparison between dextran 70, dihydroergotamine heparin and a sulfated polysaccharide. Acta Chir Scand 146:559

Bergqvist D, Hedelin H, Lindblad B (1980c) Penetrating abdominal trauma. A comparison of the development during 30 years between a rural and an urban area. Acta Chir Scand 146:417

Bergqvist G (1940) Über postoperative Thrombose. Vorläufige Mitteilung. Acta Chir Scand 83:415

Bergström K, Lahnborg G (1975) The effect of major surgery, low doses of heparin and thromboembolism on plasma anti-thrombin — comparison of immediate thrombin inhibiting capacity and the antithrombin III content. Thromb Res 6:223

Bergvall U, Hjelmstedt Å (1968) Recanalisation of deep venous thrombosis of the lower leg and thigh. A phlebographic study of fracture cases. Acta Chir Scand 134:219

Berliner AD, Lackner H (1972) Haemorrhagic diathesis after prolonged infusion of low molecular weight dextran. Am J Med Sci 263:397

Bernhard M, Gruber UF (1976) Wert der elektrischen Wadenstimulation zur Verhütung postoperativer tiefer Venenthrombosen in der allgemeinen Chirurgie. Med Welt 27:1255

Bernstein EF, Emmings DDS, Evans RL, Blum JA, Avant RF (1963) Effect of low molecular weight dextran on RBC charge during clinical extracorporeal circulation. Circulation 27:816

Bernstein IL (1956) Anaphylaxis to heparin. JAMA 161:1379

Bernstein K, Lindell S-E, Mattsson S, Ulmsten U, Åstedt B (1979) Comparison between thermography and ^{125}I-fibrinogen test for screening of post-operative thrombosis after gynaecologic surgery. Acta Thermograph 4:108

Bernstein K, Ulmsten U, Åstedt B, Jacobsson L, Mattsson S (1980) The incidence of thrombosis after gynecological surgery as evaluated by an improved ^{125}I-fibrinogen uptake test. Angiology 31:606

Bertelsen S (1971) New aspects in pulmonary embolism. Acta Chir Scand 137:415

Best LC, McGuire NB, Jones PBR, Holland TK, Martin TJ, Preston FE, Segal DS, Russel RGC (1979) Mode of action of dipyridamole on human platelets. Thromb Res 16:367

Bicher HI (1970) Anti-thrombotic effect of a heparin-like substance (SP54) preventing red cell and platelet aggregation. Arzneim-Forsch 20:379

Bick RL, Adams T, Schmalhorst WR (1976) Bleeding times, platelet adhesion, and aspirin. Am J Clin Pathol 65:69

Bieger R, Boekhout-Mussert R, Hohmann F, Loeliger E (1976) Is streptokinase useful in the treatment of deep vein thrombosis? Acta Med Scand 199:81

Biggs R, Denson KWE, Akman N, Borret R, Hadden M (1970) Antithrombin III, antifactor Xa and heparin. Br J Haematol 19:283

Bingham J, Meyer O, Pohle F (1941) Studies on the haemorrhage agent 3,3'-methylenebis (4-hydroxycoumarin) I. Its effect on the prothrombin and coagulation time of the blood of dogs and humans. Am J Med Sci 202:563

Bird AD (1972) The effect of surgery, injury, and prolonged bed rest on calf blood flow. Aust NZ J Surg 41:374

Bizzozero J (1882) Über einen neuen Formbestandteil des Blutes und dessen Rolle bei der Thrombose und der Blutgerinnung. Virch Arch Pathol Anat 90:261

Björk I, Nordenman B (1976) Acceleration of the reaction between thrombin and antithrombin III by non-stoichiometric amounts of heparin. Eur J Biochem 68:507

Björkenheim EA (1909) Early mobilization after laparotomy (In Swedish). 8th Meeting of Nordic Surgical Society 1909. Nord Kir Fören 8:e möte

Black J, Nagle CJ, Strachan CJL (1978) Prophylactic low-dose heparin by jet injection. Br Med J 2:95

Blaisdell FW (1978) Prevention of deep vein thrombosis. Surgery 83:243

Blaisdell FW (1979) Low-dose heparin prophylaxis of venous thrombosis. An editorial. Am Heart J 97:685

Bloom AL, Giddings JC, Wilks CJ (1973) Factor VIII on the vascular intima: possible importance in haemostasis and thrombosis. Nature 241:217

Bloom WL, Brewer S (1968) The independent yet synergistic effects of heparin and dextran. Acta Chir Scand [Suppl] 387:53

Bloom WL, Harmer D, Bryant M, Brewer S (1964) Coating of vascular surfaces and cells. A new concept in prevention of intravascular thrombosis. Proc Soc Exp Biol Med 115:384

Bloomfield D (1970) Fetal deaths and malformations associated with the use of coumarin derivatives in pregnancy. A critical review. Am J Obstet Gynecol 107:884

Bockslaff H, Barthels M, Stolle E, Trentz O, Wuppermann T, Zech G (1974) Frühdiagnose von Beinvenenthrombosen mit dem Radiofibrinogentest bei Patienten mit alloplastischem Hüftgelenkersatz. Muench Med Wochenschr 116:1397

Bohmansson G (1943) Discussion on the incidence of thromboembolism in the department of surgery 1932–1941 (M. Felländer) (In Swedish). Nord Med 17:182

Bohmansson G (1947) Dextran as substitute for plasma. North Med Assoc 23:129

Bohmansson G, Rosenqvist H, Thorsén G, Wilander O (1946) Clinical experiences with dextran as a plasma substitute. Acta Chir Scand 94:149

Bolton J (1978) The prevention of post-operative deep venous thrombosis by graduated compression stockings. Scot Med J 23:333

Bolton JP, Hoffman VJ (1975) Incidence of early post-operative iliofemoral thrombosis. Br Med J 1:247

Bong SC, Chow SP (1977) Mortality in fractures of the proximal end of femur in Hong Kong Chinese. J West Pacific Orthop Assoc 14:41

Bonnar J (1975) Thromboembolism in obstetric and gynaecological patients. In: Nicolaides AN (ed) Thromboembolism. Aetiology, advances in prevention and management. MTP, Lancaster

Bonnar J (1979) Venous thromboembolism and pregnancy. In: Stallworthy J, Bonone G (eds) Recent advances in obstetrics and gynaecology. No. 13. Churchill Livingstone, Edinburgh London New York

Bonnar J, Ma PTS (1979) Plasma heparin levels and patient acceptability with subcutaneous heparin sodium and heparin calcium. Thromb Haemostas 42:307

Bonnar J, Walsh J (1972) Prevention of thrombosis after pelvic surgery by British dextran 70. Lancet I:614

Borchgrevink CF (1960) A method for measuring platelet adhesiveness in vivo. Acta Med Scand 168:157

Borgström S (1950) Investigation of the effect of dicumarol and early ambulation in the prevention of postoperative thrombo-embolism in a surgical material strongly disposed to thrombosis. Acta Chir Scand [Suppl] 150

Borgström S, Gelin L-E, Zederfeldt B (1959) The formation of vein thrombi following tissue injury. Acta Chir Scand [Suppl] 247

Borgström S, Greitz T, van der Linden W, Molin J, Rudics I (1965) Anticoagulant prophylaxis of venous thrombosis in patients with fractured neck of the femur. A controlled clinical trial using venous phlebography. Acta Chir Scand 129:500

Born GVR (1962) Aggregation of blood platelets by adenosine diphosphate and its reversal. Nature 194:927

Botti RE, Ratnoff OD (1964) Studies on the pathogenesis of thrombosis: an experimental "hyper coagulable" state induced by the intravenous injection of ellagic acid. J Lab Clin Med 64:385

Böttiger LE, Westerholm B (1971) Oral contraceptives and thromboembolic disease. Acta Med Scand 190:455

Böttiger LE, Boman G, Eklund G, Westerholm B (1980) Oral contraceptives and thromboembolic disease: effect of lowering oestrogen content. Lancet I:1097

Bowald S (1979) Changes in haemodynamics and blood gases during abdominal aortic clamping and declamping. Acta Univ Ups Abstr Ups Diss Fac Med 331

Bowell RE, Marmion VJ, McCarthy CF (1970) Treatment of central retinal vein thrombosis with ancrod. Lancet I:173

Brach B, Moser K, Cedar L, Minteer M, Convery R (1977) Venous thrombosis in acute spinal cord paralysis. J Trauma 17:289

Brais M, Bertranou E, Brassard A, Stanley P, Chartrand C (1973) Effect of dextran on patency of pericardial tubular graft of the superior vena cava in the dog. J Thorac Cardiovasc Surg 65: 296

Brambel CE, Hunter RE (1950) Effect of dicumarol on the nursing infant. Am J Obstet Gynecol 59:1153

Breneman J (1963) A formula for predicting and a device for preventing postoperative thromboembolic disease. Angiology 14:437

Breneman J (1965) Postoperative thromboembolic disease. Computer analysis leading to statistical prediction. JAMA 193:576

Briel RC, Wagner U, Weselek R, Kunz S (1979) Heparin levels using the chromogenic substrate S-2222 during low dose heparin and low dose heparin-dihydroergotamine prophylaxis after gynaecological surgery. Thromb Haemost 42:380

Brinkhous K, Smith HP, Warner ED, Seegers WH (1939) The inhibition of blood clotting. An unidentified substance which acts in conjunction with heparin to prevent the conversion of prothrombin into thrombin. Am J Physiol 125:683

Brisman R, Parks LC, Haller JA (1968) Anaphylactoid reactions associated with the clinical use of dextran 70. JAMA 204:824

Brisman R, Parks L, Haller A (1971) Dextran prophylaxis in surgery. Ann Surg 174:137

Brommer EJP (1981) The effect of ticlopidine upon platelet function, haemorrhage and post-operative thrombosis in patients undergoing suprapubic prostatectomy. J Int Med Res 9:203

Bronge A, Dahlgren S, Lindquist B (1971) Prophylaxis against thrombosis in femoral neck fractures − a comparison between dextran 70 and dicumarol. Acta Chir Scand 137:29

Bronwell A, Artz C, Sako Y (1954) Evaluation of blood loss from a standardized wound after dextran. Surg Forum 5:809

Brown IK, Downie RJ, Haggart B, Littler J, Murray GH, Robb PM, Sauter GJ (1971) Pharmacological stimulation of fibrinolytic activity in the surgical patient. Lancet I:774

Brown R, Kinateder R, Rosenberg N (1980) Ipsilateral thrombophlebitis and pulmonary embolism after Cooper's ligament herniorrhaphy. Surgery 87:230

Browse NL (1962) Effect of bedrest on resting calf blood flow of healthy adult males. Br Med J 1:1721

Browse NL (1972) The ^{125}I-fibrinogen uptake test. Arch Surg 104:160

Browse NL (1978) The prevention of venous thromboembolism by mechanical methods. In: Bergan J, Yao J (eds) Venous problems. Year Book Medical Publ Chicago, London

Browse NL, Clemenson A (1974) Sequalae of an ^{125}I-fibrinogen detected thrombus. Br Med J 2:468

Browse NL, Hall JH (1969) Effect of dipyridamole on the incidence of clinically detectable deep-vein thrombosis. Lancet II:718

Browse NL, Lea Thomas M (1974) Source of non-lethal pulmonary emboli. Lancet I:258

Browse NL, Negus D (1970) Prevention of postoperative leg vein thrombosis by electrical muscle stimulation. An evaluation with ^{125}I-labelled fibrinogen. Br Med J 3:615

Browse NL, Clemenson G, Croft DN (1974a) Fibrinogen-detectable thrombosis in the legs and pulmonary embolism. Br Med J 1:603

Browse NL, Jackson BT, Mayo ME, Negus D (1974b) The value of mechanical methods of preventing postoperative calf vein thrombosis. Br J Surg 61:219

Browse NL, Clemenson G, Bateman NT, Gaunt JI, Croft DN (1976) Effect of intravenous dextran 70 and pneumatic leg compression on incidence of postoperative pulmonary embolism. Br Med J 2:1281

Browse NL, Gray L, Marland M (1977) Changes in blood fibrinolytic activity after surgery: effect of deep vein thrombosis and malignant disease. Br J Surg 64:23

Browse NL, Clemenson G, Lea Thomas M (1980) Is the postphlebitic leg always postphlebitic? Relation between phlebographic appearances of deep-vein thrombosis and late sequelae. Br Med J 2:1168

Brozovic M, Howarth DJ (1975) Factor VII in patients on oral anticoagulants. In: Hemker HC, Veltkamp JJ (eds) Prothrombin and related coagulation factors. Leiden University Press, Leiden

Brozovic M, Sterling Y, Klenerman L, Lowe, L (1973) Subcutaneous heparin and postoperative thromboembolism. Lancet II:99

Brozovic M, Sterling Y, Abbosh J (1975) Plasma heparin levels after low dose subcutaneous heparin in patients undergoing hip replacement. Br J Haematol 31:461

Brunner U (1977) Die sogenannte "Pillen-Thrombose" in chirurgischer Sicht. In: Ehringer H (ed) Akute tiefe Becken- und Beinvenenthrombosen. Hans Huber, Bern Stuttgart Vienna

Brush B, Wylie J, Block M, Beninson J, Spitzer J (1959) A device for the prevention of phlebothrombosis and pulmonary embolism. Henry Ford Hosp Med J 7:27

Bruzelius S (1945) Dicoumarin in clinical use. Studies on its prophylactic and therapeutic value in the treatment of thromboembolism. Acta Chir Scand [Suppl] 100

Bryant M, Lazenby WD, Howard JM (1958) Experimental replacement of short segments of vein. Arch Surg 76:289

Bryant M, Bloom W, Brewer S (1961) Use of dextran in preventing thrombosis of small arteries following surgical trauma. J Med Assoc Georgia 50:580

Bryant M, Bloom WL, Brewer SS (1966) Use of dextran in thrombophlebitis. Experimental and clinical studies. Am Surg 32:13

Buchanan MP, Rosenfeld J, Hirsch J (1978) The prolonged effect of sulphinpyrazone on collagen-induced platelet aggregation in vivo. Thromb Res 13:883

Buchanan MR, Rosenfeld J, Gent M, Lawrence W, Hirsh J (1979) Increased dipyridamole plasma concentrations associated with salicylate administration. Relationship to effects on platelet aggregation in vivo. Thromb Res 15:813

Bunting S, Moncada S (1980) Prostacyclin by preventing platelet activation prolongs activated clotting time in blood and platelet rich plasma and potentiates the anticoagulant effect of heparin. Br J Pharmacol 69:268P

Buonassisi V (1973) Sulfated mucopolysaccharide synthesis and secretion in endothelial cell cultures. Exp Cell Res 76:363

Burch JW, Baenzinger NL, Stanford N, Majerus PW (1978) Sensitivity of fatty acid cyclooxygenase from human aorta to acetylation by aspirin. Proc Nat Acad Sci USA 75:5181

Burdette WJ, Gehan EA (1970) Planning and analysis of clinical studies. Thomas, Springfield, Ill

Burns JJ, Yu TF, Dayton P, Berger L, Gutman A, Brodie D (1958) Relationship between pKa and uricosuric activity in phenylbutazone analogues. Nature 182:1162

Burrowes CE, Habal FM, Movat HS (1975) The inhibition of human plasma kallikrein by antithrombin III. Thromb Res 7:175

Butler MJ, Britton BJ, Smith M, Hawkey C, Irving MH (1975) Coagulation and fibrinolytic response during operative surgery. Br J Surg 62:666

Butler MJ, Matthews F, Irving MH (1977) The incidence of post-operative deep vein thrombosis after splenectomy. Clin Oncol 3:51

Butson R (1981) Intermittent pneumatic calf compression for prevention of deep venous thrombosis in general abdominal surgery. Am J Surg 142:525

Butt HR, Allen EV, Bollman JL (1941) A preparation from spoiled sweet clover [3,3'-methylene-bis-(4-hydroxycoumarin)] which prolongs coagulation and prothrombin time of the blood. Preliminary report of experimental and clinical studies. Proc Staff Mayo Clin 16:388

Buttermann G (1977) Beeinflussung des postoperativen Thromboserisikos durch Heparin und Heparin-Dihydergot. In: Pabst HW, Maurer G (eds) Postoperative Thromboembolieprophylaxe. Schattauer, Stuttgart New York

Buttermann G, Haluszcynski I, Theisinger W, Pabst HW (1981) Postoperative Thromboembolieprophylaxe mit reduziertem low-dose-Heparin-Anteil und Dihydroergotamin in fixer Kombination. Muench Med Wochenschr 123:1213

Buttermann G, Theisinger W, Oechsler H, Hör G (1975) Untersuchungen über die postoperative Thromboembolieprophylaxe nach einem neuen medikamentösen Behandlungsprinzip. Dtsch Med Wochenschr 100:2065

Buttermann G, Theisinger W, Weidenbach A, Hartung H, Welzel D, Pabst HW (1977) Quantitative Bewertung der postoperativen Thromboembolieprophylaxe. Vergleichende Untersuchungen über Thrombose- und Emboliehäufigkeiten unter Acetylsalicylsäure, Dextran, Dihydroergotamin, Heparin sowie der fixen Kombination von Heparin und Dihydroergotamine. Med Klin 72:1624

Byar D, Simon R, Friedewald W, Schlesselman J, DeMets D, Ellenberg J, Gail M, Ware J (1976) Randomized clinical trials. Perspectives on some recent ideas. N Engl J Med 295:74

Bygdeman S, Eliasson R (1966) Effect of dextrans in vitro on the adenosine diphosphate induced adhesiveness of human blood platelets. Thromb Diath Haemorrh 15:436

Bygdeman S, Eliasson R (1967) Effect of dextrans on platelet adhesiveness and aggregation. Scand J Clin Lab Invest 20:17

Bygdeman S, Tangen O (1973) Studies on the antithrombotic effect of dextran. Effect on platelet 5-hydroxytryptamine and adenosine nucleotides. Bibl Anat 12:333

Bygdeman S, Eliasson R, Gullbring B (1966) Effect of dextran infusion on the adenosine diphosphate induced adhesiveness and the spreading capacity of human blood platelets. Thromb Diath Haemorrh 15:451

Bygdeman S, Svensjö E, Tollerz G (1970) Prevention of venous thrombosis. Lancet II:419

Byrne JJ, O'Neil EE (1952) Fatal pulmonary emboli: study of 130 autopsy-proven fatal emboli. Am J Surg 83:47

Cade JF (1977) Comparison of sodium and calcium heparin in prophylaxis of venous thromboembolism. Thromb Haemost 38:110

Cade JF, Hunt D, Stubbs KP, Gallus AS (1979) Guidelines for the management of oral anticoagulant therapy in patients undergoing surgery. Med J Aust 2:292

Calnan J (1972) A new method for the assessment of tissue fluid concentrations of flavonoids. Angiologica 9:181

Calnan JS, Allenby F (1975) The prevention of deep vein thrombosis after surgery. Br J Anaesth 47:151

Calnan JS, Pflug JJ, Mills CJ (1970) Pneumatic intermittent compression legging simulating calf-muscle pump. Lancet II:502

Campion EC, Hoffman DC, Jepson RP (1968) The effects of external pneumatic splint pressure on muscle blood flow. Aust NZ J Surg 38:154

The Canadian Cooperative Study Group (1978) A randomized trial of aspirin and sulfinpyrazone in threatened stroke. N Engl J Med 299:53

Carbone JV, Furth FW, Scott R, Crosby WH (1954) A haemostatic defect associated with dextran infusion. Proc Soc Exp Biol Med 85:101

Carlin G (1980) Effect of dextran on fibrinolysis. Acta Univ Ups Abstr Ups Diss Fac Med 365

Carlin G, Saldeen T (1978) Effect of dextran on fibrinolysis inhibition activity in serum. Thromb Res 12:1165

Carlin G, Arfors K-E, Saldeen T, Tangen O (1976a) On the formation and lysis of fibrin. The effect of dextran. Forensic Sci 7:87

Carlin G, Wik KO, Arfors K-E, Saldeen T, Tangen O (1976b) Influences on the formation and structure of fibrin. Thromb Res 9:623

Carlin G, Modig J, Saldeen T (1979) Effect of infusion of dextran 70 on fibrinolysis inhibition activity in human serum. Acta Chir Scand 145:129

Carlin G, Karlström G, Modig J, Saldeen T (1980) Effect of dextran on fibrinolysis inhibition activity in the blood after major surgery. Acta Anaesth Scand 24:375

Carlsson C, Gustafsson I, Nilsson E, Nordström L, Persson P-O, Söderberg M (1972) Anaphylactoid reaction towards dextran (In Swedish). Läkartidningen 69:3690

Carlsson S, Åstedt B (1974) Oestrogenic treatment of prostatic cancer lowers the fibrinolytic activity in vein walls. Scand J Urol Nephrol 8:169

Carmichael D, Edwards S (1967) Prophylactic inferior vena caval plication. Surg Gynecol Obstet 124:785

Carson M, Reid M (1976) Warfarin and fetal abnormality. Lancet I:1356

Carter AE, Eban R (1973) The prevention of postoperative deep venous thrombosis with dextran 70. Br J Surg 60:681

Carter AE, Eban R (1974) Prevention of postoperative deep venous thrombosis in legs by orally administered hydroxychloroquine sulphate. Br Med J 3:94

Carter AE, Eban R, Perrett RD (1971) Prevention of postoperative deep venous thrombosis and pulmonary embolism. Br Med J 1:312

Cash J (1975) Physiological aspects of fibrinolysis. In: v Kaulla KN, Davidson JF (eds) Synthetic fibrinolytic thrombolytic agents. Charles & Thomas, Springfield

Cazenave J-P, Kinlough-Rathbone R, Packham M, Mustard JF (1978) The effect of acetylsalicylic acid and indomethacin on rabbit platelet adherence to collagen and the subendothelium in the presence of a low or high hematocrit. Thromb Res 13:971

Cazenave J-P, Dejana E, Kinlough-Rathbone R, Packham M, Mustard JF (1979) Platelet interactions with the endothelium and the subendothelium: the role of thrombin and prostacyclin. Haemostasis 8:183

Cegelski FC, DeWeese JA, Lund CJ (1964) Deep iliofemoral venous thrombosis during pregnancy. Am J Obstet Gynecol 89:510

Cerrato D, Ariano C, Fiacchino F (1978) Deep vein thrombosis and low-dose heparin prophylaxis in neurosurgical patients. J Neurosurg 49:378

Cerskus AL, Ali M, Zamecnik J, McDonald JWD (1978) Effects of indomethacin and sulfinpyrazone on in vivo formation of thromboxane B_2 and prostaglandin D_2 during arachidonate infusion in rabbits. Thromb Res 12:549

Chan V, Chan TK (1979) Antithrombin III in fresh and cultured human endothelial cells: A natural anticoagulant from the vascular endothelium. Thromb Res 15:209

Chandler AB (1958) In vitro thrombotic coagulation of the blood: A method for producing a thrombus. Lab Invest 7:110

Channon GM, Wiley AM (1979) Aspirin prophylaxis of venous thromboembolic disease following fracture of the upper femur. Can J Surg 22:468

Charles AF, Scott DA (1933) Studies on heparin. I. The preparation of heparin. J Biol Chem 102:425

Checketts R, Bradley J (1974) Low-dose heparin in femoral neck fractures. Injury 5:42

Cheely R, McCartney W, Perry R, Delany D, Bustad L, Wynia V, Griggs T (1981) The role of non-invasive tests versus pulmonary angiography in the diagnosis of pulmonary embolism. Am J Med 70:17

Chernoff AI (1950) Anaphylactic reactions following injection of heparin. N Engl J Med 242:315

Chesner C (1946) Hemochromatosis: a review of the literature and presentation of a case without pigmentation or diabetes. J Lab Clin Med 31:1029

Chiu WS (1976) The syndrome of retroperitoneal hemorrhage and lumbar plexus neuropathy during anticoagulant therapy. South Med J 69:595

Cho MJ, Allen MA (1978) Chemical stability of prostacyclin (PGI_2) in aqueous solutions. Prostaglandins 15:943

Choay J, Lormean J, Messmore H, Fareed J, Stulc J, Andersen Å (1981) Antithrombotic properties of low molecular weight heparin fractions from porcine muscosal heparin. Thromb Haemostas 46:186

Chu D, Owen DAA, Stürmer E (1976) Effects of ergotamine and dihydroergotamine on the resistance and capitance vessels of skin and skeletal muscle in cat. Postgrad Med J [Suppl 1] 52:32

Chu Cheng T (1981) Thrombocytopenia associated with minidose heparin therapy. Postgrad Med 70:73

Chumnijarakij T (1974) Incidence of postpartum thromboembolism in Thai women: comparison with Western experience. J Med Assoc Thailand 57:592

Chumnijarakij T, Poshyachinda V (1975) Postoperative thrombosis in Thai women. Lancet I:1357

Cifonelli JA (1974) The relationship of molecular weight and sulfate content and distribution to anticoagulant activity of heparin preparations. Carbohydr Res 37:145

Cines D, Kaywin P, Bina M, Tomaski A, Schreiber A (1980) Heparin-associated thrombocytopenia. N Engl J Med 303:788

Cipolle R, Seifert R, Neilan B, Zazke D, Hans E (1981) Heparin Kinetics: variables related to disposition and dosage. Clin Pharmacol Ther 29:387

Clagett GP, Salzman E (1975) Prevention of venous thromboembolism. Progr Cardiovasc Dis 17:345

Clagett GP, Brier DF, Rosoff CB, Schneider PB, Salzman E (1974) Effect of aspirin on postoperative platelet kinetics and venous thrombosis. Surg Forum 25:473

Clagett GP, Schneider P, Rosoff CB, Salzman E (1975) The influence of aspirin on postoperative platelet kinetics and venous thrombosis. Surgery 77:61

Clark B, Chu D, Aellig WH (1978) Actions on the heart and circulation. In: Berde B, Schild HO (eds) Ergot alkaloids and related compounds. Springer, Berlin Heidelberg New York

Clark C, Cotton LT (1968) Blood-flow in deep veins of legs. Recording technique and evaluation of methods to increase flow during operation. Br J Surg 55:211

Clark WB, Macgregor AB, Prescott RJ, Ruckley CV (1974) Pneumatic compression of the calf and postoperative deep vein thrombosis. Lancet II:5

Clayton JK, Anderson JA, McNicol GP (1976) Preoperative prediction of postoperative deep vein thrombosis. Br Med J 2:910

Clayton JK, Anderson JA, McNicol GP (1978) Effect of cigarette smoking on subsequent postoperative thromboembolic disease in gynaecological patients. Br Med J 2:402

Clayton JK, Crandon AJ, Peel KR, McNicol GP (1979) Post-operative deep vein thrombosis prophylaxis in high risk patients. Thromb Haemost 42:260

Clemmesen I (1978) Inhibition of urokinase by complex formation with human antithrombin III in absence and presence of heparin. Thromb Haemost 39:616

Coccheri S, de Rosa V, Cavallaroni K, Poggi M (1978) Activation of fibrinolysis by means of sulfated polysaccharides: present status and perspectives. In: Davidson JF, Rowan RM, Samama MM, Desnoners PC (eds) Progress in chemical fibrinolysis and thrombolysis, vol 3. Rawen press, New York, p 461

Coccheri S, de Rosa V, Pelusi G, Moretti B, Camerini T, Bernardini M (1979) The effect of some fibrinolytically active sulfated polysaccharides and a polydesoxynucleotide on the inhibition of factor Xa. In: Davidson J, Cepelak V, Samama M, Desnoyers P (eds) Progress in chemical fibrinolysis and thrombolysis, vol IV. Churchill Livingstone, Edinburgh London New York

Cockburn JS, McKenzie FN, Arfors K-E, Matheson NA (1973) The effect of surgical operation on platelet reactivity in vitro and in vivo. Bibl Anat 12:152

Cockett FB, Lea Thomas M (1965) The iliac compression syndrome. Br J Surg 52:816

Coe N, Collins R, Klein L, Bettmann M, Skillman J, Shapiro R, Salzman E (1978) Prevention of deep vein thrombosis in urological patients. A controlled, randomized trial of low-dose heparin and external pneumatic compression boots. Surgery 83:230

Cofrancesco E, Radaelli F, Pogliani E, Amici N, Torri GG, Casu B (1979) Correlation of sulphate content and degree of carboxylation of heparin and related glycosaminoglycans with anticomplement activity. Relationships to the anticoagulant and platelet-aggregating activities. Thromb Res 14:179

Cohen S, Ehrlich G, Kauffman M, Cope C (1973) Thrombophlebitis following knee surgery. J Bone Joint Surg 55-A:106

Colburn W (1976) Pharmacologic implications of heparin interactions with other drugs. Drug Metab Rev 5:281

Colby F (1948) The prevention of fatal pulmonary emboli after prostatectomy. J Urol 59:920

Colin JF, Rottcher KH, Dhall DP (1975) Venous thrombosis in Africans. Lancet I:408

Collins R, Klein L, Skillman J, Salzman E (1976) Thromboembolic problems in urologic surgery. Urol Clin North Am 3:393

Collins R, Coe N, Goldstein E, Shapiro R, Skillman J, Zervas N, Salzman E (1977) External pneumatic compression of the legs to prevent venous thromboembolism in neurosurgical patients. Thromb Haemost 38:196

Comp PC, Jacocks RM, Taylor FB, Kopta JA, Geyer JR, Kurkjian HR, Steves CR, Walters MC (1979) The dilute whole blood clot lysis assay: a screening method for identifying postoperative patients with a high incidence of deep venous thrombosis. J Lab Clin Med 93:120

Comper W, Laurent T (1978) Physiological function of connective tissue polysaccharides. Physiol Rew 58:255

Conti S (1980) Venous thromboembolism prophylaxis in the surgical patient: a regional survey. Vasc Surg 14:382

Cooke ED, Bowcock S (1979a) Further experience in the prevention of deep-vein thrombosis (DVT) after elective hip surgery using lignocaine. Thromb Haemost 42:250

Cooke ED, Bowcock S (1979b) Tocainide in the prevention of deep-vein thrombosis following elective hip surgery (Charnley arthroplasty). Thromb Haemost 42:302

Cooke ED, Bowcock S, Lloyd MJ, Pilcher MF (1977a) Intravenous lignocaine in prevention of deep venous thrombosis after elective hip surgery. Lancet II:797

Cooke ED, Dawson MH, Ibbotson RM, Path MRC, Bowcock S, Ainsworth M, Pilcher MF (1977b) Failure of orally administered hydroxychloroquine sulphate to prevent venous thromboembolism following elective hip operations. J Bone Joint Surg 59-A:496

Coon WW, Coller FA (1959) Some epidemiological considerations of thromboembolism. Surg Gynecol Obstet 109:487

Coon WW, Willis P (1966) Some side effects of heparin, heparinoids, and their antagonists. Clin Pharmacol Ther 7:379

Coon WW, Willis PW, Symous MJ (1969) Assessment of anticoagulant treatment of venous thromboembolism. Am Surg 170:559

Cooper DR, Lewis GP, Lieberman GE, Webb H, Westwick J (1979) ADP metabolism in vascular tissue, a possible thrombo-regulating mechanism. Thromb Res 14:901

Cope C, Reyes T, Skversky N (1973) Phlebographic analysis of the incidence of thrombosis in hemiplegia. Radiology 109:581

Copley AL, Robb TP (1941) The effect of heparin on the platelet count in dogs and mice. Am J Physiol 133:248

Cordier AH (1905) Phlebitis following abdominal and pelvic operations. JAMA 45:1792

Corley RD, Joseph NR (1966) Red cell charge as affected by low viscosity dextrans. Proc Soc Exp Biol 122:1171

Cornfield J, Gordon T, Smitt WW (1961) Quantal response for experimentally uncontrolled variables. Bull Int Statist Inst 38:97

Corrigan TP, Kakkar VV, Fossard DP (1974) Low dose subcutaneous heparin — optimal dose regimen. Br J Surg 61:320

Cotton LT, Sabri S, Roberts VC (1972) The dynamics of venous blood flow and the prevention of deep venous thrombosis. In: Kakkar VV, Jouhar AJ (eds) Thromboembolism: diagnosis and treatment. Churchill Livingstone, Edinburgh London

Covey TH, Sherman L, Baue AE (1975) Low-dose heparin in postoperative patients. A prospective coded study. Arch Surg 110:1021

Crafoord C (1936) Preliminary report on post-operative treatment with heparin as a preventive of thrombosis. Acta Chir Scand 79:407

Crafoord C, Jorpes E (1941) Heparin as a prophylaxis against thrombosis. JAMA 116:2831

Crandon AJ, Peel KR, Anderson JA, Thomson V, McNicol GP (1980a) Postoperative deep vein thrombosis: identifying high-risk patients. Br Med J 2:343

Crandon AJ, Peel KR, Anderson JA, Thompson V, McNicol GP (1980b) Prophylaxis of postoperative deep vein thrombosis: selective use of low-dose heparin in high-risk patients. Br Med J 2:345

Cranley JJ (1975) Venous thrombosis secondary to phlebography. In: Vascular surgery, vol 2. Harper & Row, Hagerstown Maryland

Cranley J, Canos A, Mahalingam K (1976) Non-invasive diagnosis and prophylaxis of deep venous thrombosis of the lower extremities. In: Madden J, Hume M (eds) Venous thromboembolism. Prevention and treatment. Appleton-Century-Crofts, New York

Crawford D, Dumbadze I, Ratledge W, Mulvaney W, Wendel R (1978) Deep venous thrombosis following transurethral resection of the prostate: diagnosis by phleborheography. J Urol 120:438

Cristal N, Stern J, Ronon M, Silverman C, Ho W, Bartov E (1976) Identifying patients at risk for thromboembolism. Use of ^{125}I-labeled fibrinogen in patients with acute myocardial infarction. JAMA 236:2755

Cronberg S, Belfrage S, Nilsson IM (1963) Fibrinogen-transmitted hepatitis. Lancet I:967

Cronberg S, Robertson B, Nilsson IM, Niléhn J-E (1966) Suppressive effect of dextran on platelet adhesiveness. Thromb Diath Haemorrh 16:384

Crutcher R, Daniel R (1948) Pulmonary embolism. A correlation of clinical and autopsy studies. Surgery 23:47

Culver D, Crawford JS, Gardiner JH, Wiley AM (1970) Venous thrombosis after fractures of the upper end of the femur. A study of incidence and site. J Bone Joint Surg 52-B:61

Cunningham I, Young NK (1974) The incidence of postoperative deep vein thrombosis in Malaysia. Br J Surg 61:482

Curry N, Bardana EJ, Pirofsky B (1973) Heparin sensitivity. Report of a case. Arch Intern Med 132:744

Czapek EE, Kwaan HC, Szczecinski M (1980) The effect of a sulfated polysaccharide on antithrombin III. J Lab Clin Med 95:783

Czechanowski B, Heinrich F (1981) Prophylaxe venöser Thrombosen bei frischem ischämischem zerebrovaskulärem Insult. Doppelblindstudie mit Heparin-Dihydergot. Dtsch Med Wochenschr 106:1254

Dahl-Iversen E (1945) Three years experience of postoperative thrombophlebitis and embolism in patients ambulant on the first postoperative day (In Norwegian). Nord Med 28:2085

Dahl-Iversen E, Ramberg E (1932) Investigations of postoperative phlebitis, thrombosis and embolism (In Swedish). Hospitalstidene (Copenh) 75:371

Dalen J, Alpert J (1975) Natural history of pulmonary embolism. Progr Cardiovasc Dis 17:259

D'Ambrosia RD, Lipscomb PR, McClain EJ, Wissinger A, McDowell III JH (1975) Prophylactic anticoagulation in total hip replacement. Surg Gynaecol Obstet 140:523

Damus PS, Hicks M, Rosenberg RD (1973) Anticoagulant action of heparin. Nature 246:356

Daniel WJ, Moore AR, Flanc C (1972) Prophylaxis of deep vein thrombosis (DVT) with dextran 70 in patients with a fractured neck of the femur. Aust NZ J Surg 41:289

Danishefsky I (1975) Synthesis and properties of heparin derivatives. Adv Exp Med Biol 52:105

David JL, Monfort F, Herion F, Raskinet R (1979) Compared effects of three dose-levels of Ticlopidine on platelet function in normal subjects. Thromb Res 14:35

Davidson AI, Brunt ME, Matheson NA (1972) A further trial comparing dextran 70 with warfarin in the prophylaxis of postoperative venous thrombosis. Br J Surg 59:314

Davies JA, Merrick MV, Sharp AA, Holt JM (1972) Controlled trial of ancrod and heparin in treatment of deep-vein thrombosis of lower limb. Lancet I:113

Davies JWL, Liljedahl SO, Reizenstein P (1970) Fibrinogen metabolism following injury and its surgical treatment. Injury 1:178

Davies T (1979) South Wales Multicentre Trial of prophylactic dextran 70 after surgery: a clinically oriented randomized double-blind trial. Further observations. In: Verstraete M, Vermylen J, Roberts H (eds) The challenge of clinical trials in thrombosis. FK Schattauer, Stuttgart New York

Davis FM, Quince M, Laurenson VG (1980) Deep vein thrombosis and anaesthetic technique in emergency hip surgery. Br Med J 2:1528

Dawes J, Pepper D (1979) Catabolism of low-dose heparin in man. Thromb Res 14:845

Dawidson I, Barrett J, Miller E, Litwin M (1975) Blood viscosity studies in postoperative patients. Effects of intravascular aggregate dissolution. Bibl Haematol 41:76

Dawson AA, Bennett B, Jones PF, Munro A (1981) Thrombotic risks of staging laparatomy with splenectomy in Hodkin's disease. Br J Surg 68:842

Day TK, Cowper SV, Kakkar VV, Clark GA (1977) Early venous thrombosis. A scanning electron microscope study. Thromb Haemost 37:477

De Bakey M (1954) A critical evaluation of the problem of thromboembolism. Int Abstr Surg 98:1

Dechavanne M, Saudin F, Viala J-J, Kher A, Bertrix L, de Mourgues G (1974) Prévention des thromboses veineuses. Succès de l'héparine à fortes doses lors des coxarthroses. Nouv Presse Méd 3:1317

Dechavanne M, Ville D, Viala J-J, Kher A, Fairre J, Pousset MB, Dejour H (1975) Controlled trial of platelet anti-aggregating agents and subcutaneous heparin in prevention of postoperative deep vein thrombosis in high risk patients. Haemostasis 4:94

Dejode LR, Khurshid M, Walther WW (1973) The influence of electrical stimulation of the leg during surgical operations on the subsequent development of deep-vein thrombosis. Br J Surg 60:31

de Mourgues G, Pagnier F, Clermont N, Ville D, Moyen B (1979) Etude de l'efficacité de l'héparine sous-cutanée utilisée selon deux protocoles dans la prévention de la thrombose veineuse postopératoire après prothèse totale de hanche. Rev Chir Orthop 65:74

Dencker H (1964) The frequency of postthrombotic symptoms after fractures of the femur diaphysis (In Swedish). Läkartidn 61:228

Denson KWE, Bonnar J (1973) The measurement of heparin. A method based on the potentiation of antifactor Xa. Thromb Diath Haemorrh 30:171

De Takats G (1950) Anticoagulants in surgery. JAMA 142:527

Deutsch E (1964) Antikoagulantien in der Therapie der peripheren arteriellen Durchblutungsstörungen. Wien Klin Wochenschr 76:151

DeWeese JA (1979) Interruption of the inferior vena cava for pulmonary embolism. In: May R (ed) Surgery of the veins of the leg and pelvis. Thieme, Stuttgart

DeWeese JA, Adams JT, Rogoff SM (1967) Restoration and maintenance of venous patency in venous thrombosis. Anticoagulation, thrombectomy and venous interruption. Pac Med Surg 75:77

Dhall DP, Matheson NA (1968) In vitro clumping of human platelets by dextran. Thromb Diath Haemorrh 19:70

Dhall DP, Bennett PN, Matheson NA (1967) Effect of dextran on platelet behaviour after abdominal operations. Acta Chir Scand [Suppl] 387:75

Dhall TZ, Bryce WAJ, Dhall DP (1976) Effect of dextran on the molecular structure and tensile behaviour of human fibrin. Thromb Haemost 35:737

Dick W, Matis P, Mayer W (1959) Results of alternating anticoagulant prophylaxis in surgery. Thromb Diath Haemorrh 3:11

Didisheim P (1968) Inhibition by dipyridamole of arterial thrombosis in rats. Thromb Diath Haemorrh 20:257

Diener L (1975) Origin and distribution of venous thrombi studied by postmortem intraosseous phlebography. In: Nicolaides AN (ed) Thromboembolism. Aetiology, advances in prevention and management. MTP, Lancaster

Dintenfass L (1962) Thixotrophy of blood and proneness to thrombus formation. Circ Res 11:233

Dismuke SE (1981) Declining mortality from pulmonary embolism in surgical patients. Thromb Haemostas 46:17

Dizadji H, Hammer R, Stryz B, Weisenberger J (1979) Spontaneous rupture of the liver. A complication of oral anticoagulant therapy. Arch Surg 114:734

Dodd H, Cockett F (1976) The pathology and surgery of the veins of the lower limb. Churchill Livingstone, Edinburgh London New York

Doery JC, Hirsh J, de Gruchy GC (1969) Aspirin: its effect on platelet glycolysis and release of adenosine diphosphate. Science 165:65

Dolk T, Westerborn O (1977) Complications and mortality in patients with hip fracture (In Swedish). Läkartidningen 74:3654

Dommering M (1979) Low-dose heparin prophylaxis in herniorrhaphy? A prospective trial in bleeding complications. Arch Chir Neerl 31:57

Donaldson GA, Williams C, Scannell JG (1963) A reappraisal of the application of the Trendelenburg operation to massive fatal embolism. Report of a successful pulmonary-artery thrombectomy using a cardiopulmonary by-pass. N Engl J Med 268:171

Donaldson M, Wirthlin L, Donaldson G (1980) Thirty-year experience with surgical interruption of the inferior vena cava prevention of pulmonary embolism. Ann Surg 191:367

Doran FSA, Drury M, Sivyer A (1964) A simple way to combat the venous stasis which occurs in the lower limb during surgical operations. Br J Surg 51:486

Dormandy J (1975) Abnormal blood viscosity and deep venous thrombosis. In: Nicolaides AN (ed) Thromboembolism. Aetiology, advances in prevention and management. MTP, Lancaster

Dormandy J, Edelman J (1973) High blood viscosity: an aetiological factor in venous thrombosis. Br J Surg 60:187

Dosne AM, Dupuy E, Bodevin E (1978) Production of a fibrinolytic inhibitor by cultured endothelial cells derived from human umbilical vein. Thromb Res 12:377

Douglas AS (1978) History of venous thrombo-embolic disease 1750–1900. Scot Med J 23:315

Douss TW (1976) The clinical significance of venous thrombosis of the calf. Br J Surg 63:377

Dugdale M, Nofzinger JD, Murphey F (1966) Some effects of low molecular weight dextran on coagulation. Thromb Diath Haemorrh 15:118

Ebert RV (1958) Clinical characteristics of American dextran. Bibl Haematol 7:270

Echterhoff HM, Kottmann UR, O'Koye XR, Rohner HG (1981) Ergotismus: eine wichtige Komplikation in der medikamentösen Thromboembolieprophylaxe. Deutsch Med Wochenschr 106:1717

Ecker EE, Gross P (1929) Anticomplementary power of heparin. J Infect Dis 44:250

Eckert G, Weichselbaum TE, Sights R, Miller V (1954) Study of the effect of the administration of dextran and physiologic saline solution on the colloidal osmotic pressure of the plasma in splenectomized dogs following haemorrhage. Surg Forum 4:731

Economopoulos TC, Papayannis AG, Stathakis NE, Arapakis G, Gardikas C (1977) Postoperative platelet function in patients on small subcutaneous doses of heparin. Acta Haematol 57:266

Edgar W, Prentice CRM (1973) The proteolytic action of ancrod on human fibrinogen and its polypeptide chains. Thromb Res 2:85

Editorial (1975a) Low-dose heparin and the prevention of venous thromboembolic disease. Br Med J 3:447

Editorial (1975b) Prevention of postoperative thromboembolism. Lancet II:63

Edwards DH, Steel WM, Bentley G (1975) Prophylaxis with dextran 70 against thrombosis in patients with fractures of the upper end of the femur. Injury 6:250

Egeberg CA (1845) Sudden death in the puerperium (In Norwegian). Nor Mag Laegevidensk

Egeberg O (1962) Changes in the coagulation system following major surgical operations. Acta Med Scand 171:679

Egeberg O (1965) Thrombophilia caused by inheritable deficiency of blood antithrombin. Scand J Clin Lab Invest 17:92

Ehrlich J, Stivala SS (1973) Chemistry and pharmacology of heparin. J Pharmacol Sci 62:517

Ehrly AM (1966) Wirkung von niedermolekularem Dextran auf Erythrocytenaggregate beim Sludgephänomen. Med Klin 61:989

Ehrly AM (1973) Verbesserung der Fließeigenschaften des Blutes: Ein neues Prinzip zur medikamentösen Therapie chronischer peripherer arterieller Durchblutungsstörungen. Vasa [Suppl] 1

Ehrly AM (1975) Dosis-Wirkungs-Beziehungen von subkutan applizierten Arwin bei Patienten mit chronischen arteriellen Durchblutungsstörungen. Vasa 4:161

Ehrly AM, Köhler HJ (1976) Modifiziertes Dosisschema für die subkutane Anwendung von Arwin bei Patienten mit chronischen arteriellen Durchblutungsstörungen. Vasa 5:155

Eika C (1972) The platelet aggregating effect of eight commercial heparins. Scand J Haematol 9:480

Eika C, Godal HC, Laake K, Hamborg T (1980) Low incidence of thrombocytopenia during treatment with hog mucosa and beef lung heparin. Scand J Haematol 25:19

Eisen M, Napp HE, Vock R (1975) Inhibition of platelet aggregation caused by estrogen treatment in patients with carcinoma of the prostata. J Urol 114:93

Eldor A, Weksler D (1979) Heparin and dextran sulfate antagonize PGI_2 inhibition of platelet aggregation. Thromb Res 16:617

Ellis G, Wright K, Jones S, Richardson D, Ellis C (1980) Effect of oral aspirin dose on platelet aggregation and vascular prostacyclin (PGI_2) synthesis in humans and rabbits. J Cardiovasc Pharmacol 2:387

Ellis H, Scurr JH (1982) Prophylaxis of venous thrombosis. Phlebologie 35:135

Elsner-Mackey P, Ledermair O, Schastok H, Vinazzer H (1969) Zur Wirkung von Macrodex auf die postoperative Thromboembolie-Frequenz. Wien Med Wochenschr 119:149

Emerson P, Marks P (1977) Preventing thromboembolism after myocardial infarction: effect of low-dose heparin or smoking. Br Med J 1:18

Emmons PR, Mitchell JRA (1965) Postoperative changes in platelet-clumping activity. Lancet I:71

Emmons PR, Harrison MJG, Honour AJ, Mitchell JRA (1965a) Effect of dipyridamole on human platelet behaviour. Lancet II:603

Emmons PR, Harrison MJG, Honour AJ, Mitchell JRA (1965b) Effect of pyrimidopyrimidine derivate on thrombus formation in the rabbit. Nature 208:255

Encke A, Stork C, Dumle HO (1976) Doppelblindstudie zur postoperativen Thromboembolieprophylaxe mit Dipyridamol/Acetylsalicylsäure. Chirurg 47:670

Endl VJ, Auinger W (1977) Frühdiagnose der postoperativen tiefen Beinvenenthrombose mit dem [125]Jod-Fibrinogentest an einem gynäkologisch operierten Patientgut. Wien Klin Wochenschr 89:304

Engberg A (1969) Proximal renal tubule structure and function with special reference to the effect of dextran 40. Acta Univ Ups Diss Med 77

Engberg A, Ericsson JLE (1969) Effects of dextran 40 on proximal renal tubule. Electron microscopic and cytochemical studies in the mouse. Acta Chir Scand 135:263

Engelberg H (1978) Heparin. In: Kritchevsky D, Pollak OJ, Simms H (eds) Monographs on atherosclerosis, vol 8. Karger, Basel München Paris London New York Sydney

Engeset J, Stalker AL, Matheson NA (1966) Effects of dextran 40 on erythrocyte aggregation. Lancet I:1124

Erdi A, Thomas DP, Kakkar VV, Lane DA, Dormandy JH (1976) Effect of low-dose subcutaneous heparin on whole-blood viscosity. Lancet II:342

Eriksson I, Holmberg JT (1977) Analysis of factors affecting limb salvage and mortality after embolectomy. Acta Chir Scand 143:237

Eriksson M, Saldeen T (1979) Venous macro-thromboembolism. An autopsy study. Thromb Haemostas 42:229

Eriksson M, Saldeen T (1980) Venous macrothromboembolism in an unselected autopsy material and its relation to antiplasmin activity in the vessel wall. Thromb Res 20:555

Ernst CB, Fry WJ, Kraft RO, DeWeese MS (1964) The role of low molecular weight dextran in the management of venous thrombosis. Surg Gynecol Obstet 119:1243

Eskeland G (1962) Prevention of venous thrombosis and pulmonary embolism in injured patients. Lancet I:1035

Eskeland G, Solheim K, Skjörten F (1966) Anticoagulant prophylaxis, thromboembolism and mortality in elderly patients with hip fractures. A controlled clinical trial. Acta Chir Scand 131:16

Esnouf MP, Tunnah GW (1967) The isolation and properties of the thrombin-like activity from Agcistrodon rhodostoma venom. Br J Haematol 13:581

Esquivel C, Bergqvist D, Björck C, Nilsson B (to be published a) Effect of heparin and a heparin-analogue on platelet activity and microvascular hemostasis in vivo. Thromb Res

Esquivel C, Bergqvist D, Björck C, Nilsson B, Bergentz S-E (1982 b) Effect of volume expanders on the lysability of ex vivo thrombi in the rabbit. Acta Chir Scand 148:359

Estes JW (1975) The fate of heparin in the body. Curr Ther Res 18:45

Estes JW, Poulin PF (1975) Pharmacokinetics of heparin distribution and elimination. Thromb Diath Haemorrh 33:26

Evans DS (1971) The early diagnosis of thromboembolism by ultrasound. Ann R Coll Surg Engi 49:225

Evans G, Packham MA, Nishizawa EE, Mustard JF, Murphy EA (1968) The effect of acetylsalicylic acid on platelet function. J Exp Med 128:877

Evarts C, Feil E (1971) Prevention of thromboembolic disease after elective surgery in the hip. J Bone Joint Surg [Am] 53:1271

Ewald EA, Eichelberger JW, Young AS, Weiss HJ, Crosby WH (1965) The effect of dextran on platelet factor 3 activity. In vitro and in vivo studies. Transfusion Phil 5:109

Ewart MR, Halton WWC, Barford JM, Dodgson KS (1970) The proteolytic action of arvin on human fibrinogen. Biochem J 118:603

Fahiny N, Patel D (1981) Haemostatic changes and postoperative deep vein thrombosis associated with use of a pneumatic tourniquet. J Bone Joint Surg 63-A:461

Falk V, Forkman B, Arfors K-E (1967) The permeability of the placenta to dextrans. Acta Obstet Gynecol Scand 46:414

Fanous LH, Gray A, Felmingham J (1977) Severe anaphylactoid reactions to dextran 70. Br Med J 2:1189

Faraci P, Deterling R, Stein A, Rheinlander H, Cleveland R (1978) Warfarin induced necrosis of the skin. Surg Gynecol Obstet 146:695

Fearnley GR (1965) Fibrinolysis. Arnold, London

Fearnley GR, Chakrabarti R, Hocking ED (1967) Fibrinolytic effects of diquanides plus ethyl-oestronol in occlusive vascular disease. Lancet II:1008

Feddersen C, Clausen NT, Gormsen J (1975) Effect of dextran, heparin, and split products (streptokinase-induced) on the resulting fibrin cross-linking effect in plasma clotted in vitro. In: Davidson JF, Samama MM, Desnoyers PC (eds) Progress in chemical fibrinolysis and thrombolysis. Raven Press, New York

Feigl W, Schwarz N (1977) Häufigkeit von Beinvenenthrombosen und Lungenembolien im Obduktionsgut. In: Ehringer H (ed) Akute tiefe Becken- und Beinvenenthrombosen. V H. Huber, Bern Stuttgart Vienna

Feinleib M (1972) Venous thrombosis in relation to cigarette smoking, physical activity and seasonal factors. Milbank Med Fund Q 50:123

Feinstein AR (1977) Clinical biostatistics. CV Mosby, St Louis

Feldman SA (1973) Action of muscle relaxant of the gut, the cardiovascular system, and the fetus. In: Major problems in anaesthesia. Muscle relaxants 1. WB Saunders, London Philadelphia Toronto

Felix R, Louven B (1972) Zur Vasoaktivität von Dihydroergotamin. Phlebographische Untersuchungen. Fortschr Med 90:757

Fenech A, Winter JH, Douglas AS (1979) Individualisation of oral anticoagulant therapy. Drugs 18:48

Fenech A, Winter JH, Bennett B, Smith FW. Douglas AS (1981) Preoperative frequency of deep venous thrombosis in patients with fractured neck of femur. Lancet I:1212

Fey KH, Herzfeld U, Saggau W, Oehlschläger M (1975) Postoperative Thromboseprophylaxe durch Tonisierung des kaudalen Venensystems. Med Klin 70:1553

Fidlar E, Jaques LB (1948) The effect of commercial heparin on the platelet count. J Lab Clin Med 33:1410

Field ES, Nicolaides AN, Kakkar VV, Crellin RQ (1972) Deep-vein thrombosis in patients with fractures of the femoral neck. Br J Surg 59:377

Fischer M, Wimmer H (1965) Aktivierung des fibrinolytischen Systems durch niedermolekulares Dextran. Bibl Haemat 23:1278

Flanc C, Kakkar VV, Clarke MB (1968) The detection of venous thrombosis of the legs using ^{125}I-labelled fibrinogen. Br J Surg 55:742

Flanc C, Kakkar VV, Clarke MB (1969) Postoperative deep-vein thrombosis. Effect of intensive prophylaxis. Lancet I:477

Flemma RJ, Silver D, Anlyan WG (1965) Effects of heparin, plasmin, dextran and low molecular dextran on bioelectrically induced thromboses. Surg Forum 16:123

Flessa HC, Kapstrom AB, Gluck HI (1965) Placental transport of heparin. Am J Obstet Gynecol 93:570

Fletcher AP, Alkjaersig N, O'Brien J (1972) Fibrinogen-fibrin degradation products and venous thromboembolism. In: Kakkar VV, Jouhar AJ (eds) Thromboembolism: diagnosis and treatment. Churchill Livingstone, Edinburgh London

Flicoteaux H, Kher A, Jean N, Blary M, Judet T, Honnart F, Pasteyer J (1977) Comparison of low dose heparin and low dose heparin combined with aspirin in prevention of deep vein thrombosis after total hip replacement. Pathol Biol 25:55

Florey HW, Poole JCF, Meek GA (1959) Endothelial cells and "cement" lines. J Pathol 77:625

Flotte TC, Buxton RW (1963) Reduction of serum cholesterol by dextran. Circulation 28:721

Flotte TC, Buxton RW (1965) Reduction of serum cholesterol and lipids by dextran. Circulation 31 [Suppl] II:85

Flower RJ (1974) Drugs which inhibit prostaglandin biosynthesis. Pharmacol Rev 26:33

Flower RJ, Blackwell GJ (1976) The importance of phospholipase A_2 in prostaglandin biosynthesis. Biochem Pharmacol 25:285

Flute PT, Kakkar VV, Renney JTG, Nicolaides AN (1972) The blood and venous thrombosis. In: Kakkar VV, Jouhar AJ (eds) Thromboembolism: diagnosis and treatment. Churchill Livingstone, Edinburgh London

Forconi S, Guerrini M, Di Perri T (1977) Study of the activity of a flavonoid, O-(betahydroxyethyl)-rutoside, at high dose levels on venous tone measured by "strain gauge" plethysmography. Vasa 6:279

Formolo J, Shors C (1981) Fatal pulmonary embolism from massive right atrial thrombus post-coronary artery bypass surgery. Am Heart J 101:510

Forsberg K, Törngren S (1977) Deep venous thrombosis and multiple regression analysis of the influence from various clinical factors on the fibrinogen half-life in surgical patients, using ^{125}I-fibrinogen. Thromb Res 10:235

Fossard DP, Field ES, Kakkar VV, Friend JR, Corrigan TP, Flute PT (1974a) Fibrinolytic activity and postoperative deep-vein thrombosis. Lancet I:9

Fossard DP, Kakkar VV, Higgins A (1974b) Infections and postoperative venous thrombosis. Br J Surg 61:919

Foster DP, Whipple GH (1922) Blood fibrin studies. Fibrin values influenced by cell injury, inflammation, intoxication, liver injury and the Eck fistula. Notes concerning the origin of fibrinogen in the body. Am J Physiol 58:407

Fournier A, Watchi JM, Réveillaud RJ (1968) Les nephroses dits osmotiques en vacuolication hydropiques diffuses des tubes proximaux. Actual Nephrol Hop Necker 23

Fredin H, Nillius A (1982) Fatal pulmonary embolism after total hip replacement. Acta Orthoped Scand 53:407

Fredin HO, Nillius SA, Bergqvist D (1982) Prophylaxis of deep vein thrombosis in patients with fractures of the femoral neck. A prospective comparison between dextran and a poly-sulphated saccharide. Acta Orthop Scand 53:413

Freeark R, Boswick J, Fardin R (1967) Posttraumatic venous thrombosis. Arch Surg 95:567

Freiman J, Chalmers T, Smith H, Kuebler R (1978) The importance of beta, the type II error and sample size in the design and interpretation of the randomized control trial. Survey of 71 "negative" trials. N Engl J Med 299:690

Frey C, Trollope M, Harpster W, Snyder R (1973) A fifteen-year experience with automative hepatic trauma. J Trauma 13:1039

Fried S, Barton J (1977) Synthesis of 13, 14-dehydroprostacyclin methyl ester: a potent inhibitor of platelet aggregation. Proc Natl Acad Sci USA 74:2199

Friend JR, Kakkar VV (1972) Deep vein thrombosis in obstetric and gynaecological patients. In: Kakkar VV, Jouhar AJ (eds) Thromboembolism: diagnosis and treatment. Churchill Livingstone, Edinburgh London

Fry D, Garrison N, Williams H (1980) Patterns of morbidity and mortality in splenic trauma. Am Surg 46:28

Frykholm R (1939) On the pathogenesis of venous thrombosis and mechanical prophylaxis (In Swedish). Nord Med 4:3534

Fuglsang E, Bruun P, Carlsen K (1980) Deep vein thrombosis treated with Haemaccel. A study with ^{125}I-labelled fibrinogen (In Danish). Ugeskr Laeger 142:1756

Fullen WD, Miller EH, Steele WF, McDonough JJ (1973) Prophylactic vena cava interruption in hip fractures. J Trauma 13:403

Fuller C, Willbanks O (1971) Incidental prophylactic inferior vena cava clipping. Arch Surg 102: 440

Furhoff A-K (1977) Anaphylactoid reaction to dextran – a report of 133 cases. Acta Anesthiol Scand 21:161

Galasko CBS, Edwards DH, Fearn CBD, Barber HM (1976) The value of low dosage heparin for the prophylaxis of thromboembolism in patients with transcervical and intertrochanteric femoral fractures. Acta Orthop Scand 47:276

Galle P, Muss H, McGrath K, Stuart J, Homesley H (1978) Thrombocytopenia in two patients treated with low-dose heparin. Obstet Gynecol 52 [Suppl] 9S

Gallus A, Darby T (1981) Intermittent calf compression; a randomized trial in elective hip replacement. Thromb Haemost 46:93

Gallus AS, Hirsh J (1975) Small doses subcutaneous heparin in preventing deep venous thrombosis. In: Nicolaides AN (ed) Thromboembolism. Aetiology, advances in prevention and management. MTP, Lancaster

Gallus AS, Hirsh J (1976a) Antithrombotic drugs. Med Prog 12:63

Gallus AS, Hirsh J (1976b) Prevention of venous thromboembolism. Sem Thromb Haemostas 2: 232

Gallus AS, Hirsh J, Gent M (1973a) Relevance of preoperative and postoperative blood tests to postoperative leg-vein thrombosis. Lancet II:806

Gallus AS, Hirsh J, Tuttle R, Trebilcock R, O'Brien S, Carroll J, Minden J, Hudecki S (1973b) Small subcutaneous doses of heparin in prevention of venous thrombosis. N Engl J Med 288: 545

Gallus AS, Hirsh J, O'Brien S, McBride J, Tuttle R, Gent M (1976) Prevention of venous thrombosis with small, subcutaneous doses of heparin. JAMA 235:1980

Gazzaniga AG, Cahill JL, Replogle RL, Tilney NL (1967) Changes in blood volume and renal function following ligation of the inferior vena cava. Surgery 62:417

Gelin L-E (1956) Studies in anemia of injury. Acta Chir Scand [Suppl] 210

Gelin L-E (1962) Rheologic disturbances and the use of low viscosity dextran in surgery. Rev Surg 19:385

Gelin L-E (1966) Use and misuse of Rheomacrodex (In Swedish). Sven Läkartidn 63:1377

Gelin L-E, Ingelman B (1961) Rheomacrodex — a new dextran solution for rheological treatment of impaired capillary flow. Acta Chir Scand 122:294

Gelin L-E, Shoemaker WC (1961) Hepatic blood flow and microcirculatory alterations induced by dextran of high and low viscosity. Surgery 49:753

Gelin L-E, Thorén O (1961) Influence of low viscous dextran on peripheral circulation in man. Acta Chir Scand 122:303

Gelin L-E, Zederfeldt B (1960) Low molecular weight dextran — a rheologic agent counteracting capillary stagnation. Acta Chir Scand 119:168

Gelin L-E, Zederfeldt B (1961) Experimental evidence of the significance of disturbances in the flow properties of blood. Acta Chir Scand 122:336

Gelin L-E, Korsan-Bengtsen K, Ygge J, Zederfeldt B (1961) Influence of low viscous dextran on the hemostatic mechanism. Acta Chir Scand 122:324

Gelpi AP, Ende N (1958) A hereditary anemia with hemochromatosis. Studies of an unusual hemopathic syndrome resembling thalassemia. Am J Med 25:303

Gent M (1979) The Canadian cooperative study of platelet suppressant therapy in threatened stroke. In: Verstraete M, Vermylen J, Roberts H (eds) The challenge of clinical trials in thrombosis. FK Schattauer, Stuttgart New York

Gent M, Sackett DL (1979) The qualification and disqualification of patients and events in long-term cardiovascular clinical trials. In: Verstraete M, Vermylen J, Roberts H (eds) The challenge of clinical trials in thrombosis. FK Schattauer, Stuttgart New York

Genton E (1974) Guidelines for heparin therapy. Ann Intern Med 80:77

Genton E, Gent M, Hirsh J, Harker L (1975) Platelet-inhibiting drugs in the prevention of clinical thrombotic disease (I). N Engl J Med 293:1174

Genton E, Barnett HJM, Fields WS, Gent M, Heak IC (1977) Cerebral ischemia: The role of thrombosis and of antithrombotic therapy. Stroke 9:147

Gerrard JM, White JG (1978) Prostaglandins and thromboxanes. "Middlemen" modulating platelet function in haemostasis and thrombosis. In: Spaet T (ed) Progress in haemostasis and thrombosis, vol 4. Grune & Stratton, New York

Getzen JH, Speiggle W (1963) Anaphylactic reaction to dextran. Arch Intern Med 112:168

Giacommetti N, Chervet D, Bouvier CA (1975) Effets sur la coagulabilité sanguine de trois types differentes d'héparine pour administration sous-cutanée. Schweiz Apoth Ztg 113:126

Gibbard FB, Gould SR, Marks P (1976) Incidence of deep vein thrombosis and leg oedema in patients with strokes. J Neurol Neurosurg Psychiatry 39:1222

Gibbs NM (1957) Venous thrombosis of the lower limbs with particular reference to bed-rest. Br J Surg 45:209

Giddon DB, Lindhe J (1972) In vivo quantification of local anesthetic suppression of leukocyte adherence. Am J Pathol 68:327

Ginsberg M, Miller J, McElfatrick G (1967) The use of inflatable plastic splints. JAMA 200:180

Girolami A, Patrassi GM, Celle G, Burul A, Dal Bo Zanon R (1978) Failure of heparin treatment to affect blood or plasma viscosity. In: Coccheri (ed) Fifth International Congress on Thromboembolism. Bologne 1978. Quaderni della Coagulazione Periodic di Informatione medica, p 126

Gitel S, Salvati E, Wessler S, Robinson H, Worth M (1979) The effect of total hip replacement and general surgery on antithrombin III in relation to venous thrombosis. J Bone Joint Surg 63-A: 653

Gjønnaess H, Abildgaard U (1976) Bleeding in gynecological surgery: influence of low dose heparin. Int J Gynaecol Obstet 14:9

Gjöres JE (1956) The incidence of venous thrombosis and its sequelae in certain districts of Sweden. Acta Chir Scand [Suppl] 206

Glimelius B, Busch C, Höök M (1978) Binding of heparin on the surface of cultured human endothelial cells. Thromb Res 12:773

Godal HC (1962) Quantitative and qualitative changes in fibrinogen following major surgical operations. Acta Med Scand 171:687

Godal HC (1980) Report of the international committee on thrombosis and haemostasis. Thrombocytopenia and heparin. Thromb Haemost 43:222

Godal HC, Rygh M, Laake K (1974) Progressive inactivation of purified factor VII by heparin and antithrombin III. Thromb Res 5:773

Golden G (1978) Eine Übersicht über neue pharmakologische Effekte und klinische Resultate von 0-(β-Hydroxyethal)-rutosiden. In: Voelter W, Jung G (eds) 0-(β-Hydroxyethyl)-rutoside – experimentelle und klinische Ergebnisse. Springer, Berlin Heidelberg New York

Goldsmith H (1966) The prophylaxis of thromboembolism. Surg Gynecol Obstet 122:799

Gollub G, Schaefer C (1968) Structural alterations in canine fibrin produced by colloid plasma expanders. Surg Gynecol Obstet 127:783

Gollub S, Ulin AW (1962) Heparin-induced thrombocytopenia in man. J Lab Clin Med 59:430

Gordon RR, Dean T (1955) Fetal deaths from antenatal anticoagulant. Br Med J 2:719

Gordon-Smith IC, Grundy DJ, Le Quesne LP, Newcombe JF, Bramble FJ (1972a) Controlled trial of two regimens of subcutaneous heparin in prevention of postoperative deep-vein thrombosis. Lancet I:1134

Gordon-Smith IC, Hickman JA, El Masri SH (1972b) The effect of the fibrinolytic inhibitor epsilon-aminocaproic acid on the incidence of deep-vein thrombosis after prostatectomy. Br J Surg 59:522

Gordon-Smith IC, Hickman JA, LeQuesne LP (1974) Postoperative fibrinolytic activity and deep-vein thrombosis. Br J Surg 61:213

Gore I, Hirst A, Tanaka K (1964) Myocardial infarction and thromboembolism. A comparative study in Boston and in Kyushu, Japan. Arch Intern Med 113:323

Gorman RR, Bunting S, Miller OV (1977) Modulation of human platelet adenyl cyclase by prostacyclin (PGX). Prostaglandins 13:377

Gormsen J, Feddersen C, Clausen N (1974) Low-dose heparin. Theoretical and practical evaluation. (In Danish). Ugeskr Laeger 136:865

Gotz A (1951) Severe spontaneous hypersensitivity to heparin. Ann Intern Med 35:919

Graham J, Mattox K, Vaughan D, Jordan G (1979) Combined pancreatoduodenal injuries. J Trauma 19:340

Gralnick H, Greipp P (1971) Thrombosis with epsilon aminocaproic acid therapy. Am J Clin Path 56:151

Green D, Harris K, Reynolds N, Roberts M, Patterson R (1978) Heparin immune thrombocytopenia. Evidence for a heparin-platelet complex as the antigenic determinant. J Lab Clin Med 91:167

Greiss F (1978) Deaths from pulmonary thromboembolism after induced abortion. Am J Obstet Gynecol 132:173

Greten H, Schettler G, Mordasini R, Zipperle G, Klar E, Laible V (1978) Der Wirkungsmechanismus synthetischer Heparinoide. Resultate bei Patienten mit Hypertriglyceridämie. Dtsch Med Wochenschr 103:204

Griffith G, Boggs R (1964) The clinical usage of heparin. Am J Cardiol 14:39

Griffith GC, Nichols G, Asher JD, Flanagan B (1965) Heparin osteoporosis. JAMA 193:91

Grönwall A (1959) Antigenicity in Swedish clinical dextran. Acta Soc Med Upsal 64:244

Grönwall A (1966) Dextran: Plasma volume expanders – chemistry and biological activities. Med Postgrad 4:1

Grönwall A, Ingelman B (1944) Untersuchungen über Dextran und sein Verhalten bei parenteraler Zufuhr. Acta Physiol Scand 7:97

Grönwall A, Hint H, Ingelman B (1968) Dextran plasma volume expanders: chemistry and biological activities. Bibl Haemat 29:874

Groote Schuur Hospital Thromboembolus Study Group (1979) Failure of low-dose heparin to prevent significant thromboembolic complications in high-risk surgical patients. Interim report of a prospective trial. Br Med J 1:1447

Groth C-B, Löfström B (1966) The effect of infused high and low molecular weight dextran on the tissue oxygenation. Acta Chir Scand 131:275

Grotte G (1956) Passage of dextran molecules across the blood-lymph barrier. Acta Chir Scand [Suppl] 211

Gruber UF (1968) Blutersatz. Springer, Berlin Heidelberg New York

Gruber UF (1975) Dextran and the prevention of postoperative thromboembolic complications. Surg Clin North Am 55:679

Gruber UF (1977) Prevention of thromboembolic complications. The problem and alternatives. Acta Univ Ups. Symp Univ Ups Ann 500 Celebrantis 3, Uppsala

Gruber UF (1982) Prevention of fatal postoperative pulmonary embolism by heparin dihydro-ergotamine or Dextran 70. Br J Surg 69:S 54

Gruber UF, Bergentz S-E (1966) The antithrombotic effect of dextran. J Surg Res 6:379

Gruber UF, Messmer K (1977) Colloids for blood volume support. Progr Surg 15:49

Gruber UF, Gorgerat J-F, Torhorst J (1981) Prevention of fatal postoperative pulmonary embolism with heparin-DHE or dextran. Thromb Haemost 46:92

Gruber UF, Hohl M, Sturm V (1975a) Intra- und postoperative Thromboseprophylaxe. In: Ahnfeld FW, Bergmann H, Burri C, Dick W, Halmagyi M, Rügheimer E (eds) Klinische Anästhesiologie und Intensivtherapie. Band 9. Springer, Berlin Heidelberg New York, p 17

Gruber UF, Sturm V, Rem J, Schaub N, Rittman WW (1975b) The present state of prevention of postoperative thromboembolic complications. Bibl Haematol 41:98

Gruber UF, Bauser P, Frick J, Loosli J, Matt E, Segesser D (1977a) Sulfinpyrazone and postoperative deep vein thrombosis. Eur Surg Res 9:303

Gruber UF, Fridrich R, Duckert F, Torhorst J, Rem J (1977b) Prevention of postoperative thromboembolism by dextran 40, low-doses of heparin, or xantinol nicotinate. Lancet I:207

Gruber UF, Brun M, Brunner R, Gaugler U, Müller J, Schumacher S, Tichy J, Hohl M (1979) S.c. Heparin oder i.v. Dextran? Helv Chir Acta 46:65

Gruber UF, Saldeen T, Brokop T, Eklöf B, Eriksson I, Goldie I, Gran L, Hohl M, Jonsson T, Kristersson S, Ljungström KG, Lund T, Maartman Moe H, Svensjö E, Thomson D, Torhorst J, Trippestad A, Ulstein M (1980) Incidences of fatal postoperative pulmonary embolism with dextran 70 and low-dose heparin. An International Multicentre Study. Br Med J 280:69

Gryglewski RJ, Bunting S, Moncada S (1976) Arterial walls are protected against deposition of platelet thrombi by a substance (prostaglandin-X) which they make from prostaglandin endoperoxides. Prostaglandins 12:685

Gryglewski RJ, Korbut R, Ocetkiewicz A (1978) Generation of prostacyclin by lungs in vivo and its release into the arterial circulation. Nature 273:765

Gunn I (1979) Anti-Xa factor as a predictor of postoperative deep vein thrombosis in general surgery. Br J Surg 66:636

Gurewich V, Nunn T, Kuriakose T, Hume M (1978) Hemostatic effects of uniform, low-dose subcutaneous heparin in surgical patients. Arch Intern Med 138:41

Gurland HJ, Brunner FP, von Dahn H, Härlen H, Parsons FM, Schärer K (1973) Combined report on regular dialysis and transplantation in Europe, III, 1972. Proc Eur Dial Transplant Assoc 10:177

Gustafsson L, Appelgren L, Myrvold HE (1977) Flow improvement after defibrinogenation. J Surg Res 22:113

Hæger K (1965) The unreliability of clinical diagnosis of deep vein thrombosis. Läkartidningen 62:1067

Haeger K, Nylander G (1971) Leg vein thrombosis (In Swedish). Läkartidningen 68:4625

Haglind E (1981) Intestinal vascular obstruction. Pathophysiological mechanisms in a shock model. Thesis, University of Göteborg

Haining CG (1955) Histamine release in rabbit blood by dextran and dextran sulphate. Br J Pharmacol 10:87

Hall J, Pauli R, Wilson K (1980) Maternal and fatal sequelae of anticoagulation during pregnancy. Am J Med 63:122

Hallböök T (1978) Varicose veins (In Swedish). SPRI-rapport 3, Svenska Läkaresällskapets Handlingar 87:108

Ham JM, Slack WW (1967) Platelet adhesiveness after operation. Br J Surg 54:385

Ham JM, Slack WW (1968) The effect of small doses of heparin on platelet adhesiveness and lipoprotein-lipase activity before and after operation. Br J Surg 55:227

Hamberg M, Svensson J, Wakabayashi T, Samuelsson B (1974) Isolation and structure of two prostaglandin endoperoxides that cause platelet aggregation. Proc Natl Acad Sci USA 71:345

Hamberg M, Svensson J, Samuelsson B (1975) Thromboxanes: a new group of biologically active compounds derived from prostaglandin endoperoxides. Proc Natl Acad Sci USA 72:2994

Hamer JD (1972) Investigation of oedema of the lower limb following successful femoropopliteal bypass surgery: the role of phlebography in demonstrating venous thrombosis. Br J Surg 59:979

Hamer JD, Malone PC, Silver IA (1981) The PO_2 in venous value pockets; its possible bearing on thrombogenesis. Br J Surg 68:166

Hamilton HW, Crawford JS, Gardiner JH, Wiley AM (1970) Venous thrombosis in patients with fracture of the upper end of the femur. A phlebographic study of the effect of prophylactic anticoagulation. J Bone Joint Surg 52-B:268

Hammarsten JE, Heller B (1952) The effect of dextran in subjects with normal blood volumes and in subjects after bleeding. J Lab Clin Med 40:807

Hammarsten JE, Heller BI, Ebert RV (1953) The effects of dextran in normovolemic and oligemic subjects. J Clin Invest 32:340

Hampson WGJ, Harris BC, Lucas K, Roberts PH, McCall IW, Jackson PC, Powell NL, Staddon GE (1974) Failure of low-dose heparin to prevent deep-vein thrombosis after hip-replacement arthroplasty. Lancet II:795

Hampton JR, Harris MJG, Honour AJ, Mitchell JRA, Prichard JS (1972) Assessment of antithrombotic agents: effects of dipyridamole analogues on platelet behaviour. Cardiovasc Res 6:696

Han P, Ardlie NG (1974) Heparin, platelets and blood coagulation: implications for low-dose heparin prophylactic regimens in venous thrombosis. Br J Haematol 27:253

Handley A (1972) Low-dose heparin after myocardial infarction. Lancet II:623

Handley A, Emerson P, Fleming PR (1972) Heparin in the prevention of deep vein thrombosis after myocardial infarction. Br Med J 2:436

Hanley SP, Bevan J, Cockbill SR, Heptinstall S (1981) Differential inhibition by low-dose aspirin of human venous prostacyclin synthesis and platelet thromboxane synthesis. Lancet I:969

Hansen E, Jessing P, Lindewald H, Østergaard P, Olesen T, Malver E (1976) Hydroxychloroquine sulphate in prevention of deep venous thrombosis following fracture of the hip, pelvis, or thoraco-lumbar spine. J Bone Joint Surg [Am] 58:1089

Hargreaves T, Howell M (1965) Phenindione jaundice. Br Heart J 27:932

Harjola P, Meurala H, Frick MH (1981) Prevention of early reocclusion by Dipyridamole and ASA in arterial reconstructive surgery. J Cardiovasc Surg 22:141

Harker LA, Slichter SJ (1972a) The bleeding time as a screening test for evaluation of platelet function. N Engl J Med 287:155

Harker LA, Slichter SJ (1972b) Platelet and fibrinogen consumption in man. N Engl J Med 287:999

Harker L, Hirsh J, Gent M, Genton E (1975) Critical evaluation of platelet-inhibiting drugs in thrombotic disease. Prog Haematol 9:229

Harker LA, Wall RT, Haslam JM, Ross R (1978) Sulfinpyrazone prevention of homocystein-induced endothelial cell injury and arteriosclerosis. Clin Res 26:554A

Harlan J, Harker L (1981) Hemostasis, thrombosis and thrombembolic disorder. The role of arachidonic acid metabolites in platelet vessel wall interactions. Med Clin North Am 65:855

Harper DR, Dhall DP, Woodruff WH (1973) Prophylaxis in iliofemoral venous thrombosis. The major amputee as a clinical research model. Br J Surg 60:831

Harris WH, Salzman EW, Athanasoulis C (1974) Comparison of warfarin, low-molecular-weight dextran, aspirin, and subcutaneous heparin in prevention of venous thromboembolism following total hip replacement. J Bone Joint Surg [Am] 56:1552

Harris WH, Salzman E, Athanasoulis C, Waltman A, Baum S, DeSanctis R, Potsaid M, Sise H (1975) Comparison of ^{125}I-fibrinogen count scanning with phlebography for detection of venous thrombi after elective hip surgery. N Engl J Med 292:665

Harris WH, Raines J, Athanasoulis C, Waltman E, Salzman E (1976) External pneumatic compression versus warfarin in reducing thrombosis in high-risk patients. In: Madden J, Hume M (eds) Venous thromboembolism. Prevention and treatment. Appleton-Century-Crafts, New York

Harris WH, Salzman E, Athanasoulis C, Waltman A, DeSanctis R (1977) Aspirin prophylaxis of venous thromboembolism after total hip replacement. N Engl J Med 297:1246

Harris W, Athanasoulis C, Waltman A, Salzman E (1982) High and low-dose aspirin prophylaxis against venous thromboembolic disease in total hip replacement. J Bone Joint Surg 64-A:63

Hartman T, Altner P, Freeark R (1970) The effect of limb elevation in preventing venous thrombosis. A venographic study. J Bone Joint Surg 52:1618

Hartshorn J, Teale S, Faiz M (1969) Dextran 75 and postoperative phlebitis. Evaluation of dextran 75 in the prophylaxis of postoperative thrombophlebitis, pulmonary embolism and myocardial infarction. Arch Surg 98:694

Hartsuck J, Greenfield L (1973) Postoperative thromboembolism. A clinical study with ^{125}I-fibrinogen and pulmonary scanning. Arch Surg 107:733

Hassan MA, Rahman EA, Rahman IA (1973) Postoperative deep vein thrombosis in Sudanese patients. Br Med J 1:515

Hassan MA, Rahman EA, Rahman IA (1974) Prostatectomy and deep vein thrombosis in Sudanese patients. Br J Surg 61:650

Hatton MWC, Berry LR, Regoeczi E (1978) Inhibition of thrombin by antithrombin III in the presence of certain glycosaminoglycans found in the mammalian aorta. Thromb Res 13:655

Havig Ö (1977) Deep vein thrombosis and pulmonary embolism. An autopsy study with multiple regression analysis of possible risk factors. Acta Chir Scand [Suppl] 478

Heaf DJ, Kaijser L, Eklund B, Carlson LA (1977) Differences in heparin-released lipolytic activity on the superficial and deep veins of the human forearm. Eur J Clin Invest 7:195

Heather B, Jennings S, Greenhalgh R (1980) The saline dilution test − a preoperative predictor of DVT. Br J Surg 67:63

Heatley RV, Hughes LE, Morgan A, Okwonga W (1976) Preoperative or postoperative deep-vein thrombosis? Lancet I:437

Hedblom C (1925) Diaphragmatic hernia. A study of three hundred and seventy-eight cases in which operation was performed. JAMA 85:947

Hedin H (1977) Dextran-induced anaphylactoid reactions in man. Immunological in vitro and in vivo studies. Acta Univ Ups Abst Ups Diss Fac Med 432

Hedin H, Smedegård G (1979) Complement profiles in monkeys subjected to aggregate (immune complex) anaphylaxis, and following injection of soluble and particulate polysaccharides. Int Arch Allergy Appl Immunol 60:286

Hedin H, Richter W, Ring J (1976) Dextran-induced anaphylactoid reactions in man. Role of dextran reactive antibodies. Int Arch Allergy Appl Immunol 52:145

Hedlund PO (1975) Postoperative venous thrombosis in benign prostatic disease. A study of 316 patients with the ^{125}I-fibrinogen uptake test. Scand J Urol Nephrol [Suppl] 27

Hedlund PO, Blombäck M (1979) The effect of prophylaxis with low dose heparin on blood coagulation parameters. A double blind study in connection with transvesical prostatectomy. Thromb Haemost 41:337

Hedlund PO, Blombäck M (1981) The effects of low dose heparin treatment in patients undergoing transvesical prostatectomy. Urol Res 9:147

Hedner U, Martinsson G (1978) Inhibition of activated Hageman factor (Factor XIIa) by an inhibitor of the plasminogen activation (PA inhibitor). Thromb Res 12:1015

Hedner U, Nilsson IM (1973) Antithrombin III in a clinical material. Thromb Res 3:631

Hedner U, Martinsson G, Bergqvist D (1983) Influence of operative trauma on F XII and inhibitor of plasminogen activator

Hehre EJ, Sugg JY, Neill JM (1952) The serological activity of dextran. NY Acad Sci 55:467

Heidrich H, Wachta T (1978) Blutviskosität unter intravenöser Langzeitinfusion von niedermolekularem Dextran (Rheomacrodex® 10%). Dtsch Med Wochenschr 103:298

Heistø H, Lund I (1953) Studies on allergic reactions following administration of dextran. J Oslo City Hosp 3:159

Hellem A (1960) The adhesiveness of human blood platelets in vitro. Scand J Clin Lab Invest [Suppl] 51:117

Hellem A, Ödegaard AE, Skålhegg BA (1963) Investigations on adenosine diphosphate (ADP) induced platelet adhesiveness in vitro. I: The ADP-platelet reaction in various experimental conditions. Thromb Diath Haemorrh 10:61

Hellgren M, Hägnevik K, Blombäck M (1979) Inhalation of heparin and its effect on blood coagulation. Thromb Haemost 42:305

Hellgren M, Hägnevik K, Blombäck M (1981) Heparin aerosol effect on blood coagulation and pulmonary function. Thromb Res 21:493

Hellgren U, Scheibe O (1975) Thromboemboliprophylaxe mit Acetyl-salicylsäure (Colfarit). Wirkung und Nebenwirkung. Chirurg 46:173

Hemker HC (1977) Drugs affecting coagulation factor synthesis. In: Ogston D, Bennett B (eds) Haemostasis: biochemistry, physiology, and pathology. Wiley & Sons, London New York Sydney Toronto

Hemker HC, Veltkamp JJ, Hensen A, Loeliger EA (1963) Nature of prothrombin biosynthesis pre-prothrombinaemia in vitamin K-deficiency. Nature 200:589

Henderson HP, Cooke ED, Bowcock S, Hackett MEJ (1978) After-exercise thermography predicting postoperative deep vein thrombosis. Br Med J 1:1020

Henderson SR, Lund CJ, Cresman WT (1972) Antepartum pulmonary embolism. Am J Obstet Gynecol 112:475

Hendolin H (1980) The influence of continuous epidural analgesia and general anaesthesia on the peri- and postoperative course of patients subjected to retropubic prostatectomy. Thesis, University of Kuopio

Hendolin H, Mattila MAK, Poikolainen E (1981) The effect of lumbar epidural analgesia on the development of deep vein thrombosis of the legs after open prostatectomy. Acta Chir Scand 147:425

Henley EE, McPhaul JJ, Albert SN (1957) Anaphylactic reaction to dextran. Med Ann D C 27:21

Henry M (1975) Pulmonary embolism and maternal mortality 1966–1973. J Ir Med Assoc 68:175

Henry R (1971) Methods for the experimental study of intravascular thrombus formation. In: Bang N, Beller F, Deutsch E, Mammen E (eds) Thrombosis and bleeding disorders. Theory and methods. Academic Press, New York London

Hensby CN, Barnes PJ, Dollery CT, Dargie H (1979) Production of 6-0X0-PGF$_1\alpha$ by human lung in vivo. Lancet II:1162

Herbert DC (1968) Anticoagulant therapy and the acute abdomen. Br J Surg 55:353

Hergt K (1972) Blood levels of thrombocytes in burned patients: observations on their behavior in relation to the clinical condition of the patients. J Trauma 12:599

Herlev Hospital Study Group (1979) Diagnostic decision-process in suspected pulmonary embolism. Lancet I:1336

Hermann RE, Davis JH, Holden WD (1961) Pulmonary embolism: a clinical and pathologic study with emphasis on the effect of prophylactic therapy with anticoagulants. Am J Surg 102:19

Hewson W (1771) Experimental inquiries. 1. An inquiry into the properties of the blood, with some remarks on some of its morbid appearances, and an appendix relating to the discovery of the lymphatic system in birds, fish and the animals called amphibians. T Cadell, London

Heyns AP, Badenhorst CJ, Retief FP (1977) ADPase activity of normal and atherosclerotic human aorta intima. Thromb Haemost 37:429

Heyns AP, van den Berg DJ, Potgieler GM, Retief FP (1974) The inhibition of platelet aggregation by an aorta intima extract. Thromb Diath Haemorrh 32:417

Hickman JA (1971) A study of the metabolism of fibrinogen after surgical operations. Clin Sci 41:141

Hicks BH, Hazell J (1973) Safe use of ^{125}I-fibrinogen. Lancet II:931

Hiebert LM, Jaques LB (1976) The observation of heparin on endothelium after injection. Thromb Res 8:195

Highsmith RF, Rosenberg RD (1974) The inhibition of human plasmin by human antithrombin-heparin cofactor. J Biol Chem 249:4335

Higgs EA, Moncada S, Vane JR (1978) Effect of prostacyclin (PGI$_2$) on platelet adhesion to rabbit arterial subendothelium. Prostaglandins 16:17

Hiilesmaa V (1960) Occurrence and anticoagulant treatment of thromboembolism in gravidae, parturients and gynaecologic patients. A study of 678 cases treated in the Women's Clinic of the University of Helsinki in 1953–1957. Acta Obstet Gynaecol Scand [Suppl] 2

Hill J, Caprini J, Robbins J (1976) An unusual complication of minidose heparin therapy. Clin Orthop 118:130

Hill R, Dahrling B, Starzl T, Rifkind O (1967) Death after transplantation. An analysis of sixty cases. Am J Med 42:327

Hills NH, Pflug JJ, Jeyasingh K, Boardman L, Calnan JS (1972) Prevention of deep vein thrombosis by intermittent pneumatic compression of calf. Br Med J 1:131

Hint H (1964) The flow properties of erythrocyte suspensions in isolated rabbit's ear, the effects of erythrocyte aggregation, haematocrit and perfusion pressure. Bibl Anat 4:112

Hint H (1965) Colloid osmotic effect in isolated perfused rabbit's ear. Bibl Anat 7:250

Hint H (1968) The pharmacology of dextran and the pathophysiological background for the clinical use of Rheomacrodex and Macrodex. Acta Anaesthiol Belg 19:119

Hirsh J, Dacie JV (1966) Persistent post-splenectomy thrombocytosis and thrombo-embolism: a consequence of continuing anaemia. Br J Haematol 12:44

Hirsh J, Gallus AS (1975) ^{125}I-fibrinogen labelled fibrinogen scanning. Use in the diagnosis of venous thrombosis. JAMA 233:970

Hirsh J, Street D, Cade JF, Amy H (1973) Relation between bleeding time and platelet connective tissue reactions after aspirin. Blood 41:369

Hirsh J, Gallus AS, Cade JF (1974) Diagnosis of thrombosis. Evaluation of ^{125}I-fibrinogen scanning and blood tests. Thromb Diath Haemorrh 32:11

Hirsjärvi E, Palmborg S, Lepäntalo MJA (1974) Deep vein thrombosis in hip-joint surgical geriatric patients diagnosed by radioiodinated fibrinogen. Gerontology 20:58

Hjelmstedt Å (1968) Deep venous thrombosis in tibial fracture. A clinical phlebographic and physiological study. Thesis. Almquist and Wiksell, Uppsala

Hladovec J (1977) Antithrombotic effects of some flavonoids alone and combined with acetylsalicylic acid. Arzneim Forsch 27:1989

Hobbs J (1974) Surgery and sclerotherapy in the treatment of varicose veins. Arch Surg 109:793

Hobbs J (1978) Compression sclerotherapy of varicose veins. In: Bergan J, Yao J (eds) Venous problems. Year Book Med Publ, Chicago London

Hobson R, Croom R, Rich N (1973) Influence of heparin and low molecular weight dextran on the patency of autogenous vein grafts in the venous system. Ann Surg 178:773

Hodgson DC (1964) Venous stasis during surgery. Anaesthiol 19:96

Hodgson J, Portmann K (1974) Complications of 10453 consecutive first trimester abortions: a prospective study. Am J Obstet Gynaecol 120:802

Hodin E, Dass J (1960) Spontaneous retroperitoneal haemorrhage complicating anticoagulant therapy. Ann Surg 170:848

Hohl M, Lüscher P, Annaheim M, Fridrich R, Gruber UF (1980) Dihydroergotamine and heparin or heparin alone for the prevention of postoperative thrombosis in gynecology. Arch Gynecol 230:15

Hohl M, Lüscher K, Tichy J, Stiner M, Fridrich R, Gruber U, Käser O (1980) Prevention of postoperative thromboembolism by dextran 70 or low-dose heparin. Obstet Gynaecol 55:497

Holford CP (1976) Graded compression for preventing deep venous thrombosis. Br Med J 2:969

Holleman WH, Coen LJ (1970) Characterization of peptides released from human fibrinogen by arvin. Biochim Biophys Acta 200:587

Holmberg L, Mannucci BM, Turesson I, Ruggeri ZM, Nilsson IM (1974) Factor VIII antigen in the vessel wall in von Willebrand's disease and haemophilia A. Scand J Haematol 13:33

Holmer E (1979) Heparin – chemical and biological properties (In Swedish). Ronden 12:161

Holmer E (1980) Anticoagulant properties of heparin and heparin fractions. Scand J Haematol [Suppl] 36:25

Holmer E, Lindahl U, Bäckström G, Thunberg L, Sandberg H, Söderström G, Andersson L-O (1980) Anticoagulant activities and effects on platelets of a heparin fragment with high affinity for antithrombin. Thromb Res 18:861

Holmer E, Mattsson C, Nilsson S, Söderström G, Svahn CM (1981) Antithrombotic properties of a low molecular weight heparin. Thromb Haemost 46:117

Holmer E, Söderström G, Andersson L-O (1979) Studies on the mechanism of the rate enhancing effect of heparin on the thrombin-antithrombin III reaction. Eur J Biochem 93:1

Holmes I, Smith G, Freuler F (1977) The effect of intravenous adenosine diphosphate on the number of circulating platelets in experimental animals inhibition by prostaglandin E_1, dipyridamole, SH-869 and VK-774. Thromb Haemost 37:36

Holmsen H, Day HJ, Stormorken H (1969) The blood platelet release reaction. Scand J Haematol [Suppl] 8:3

Holt PJL, Bennett RM (1972) Pneumatic stockings to treat "rheumatic oedema". Lancet II:688

Holtgrewe HL, Valk WL (1962) Factors influencing the mortality and morbidity of transurethral prostatectomy: a study of 2015 cases. J Urol 87:450

Homan JDH, Lens J (1948) A simple method for the purification of heparin. Biochim Biophys Acta 2:333

Homans J (1934) Thrombosis of the deep veins of the lower leg causing pulmonary embolism. N Engl J Med 211:993

Hongler T, Schmitt HE, Fridrich R, Duckert F, Gruber UF (1976) Das Verhalten intraoperativ entstandener tiefer Venenthrombosen, beurteilt anhand wiederholter Phlebographien. Klin Wochenschr 54:521

Höör G, Buttermann G, Theisinger W, Pabst HW (1976) Prevention of postoperative thromboembolism by various treatments. Eur J Nuclear Med 1:197

Hopwood J, Höök M, Linker A, Lindahl U (1976) Anticoagulant activity of heparin. Isolation of antithrombin-binding sites. FEBS Lett 69:51

Horner AA (1971) Macromolecular heparin from rat skin: isolation characterization and depolymerisation with ascorbate. J Biol Chem 246:231

Houghton GR, Papadakis EG, Rizza CR (1978) Changes in blood coagulation during total hip replacement. Lancet I:1336

Hovig T (1963) Release of platelet-aggregating substance (adenosine diphosphate) from rabbit blood platelets induced by saline "extract" of tendons. Thromb Diath Haemorrh 9:264

Hovig T, McKenzie FN, Arfors K-E (1974) Measurement of the platelet response to laser-induced micorvascular injury. Ultrastructural studies. Thromb Diath Haemorrh 32:695

Howard JM, Teng CT, Loeffler RK (1956) Studies on dextran of various molecular sizes. Ann Surg 143:369

Howell WH, Holt E (1918) Two new factors in blood coagulation: heparin and proantithrombin. Am J Physiol 47:328

Howie PW (1979) Blood clotting and fibrinolysis in pregnancy. Postgrad Med J 55:362

Hoyt RK, Domanig E, Hahnloser P, Delin NA, Schenk WG (1964) Blood viscosity alteration following haemorrhage and after volume restitution with saline, plasma, dextrans, or shed blood. Surg Forum 15:34

Hrushesky W (1978) Subcutaneous heparin-induced thrombocytopenia. Arch Intern Med 138:1489

Hull R, Delmore TJ, Hirsh J, Gent M, Armstrong P, Lofthouse R, MacMillan A, Blackstone I, Reed-Davis R, Detwiler RC (1979a) Effectiveness of intermittent pulsative elastic stockings for the prevention of calf and thigh vein thrombosis in patients undergoing elective knee surgery. Thromb Res 16:37

Hull R, Hirsh J, Sackett DL, Powers P, Turpie AGG, Walker I, McBride J (1979b) The value of adding impedance phletysmography to ^{125}I-fibrinogen leg scanning for the detection of deep vein thrombosis in high risk surgical patients: a comparative study between patients undergoing general surgery and hip surgery. Thromb Res 15:227

Hume M, Glancy JJ, Chan YK (1969) Blood tests and Doppler flowmeter examination. Arch Surg 97:894

Hume M, Sevitt S, Thomas LP (1970) Venous thrombosis and pulmonary embolism. Harvard Univ Press, Cambridge

Hume M, Kuriakose T, Xavier ZL, Turner RH (1973) ^{125}I-fibrinogen and the prevention of venous thrombosis. Arch Surg 107:803

Hume M, Turner RH, Kuriakose TX, Surprenant J (1976) Venous thrombosis after total hip replacement. Combined monitoring as a guide for prophylaxis and treatment. J Bone Joint Surg 58:933

Humphreys WV, Walker A, Charlesworth D (1976) Altered viscosity and yield stress in patients with abdominal malignancy: relationship to deep vein thrombosis. Br J Surg 63:559

Hunter WC, Krygier JJ, Kennedy JC, Sneeden VD (1945) Etiology and prevention of thrombosis of deep leg veins. A study of 400 cases. Surgery 17:178

Hurson B, Ennis JT, Corrigan TP, Macauley P (1979) Dextran prophylaxis in total hip replacement: a scintigraphic evaluation of the incidence of deep vein thrombosis and pulmonary embolus. Ir J Med Sci 148:140

Husni EH (1967) The oedema of arterial reconstruction. Circulation [Suppl 1] 35:169

Husni E, Pena L, Lanhert E (1967) Thrombophlebitis in pregnancy. Am J Obstet Gynaecol 97:901

Hussey C, Bernhard V, McLean M, Fobian J (1979) Heparin induced platelet aggregation: in vitro confirmation of thrombotic complications associated with heparin therapy. Ann Clin Lab Sci 9:487

Hutter O, Duckert F, Fridrich R, Gruber UF (1976) Dextran 40 zur Prophylaxe tiefer Venenthrombosen in der Chirurgie. Dtsch Med Wochenschr 101:1834

Huttunen H, Mattila MAK, Hakalehto J, Kettunen K, Rehnberg V, Babinski M (1971) Single infusion of dextran 70 in the prophylaxis of postoperative deep venous thrombosis. Ann Chir Gynecol Fenn 60:119

Huttunen H, Mattila MAK, Alhava EM, Kettunen K, Karjalainen P, Poikolainen P, Huttunen K (1977) Preoperative infusion of dextran 70 and dextran 40 in the prevention of postoperative deep venous thrombosis as confirmed by the ^{125}I-labelled fibrinogen uptake method. Ann Chir Gynecol Fenn 66:79

Hwang WS (1969) The rarity of pulmonary thromboembolism in Asians. Singapore Med J 9:276

Immelman EJ, Jeffery P, Benatar SR, Elliot MS, Ferguson AD, Smith JS, Shepstone BJ, Furnston MR, Jacobs R, Louw JH (1981) The prevention of post-operative thromboembolic disease — a prospective trial. International Vascular Symposium. Abstract 073, London. Groote Schuur Thromboembolus Study Group, Cape Town, South Africa

Inagaki A (1968) An experimental study on the role of microthrombi in the formation of venous thrombosis. Jap Circ J 32:715

Ingelman B, Siegbahn K (1944) An electron microscopic study of dextran molecules. Arch Kemi 186:1

Inman WHW, Vessey MP, Westerholm B, Engelund A (1970) Thromboembolic disease and the steroidal content of oral contraceptives. A report to the Committee on Safety of Drugs. Br Med J 2:203

Innes D, Sevitt S (1964) Coagulation and fibrinolysis in injured patients. J Clin Pathol 17:1

An International Multicentre Trial (1975) Prevention of fatal postoperative pulmonary embolism by low doses of heparin. Lancet II:45

Isacson S, Nilsson IM (1972a) Coagulation and platelet adhesiveness in recurrent "idiopathic" venous thrombosis and thrombophlebitis. Acta Chir Scand 138:263

Isacson S, Nilsson IM (1972b) Defective fibrinolysis in blood and vein walls in recurrent "idiopathic" venous thrombosis. Acta Chir Scand 138:313

Ishak M, Morley K (1981) Deep venous thrombosis after total hip arthroplasty: a prospective controlled study to determine the prophylactic effect of graded pressure stockings. Br J Surg 68:429

Jackaman FR, Perry BJ, Siddons H (1978) Deep vein thrombosis after thoracotomy. Thorax 33:761

Iverius PH, Laurent TC (1966) Precipitation of some plasma proteins by the addition of dextran or polyethylene glycol. Biochim Biophys Acta 133:371

Jackson AM, Pollock AV (1981) Skin necrosis after heparin injection. Br Med J 283:1087

Jackson P (1972) Puerperal thromboembolic disease in "high-risk" cases. Br Med J 1:263

Jacobaeus U (1957) Studies on the effect of dextran on the coagulation of blood. Diss Med Karolinska Inst Stockh

Jacobsen CD, Chandler AB (1965) Thrombolysis in vitro. I. Method, comparison of various thrombolytic agents and factors influencing thrombolysis. Scand J Clin Lab Invest 17:209

Jacobsson B (1969) Effect of pretreatment with dextran 70 on platelet adhesiveness and thromboembolic complications following percutaneous arterial catheterization. Acta Radiol 8:289

Jacobsson L, Mattsson S, Bernstein K, Ulmsten U, Åstedt B (1980) A method for determination of the depth of thrombi after injection of fibrinogen labelled with iodine 125. Br J Radiol 53: 668

Jaenike JR, Waterhouse C (1955) Metabolic and haemodynamic changes induced by the prolonged administration of dextran. Circulation 11:1

Jaffe EA, Hoyer LW, Nachman RL (1973) Synthesis of antihemophilic factor antigen by cultured human endothelial cells. J Clin Invest 52:2757

Jaffe MD, Willis PW (1965) Multiple fractures associated with long-term sodium heparin therapy. JAMA 193:158

Jansen H (1972) Postoperative thromboembolism and its prevention with 500 ml dextran given during operation. With a special study of the venous flow pattern in the lower extremities. Acta Chir Scand [Suppl] 427

Janvrin SB, Davies G, Greenhalgh RM (1980a) Ultra-low-dose intravenous heparin. Lancet I:1303

Janvrin SB, Davies G, Greenhalgh RM (1980b) The pelvic phlebolith — a marker of venous thrombosis. Br J Surg 67:367

Janvrin SB, Davies G, Greenhalgh RM (1980c) Postoperative deep vein thrombosis caused by intravenous fluids during surgery. Br J Surg 67:690

Jaques LB (1949) A study of the toxicity of the protamine salmine. Br J Pharmacol 4:135

Jaques LB (1967) The pharmacology of heparin and heparinoids. In: Progress Med Chem 5:139

Jaques LB (1976) Identification of heparin in publications. Thromb Res 8:115

Jaques LB (1978a) The nature of mucopolycaccharides. Med Hypothes 4:123

Jaques LB (1978b) Simplified and rational nomenclature for heparins, glucosaminoglycans and sulfated mucopolysaccharides. Artery 4:144

Jaques LB (1979) Heparin: an old drug with a new paradigm. Science 206:528

Jaques LB, Kavanaugh LW (1973) Variability of heparin preparations in clinical use. Thromb Haemost 56:171

Jaques LB, Mahadoo J (1978) Pharmacodynamics and clinical effectiveness of heparin. Semin Thromb Haemost 4:298

Jaques LB, Charles AF, Best CH (1938) The administration of heparin. Acta Med Scand [Suppl] 90:190

Jaques LB, Mahadoo J, Kavanaugh LW (1976) Intrapulmonary heparin. A new procedure for anticoagulant therapy. Lancet II:1157

Jardon L (1976) Deep vein thrombosis in surgery. Detection by the method using labelled fibrinogen. Acta Anaesthiol Belg 27:193

Järhult J, Mårtensson O (1980) Mesenteric vein occlusion as a complication in estrogen treatment in prostatic carcinoma (In Swedish). Läkartidn 77:2911

Järvinen P, Asp K (1975) Clinical diagnosis and prognosis of deep venous thrombosis. Ann Chir Gynecol Fenn 64:96

Jaswig EH, Jaswig-Priewe H (1973) Thromboembolieprophylaxe bei der Radiumtherapie des Kollum-Karzinoms. Geburtshilfe Frauenheilkd 33:988

Jeanloz RW (1965) Heparin enzymatic deproteinization and preparation of crystalline barium and benzidine salts. In: Whistler RL, Bemiller JN, Wolfram NL (eds) Methods in carbohydrate chemistry. Vol 5. Academic Press, New York

Jeffcoate TNA, Wilson JK (1955) The effect of hydergine on uterine action. Lancet I:1187

Jennings G, Esler M, Holmes R (1979) Treatment of orthostatic hypotension with dihydroergotamine. Br Med J 2:307

Jick H, Porter J (1978) Thrombophlebitis of the lower extremities and ABO blood type. Arch Int Med 38:1566

Jick HJ, Sloane D, Borda IT, Shapiro S (1968) Efficacy and toxicity of heparin in relation to age and sex. N Engl J Med 279:284

Jick H, Sloane D, Westerholm B, Inman WHW, Vessey MP, Shapiro S, Lewis GP, Worcester J (1969) Venous thromboembolic disease and ABO blood type. Lancet I:539

Jipp P (1962) Subkutane Fettgewebsnekrosen nach Antikoagulantientherapie. Chirurg 33:481

Joffe SN (1974) Racial incidence of postoperative deep vein thrombosis in South Africa. Br J Surg 61:982

Joffe SN (1975a) The incidence of postoperative deep vein thrombosis. Thromb Res 7:141

Joffe SN (1975b) Incidence of postoperative deep vein thrombosis in neurosurgical patients. J Neurosurg 42:201

Joffe SN (1975c) Postoperative deep vein thrombosis in children. J Pediat Surg 10:539

Joffe SN (1976) Drug prevention of postoperative deep vein thrombosis. A comparative study of calcium heparinate and sodium pentosan polysulphate. Arch Surg 111:37

Joffe SN, Immelman EJ, Louw JH (1973) The incidence of postoperative deep vein thrombosis. S Afr J Surg 11:107

Johansson E, Forsberg K (1976) Thromboprophylaxis with hydroxychloroquine in patients undergoing total limb replacement (In Swedish). Sven Läkaressällsk Förh 85:24

Johansson E, Ericson K, Åsard P (1975) Postoperative leg vein thrombosis and pulmonary embolism after upper abdominal operations. A prospective study with ^{125}I-fibrinogen test and pulmonary scintigraphy. Acta Chir Scand 141:522

Johansson E, Forsberg K, Johnsson H (1981) Clinical and experimental evaluation of the thromboprophylactic effect of hydroxychloroquine sulfate after total hip replacement. Haemostasis 10:89

Johansson S, Holmdahl S (1945) On thromboembolism. A summary from a 20-year period (In Swedish). Nord Med 25:524

Johnson EA, Kirkwood TBL, Stirling Y, Perez-Requejo JL, Ingram CIC, Bangham DR, Brozovic M (1976) Four heparin preparations: anti-Xa potentiating effect of heparin subcutaneous injection. Thromb Haemost 35:586

Johnson P (1971) The role of lung scanning in pulmonary embolism. Semin Nucl Med 1:161

Johnson RH, Mansfield A (1978) A new method for the detection of plasminogen activator content of vein walls. Acta Haematol 60:243

Johnson SR, Bygdeman S, Eliasson R (1968) Effect of dextran on postoperative thrombosis. Acta Chir Scand [Suppl] 387:80

Johnson W, Eiseman B (1969) Evaluation of arteriovenous shunts to maintain patency of venous autograft. Am J Surg 118:915

Johnsson K-Å, Göthman B, Nordström S (1974) The iliac compression syndrome. Acta Radiol 15: 539

Jönsson G (1951) Venous circulation in the lower half of the body. A clinico-experimental study with special reference to the postoperative phase. Acta Chir Scand [Suppl] 161

Jørgensen L, Hovig T, Rowsell HC, Mustard JF (1970) Adenosine diphosphate-induced platelet aggregation and vascular injury in swine and rabbits. Am J Pathol 61:161

Jorpes E (1935) The chemistry of heparin. Biochem J 29:1817

Jorpes E (1936) Chemistry of heparin and its medical application. Hygiea 98:218

Jorpes E (1946) Heparin in the treatment of thrombosis. 2nd ed. Oxford Med, London

Jorpes E, Holmgren H, Wilander O (1937) Über das Vorkommen von Heparin in den Gefäßwänden und in den Augen. Ein Beitrag zur Physiologie der Ehrlichschen Mastzellen. Z Mikro Anat Forsch 42:79

Jorpes JE, Boström H, Mutt V (1950) The linkage of the aminogroup in heparin. J Bibl Chem 183: 607

Josa M, Lie JT, Bianco R, Kaye M (1981) Reduction of thrombosis in canine coronary bypass vein grafts with dipyridamole and aspirin. Am J Cardiol 47:1248

Jung W, Fridrich R, Duckert F, Gruber UF (1975) Der Radiofibrinogentest zur Diagnose frischer tiefer Venenthrombosen. Schweiz Med Wochenschr 105:391

Kabat EA, Bezer AE (1958) The effect of variation in molecular weight on the antigenicity of dextran in man. Arch Biochem Biophys 78:306

Kabat EA, Turino GM, Tarrow AB, Maurer PB (1957) Studies on the immunochemical basis of allergic reactions to dextran in man. J Clin Invest 36:1160

Kaegi A, Pineo GF, Shimizu A, Trivedi H, Hirsh J, Gent M (1975) The role of sulfinpyrazone in the prevention of arterio-venous shunt thrombosis. Circulation 52:497

Kahlé LH, Dannijs GJ, ten Cate JW (1975) Effects of some semisynthetic rutoside derivates on human platelets. Bibl Anat 13:263

Kaij K (1959) The frequency of thromboembolism in autopsy material (In Swedish). Sven Läkartidn 56:1437

Kakkar VV (1973) Low-doses of heparin in the prevention of deep vein thrombosis. Bull Schweiz Akad Med Wiss 29:235

Kakkar VV (1975a) Efficacy of low-dose heparin prophylaxis. Curr Ther Res 18:6

Kakkar VV (1975b) Deep vein thrombosis. Detection and prevention. Circulation 51:8

Kakkar VV (1977) Fibrinogen uptake test for detection of deep vein thrombosis – a review of current practice. Semin Nucl Med 7:229

Kakkar VV (1978) The current status of low-dose heparin in the prophylaxis of thrombophlebitis and pulmonary embolism. World J Surg 2:3

Kakkar VV (1979a) The logistic problems encountered in the multicenter trial of low-dose heparin prophylaxis. In: Verstraete M, Vermylen J, Roberts H (eds) The challenge of clinical trials in thrombosis. Schattauer, Stuttgart New York

Kakkar VV (1979b) Preventing postoperative thromboembolism. Br Med J 2:127

Kakkar VV (1979c) The surgeon's comments II. In: Verstraete M, Vermylen J, Roberts H (eds) The challenge of clinical trials in thrombosis. Schattauer, Stuttgart New York

Kakkar VV (1981) Knowledge and prospective of thromboembolic research. In: Tscherne H, Deutsch E (eds) Postoperative Thromboembolie-Prophylaxe aus aktueller Sicht. Thieme, Stuttgart New York

Kakkar VV, Corrigan T, Spindler J, Fossard DP, Flute PT, Crellin RQ, Wessler S, Yin ET (1972) Efficacy of low doses of heparin in prevention of deep-vein thrombosis after major surgery. Lancet II:101

Kakkar VV, Corrigan TP, Fossard DP, Sutherland K, Thirwell J (1977) Prevention of fatal postoperative pulmonary embolism by low doses of heparin. Reappraisal of results. Int Multicentre Trial. Lancet I:567

Kakkar VV, Djazaeri B, Scully M, Weerasinghe K (1981a) Synthetic heparin analogue and prothrombin time. Lancet I:1167

Kakkar VV, Djazaeri B, Webb P, Scully M, Westwick J, Mac Gregor I (1981b) Low molecular weight heparin and postoperative deep vein thrombosis. Thromb Haemost 46:116

Kakkar VV, Djazaeri B, Fox J, Fletcher M, Scully MF, Westwick J (1982) Low-molecular-weight heparin and prevention of postoperative deep vein thrombosis. Br Med J 1:375

Kakkar VV, Flanc C, Howe CT, O'Shea M, Flute PT (1969a) Treatment of deep vein thrombosis. A trial of heparin, streptokinase and arvin. Br Med J 1:806

Kakkar VV, Howe CT, Flanc C, Clarke MB (1969b) Natural history of postoperative deep-vein thrombosis. Lancet II:230

Kakkar VV, Howe CT, Nicolaides AN, Renney JTG, Clarke MB (1970) Deep vein thrombosis of the leg: Is there a "high-risk" group? Am J Surg 120:527

Kakkar VV, Nicolaides AN, Field ES, Flute PT, Wessler S, Yin ET (1971) Low doses of heparin in prevention of deep-vein thrombosis. Lancet II:669

Kakkar VV, Lawrence D, Bentley PG, de Haas HA, Ward V, Scully MF (1978) A comparative study of low doses of heparin and a heparin analogue in the prevention of postoperative deep vein thrombosis. Thromb Res 13:111

Kakkar VV, Stamatakis J, Bentley P, Lawrence D, de Haas H, Ward V (1979) Prophylaxis for postoperative deep-vein thrombosis. Synergistic effect of heparin and dihydroergotamine. JAMA 241:39

Kamm R, Shapiro A (1976) Hemodynamics of external pneumatic compression. In: Madden J, Hume M (eds) Venous thromboembolism. Prevention and treatment. Appleton-Century-Crofts, New York

Kapsch D, Silver D (1981) Heparin-induced thrombocytopenia with thrombosis and haemorrhage. Arch Surg 116:1423

Kapsch D, Adelstein E, Rhodes G, Silver D (1979) Heparin-induced thrombocytopenia, thrombosis and haemorrhage. Surgery 86:148

Karaca M, Nilsson IM (1971) Fibrinolytic activity in hemiplegic patients. Acta Med Scand 189:325

Karino T, Motomiya M (1981) Vortices in the pockets of a venous valve. Microvasc Res 21:247

Kasimis B, Spiers A (1979) Thrombotic complications in patients with advanced prostatic cancer treated with chemotherapy. Lancet I:159

Kelsey J, Wood P, Charnley J (1976) Prediction of thromboembolism following total hip replacement. Clin Orthop Rel Res 114:247

Kelton J, Blajchman M (1980) Prostaglandin I_2 (prostacyclin). Can Med Assoc Journal 122:175

Kelton JG, Hirsh J, Carter CJ, Buchanan MR (1978a) Sex differences in the antithrombotic effects of aspirin. Blood 52:1073

Kelton JG, Hirsh J, Carter CJ (1978b) Thrombogenic effect of high-dose aspirin in rabbits. J Clin Invest 62:892

Kemble JV (1971) The effect of surgical operation on leg venous flow measured with radioactive hippuran. Postgrad Med J 47:773

Kerber I, Warr O, Richardson C (1968) Pregnancy in a patient with a prosthetic mitral valve associated with a fetal anomaly attributed to warfarin sodium. JAMA 203:223

Kerr MG, Scott DB, Samuel E (1964) Studies of the inferior vena cava in late pregnancy. Br Med J 1:532

Kettunen K (1981) Prophylaxis against postoperative thromboembolism in Finland (In Finnish). Suom Lääkärilehti 36:2907

Kettunen K, Poikolainen E, Karjalainen P, Oksala I, Alhava E, Rehnberg V, Huttunen H, Mattilla M (1974) Low-dose heparin as prophylaxis against postoperative deep vein thrombosis (In Finnish). Duodecim 90:834

Kidess E, Miller H, Briel R, Kunz S (1978) Thrombozytenaggregation nach abdominaler Hysterektomie unter kombinierter Thromboemboliprophylaxe mit Macrodex 6% und Sintrom. Infusionsther 5:86

Kierkegaard A (1980) Incidence of acute deep vein thrombosis in two districts. A phlebographic study. Acta Chir Scand 146:267

Kiesselback TH, Wagner RH (1966) Fibrin-stabilizing factor. A thrombin-labile platelet protein. Am J Physiol 211:1472

Kiil J, Møller JC (1979) Postoperative deep vein thrombosis of the lower limb and prophylactic value of heparin evaluated by phlebography. Acta Radiol [Diagn] (Stockh) 20:507

Kiil J, Taagehøj-Jensen F (1978) Pulmonary embolism associated with elective surgery, detected by ventilation-perfusion scintigraphy. Acta Chir Scand 144:427

Kiil J, Kiil J, Axelsen F, Andersen D (1978) Prophylaxis against postoperative pulmonary embolism and deep-vein thrombosis by low-dose heparin. Lancet I:1115

Kimball AM, Hallum A, Cates W (1978) Deaths caused by pulmonary thromboembolism after legally induced abortion. Am J Obstet Gynaecol 132:169

Kincaid-Smith P (1969) Modification of the vascular lesions of rejection in cadaveric renal allografts by dipyridamole and anticoagulants. Lancet II:920

Kindness G, Williamson FB, Long WF (1979) Effects of a sulphated xylan on aggregation of human blood platelets. Thromb Res 16:97

King JB, Joffe SN (1974) The prediction of postoperative deep vein thrombosis, using a newly described test of platelet function. Thromb Diath Haemorrh 32:502

King R, Daly A (1975) The prevention of postoperative pulmonary emboli with low-molecular-weight dextran. Am J Obstet Gynecol 123:46

Kipen CS (1961) Gangrene of the breast, a complication of anticoagulant therapy. N Engl J Med 265:638

Kirstein P, Jogestrand T, Johnsson H, Olsson AG (1980) Antiaggregatory, physiological and clinical effect of Ticlopidine in subjects with peripheral atherosclerosis. Atherosclerosis 36:471

Kiss J (1973) Chemical structure of heparin. In: Kakkar VV, Thomas DP (eds) Heparin. Chemistry and clinical usage. Acad Press, London

Kistner RL, Bell JJ, Nordyke RA, Freeman GC (1972) Incidence of pulmonary embolism in the course of thrombophlebitis of the lower extremities. Am J Surg 124:169

Kitianik E, Quiros RS (1972) Thrombectomy and caval interruption. Indications and results. J Cardiovasc Surg 13:440

Kivikoski J, Lundbom S, Airaksinen JT (1966) The dextran concentration in the umbilical cord of a newborn infant. Acta Anaesth Scand [Suppl] 24:33

Kiviluoto O, Julkanen H, Honkonen K (1979) Vorbeugung venöser Thromboembolien durch niedrig dosiertes Heparin bei Patienten mit proximalen Femurbrüchen. Zentralbl Chir 105:460

Kladetzky RG, Popov-Cenic S, Müller N, Hack G, Lang U (1977) The effect of dextran 70 on the intra- and postoperative behaviour of haemostasis. Bibl Anat 16:463

Klein MD, Bell WR, Nasser N, Lown B (1969) The effect of arvin upon cardiac function. Proc Soc Exp Biol Med 132:1123

Klenerman L, Chakrabarti R, Mackie I, Brozovic M, Stirling M (1977) Changes in haemostatic system after application of a tourniquet. Lancet I:970

Kline A, Hughes LE, Campbell H, Williams A, Zlosnick J, Leach KG (1975) Dextran 70 in prophylaxis of thromboembolic disease after surgery: a clinically oriented randomized double-blind trial. Br Med J 2:109

Knight MTN, Dawson R (1976) Effect of intermittent compression of the arms on deep venous thrombosis in the legs. Lancet II:1265

Knight MTN, Metrewelli C (1977) Postoperative pulmonary perfusion defects: their natural history, origin and significance. Br J Surg 64:712

Knight MTN, Dawson R, Melrose DG (1977) Fibrinolytic response to surgery. Labile and stable patients and their relevance to post-operative deep venous thrombosis. Lancet II:370

Koch-Weser J (1968) Coumarin necrosis. Editorial notes. Ann Intern Med 68:1365

Kockum-Ivemark C (1979) Fibrinopeptide A — radioimmunoassay and clinical implications. Thesis. University of Stockholm

Kocsis JJ, Hernandovich J, Silver MJ, Smith JB, Ingerman C (1973) Duration of inhibition of platelet prostaglandin formation and aggregation by ingested aspirin or indomethacin. Prostaglandins 3:141

Koekenberg LJL (1961) Experimental use of macrodex as a prophylaxis against postoperative thromboembolism. Exp Med Amst 40:123

Koekenberg LJL (1962) Experimental use of macrodex as a prophylaxis against post-operative thromboembolism. Bull Soc Int Chir 21:501

Köster KH, Schwartz M, Gele V, Sindrup E (1957) Blood volume changes after infusion of dextran solutions. Lancet II:262

Kohen M, Mattikow M, Middleton E, Butsch DW (1970) A study of three untoward reactions to dextran. J Allergy 46:309

Kohn P, Zakert F, Vormittag E, Havelec L (1974) Die tödliche Lungenembolie in der Allgemeinchirurgie: Häufigkeit, Risikofaktoren, Diagnostik. Acta Chir Austriaca 6:122

Kokores JA, Economopoulos TC, Alexopoulos C, Pyrovolakis J, Papayannis AG (1977) Platelet function tests during major operation for gastrointestinal carcinoma. Br J Surg 64:147

Koppenhagen K, Häring R (1981) Thromboembolieprophylaxe mit vermindertem Blutungsrisiko. Untersuchungen mit Heparin-Dihydergot 2500. Med Welt 32:1020

Koppenhagen K, Wiechmann A, Frey E, Wenig HG, Latka H, Zühlke H-V, Tank H, Hardieck J, Ernst H, Häring R (1977) Klinisch-experimentelle Ergebnisse mit Heparin-Dihydroergotamin. Dtsch Med Wochenschr 102:1374

Koppenhagen K, Vogt L, Wenig HG (1979a) Dihydroergotamin-Wirkung auf die Lungenperfusion im Akzelerationsstress. Dtsch Med Wochenschr 104:1208

Koppenhagen K, Wiechmann A, Zühlke H-V, Wenig HG, Häring R (1979b) Leistungsfähigkeit und Risiko der Thromboembolieprophylaxe in der Chirurgie. Eine vergleichende Untersuchung von Heparin-Dihydergot und "low-dose"-Heparin. Therapiewoche 29:5920

Korvald E, Støren E, Ongre A (1973) Simultaneous use of warfarin-sodium and dextran 70 to prevent post-operative venous thrombosis in patients with hip fractures. J Oslo City Hosp 23:25

Korvald E, Abildgaard U, Fagerhol MK (1974) Major operations, hemostatic parameters and venous thrombosis. Thromb Res 4:147

Kraemer PM (1977) Heparin releases heparan sulfate from the cell surface. Biochem Biophys Res Commun 78:1334

Kraemmer-Nielsen H, Bechgaard P, From-Nielsen P, Elbjaer-Husted S, Geday E (1981) 178 fatal cases of pulmonary embolism in a medical department. Acta Med Scand 209:351

Kraytman M, Kutnowski M, Ansay J, Fastrez R (1976) Prophylaxie par l'heparine sous-cutanée à faibles doses des thromboses veineuses postopératoires. Acta Chir Belg 5:519

Kremer H, Narik G (1955) Die pharmakodynamische Beeinflußbarkeit der Uterusmotorik sub partu. Geburtsh Frauenheilkd 15:433

Kristiansen P, Bergentz S-E, Bergqvist D, Nylander G (1981) Thrombosis after elective phlebography as demonstrated with the ^{125}I-fibrinogen test. Acta Radiol [Diagn] (Stockh) 22:577

Kroese A, Doblaug I (1976) Subcutaneous low dose heparin in the prevention of postoperative thromboembolic complications. J Oslo City Hosp 26:45

Kroese AJ, Stiris G (1976) The risk of deep vein thrombosis after operations on a bloodless lower limb. A venographic study. Injury 7:271

Kruse-Blinkenberg HO, Bech-Jansen P, Jensen J, Schmidt A, Gormsen J (1977a) Low dose heparin in major surgery: clinical relevance of plasma heparin concentration. Haemostasis 6:252

Kruse-Blinkenberg HO, Bech-Jansen P, Gormsen J (1977b) Plasma heparin concentrations in thoracic surgery. Low-dose heparin prophylaxis. Scand J Thor Cardiovasc Surg 11:229

Kruse-Blinkenberg HO, Gormsen J (1980) The influence of low-dose heparin in elective surgery on blood coagulation, fibrinolysis, platelet function, antithrombin III and antiplasmin. Acta Chir Scand 146:375

Kruse-Blinkenberg HO, Gormsen J, Jensen J, Thomsen F, Wille-Jørgensen P (1980) Low-dose heparin in elective abdominal surgery. Correlation between concentrations of heparin, antithrombin III and antiplasmin in patients with and without DVT. Acta Chir Scand 146:383

Kümmel H (1908) Abkürzung des Heilungsverlaufs Laparatomierter durch frühzeitiges Aufstehen. Verh Dtsch Ges Chir 1

Kumuda T, Ishihara M, Ogawa H, Abiko Y (1980) Experimental model of venous thrombosis in rats and effect of some agents. Thromb Res 18:189

Kunz S, Briel RC, Drähne A (1979) Das Thromboserisiko nach abdominaler und vaginaler Hysterektomie. Effektivität und Praktikabilität verschiedener Arten medikamentöser Prophylaxe. Geburtshilfe Frauenheilkd 39:932

Kunz S, Drähne A, Briel RC (1977) Prophylaxe der postoperativen Thromboembolie. Erfahrungen mit Heparin-Dihydergot in der Gynäkologie. In: Pabst HW, Maurer G (eds) Postoperative Thromboembolieprophylaxe. Schattauer, Stuttgart New York, p 133

Kutnowski M, Vandendris M, Steinberger B, Kraytman M (1977) Prevention of postoperative deep-vein thrombosis by low-dose heparin in urological surgery. A double-blind, randomized study. Urol Res 5:123

Kwaan H, Barlow G (1971) The mechanism of action of arvin and reptilase. Thromb Diath Haemorrh 47:361

Kwaan H, Barlow G, Suwanwela N (1973) Fibrinogen and its derivatives in relationship to ancrod and reptilase. Thromb Res 2:123

Laaksonen VO, Arola MKJ, Hannelin M, Inberg MV, Kiivisaari A (1973) Effect of anaesthesia on the incidence of postoperative lower limb thrombosis. Ann Chir Gynecol Fenn 62:304

Laaksonen VO, Arola MKJ, Kivisaari A, Hannelin M (1974) Effect of different modes of operative anaesthesia on the clearance time of ^{125}I-fibrinogen from calf veins. Ann Chir Res 6:356

Lagarde M, Byron PA, Vargaftig B, Dechaunne M (1978) Impairment of platelet thromboxane A_2 generation and of the platelet release reaction in two patients with congenital deficiency of platelet cyclooxygenase. Br J Haematol 38:251

Lahnborg G (1978) Prophylaxis with heparin and oral anticoagulants (In Swedish). In: Thorén L (ed) Anticoagulants and coagulants. Symposium. The Swedish Health Anthorotics Committee on Drug Information, No 3

Lahnborg G (1980) Effect of low-dose heparin and dihydroergotamine prophylaxis on frequency of postoperative deep-vein thrombosis in patients undergoing post-traumatic hip surgery. Acta Chir Scand 146:319

Lahnborg G, Bergström K (1975) Clinical and haemostatic parameters related to thromboembolism and low-dose heparin prophylaxis in major surgery. Acta Chir Scand 141:590

Lahnborg G, Bergström K, Friman L, Lagergren H (1974) Effect of low-dose heparin on incidence of postoperative pulmonary embolism detected by photoscanning. Lancet I:329

Lahnborg G, Berghem L, Lagergren H, Schildt B (1976a) Effect of low-dose heparin on the phagocytic and catabolic function of the reticuloendothelial system in man during surgery. Ann Chir Gynecol Fenn 65:376

Lahnborg G, Lagergren H, Hedenstierna G (1976b) Effects of low-dose heparin prophylaxis on arterial oxygen tension after high laparatomy. Lancet I:54

Lahnborg G, Brundin T, Schildt B (1974) Does epidural analgesia work as prophylaxis against postoperative venous thrombosis? (In Swedish). Sven Läkaresällsk Förh 86:74

Laiwah H, Goudie RB, Goldberg DM, Davidson JF, Murray TS (1970) Australia antigen in west of Scotland and north of England. Lancet II:121

Lam LG, Gilbert JE, Rosenberg RD (1976) The separation of active and inactive forms of heparin. Biochem Biophys Res Commun 69:570

Lambie JM, Barber DC, Dhall DP, Matheson NA (1970a) Dextran 70 in prophylaxis of postoperative venous thrombosis. A controlled trial. Br Med J 2:144

Lambie JM, Mahaffy RG, Barber DC, Karmody AM, Schott MM, Matheson NA (1970b) Diagnostic accurancy in venous thrombosis. Br Med J 2:142

Lamke L-O, Liljedahl S-O (1977) Alterations in the plasma volume after replacement with different solutions (In Swedish). Sven Läkartidn 74:1486

Lane DA, Michalski R, van Ross M, Kakkar VV (1977) Comparison of heparin and a semi-synthetic heparin analogue, A73025. I: Kinetics of clearance from the circulation of man following intravenous injection. Br J Haematol 37:239

Lane DA, MacGregor R, Cella G, Kakkar VV (1979) Administration of fractionated heparins to man. Thromb Haemost 42:419

Langdell RD, Adelson E, Furth FW, Crosby WH (1958) Dextran and prolonged bleeding time. JAMA 25:346

Lange H-J (1977) Multivariate Ansätze in der medizinischen Prognostik. In: Pabst HW, Maurer G (eds) Postoperative Thromboembolie-Prophylaxe. Schattauer, Stuttgart New York

Lange L, Echt M (1972a) Vergleichende Untersuchungen über venentonisierende Pharmaka. Fortschr Med 90:1161

Lange L, Echt M (1972b) Vergleichende Untersuchungen über venentonisierende Pharmaka mit Noradrenalin, Äthyladrianol, Dihydroergotamin und Roßkastanienextrakt. Fortschr Therapie 90:1

Langsjoen P, Murray R (1971) Treatment of postsurgical thromboembolic complications. JAMA 218:855

Lansing AM, Davis WM (1968) Five-year follow-up study of iliofemoral venous thrombectomy. Ann Surg 168:620

Lapetina EG, Schmitges CJ, Chandrabose K, Cuatrecasas P (1977) Cyclic AMP and PG inhibit membrane phospholipase activity in platelets. Biochem Biophys Res Commun 76:828

Larsson J, Risberg B (1977) Fibrinolytic activity in human legs in tourniquet ischemia. Thromb Res 11:817

Lasker SE, Stivala SS (1966) Physiochemical studies of fractionated bovine heparin. 1. Some dilute solution properties. Arch Biochem Biophys 115:360

Latto C (1979) Postoperative deep vein thrombosis in Nigerians on high-fibre diets. Br Med J 1:199

Laube L, Reichelt W, Arndt JO (1977) Vergleichende Untersuchungen über die Venenwirksamkeit des ADH-Abkömmlings Ornithin-9-Vasopressin sowie von Dihydroergotamin am kreislaufgesunden Menschen. Herz-Kreislauf 9:295

Laurell AB (1951) Influence of dextran on the conversion of fibrinogen to fibrin. Scand J Clin Lab Invest 3:262

Laurent TC (1963) The interaction between polysaccharides and other macromolecules. 5. The solubility of proteins in the presence of dextran. Biochem J 89:253

Laurent TC, Tengblad A, Thunberg L, Höök M, Lindahl U (1978) The molecular-weight-dependence of the anti-coagulant activity of heparin. Biochem J 175:691

Lawrence D, Kakkar VV (1980) Post-phlebitic syndrome — a functional assessment. Br J Surg 67: 686

Lawrence JC, Xabregas A, Gray L, Ham JM (1977) Seasonal variation in the incidence of deep vein thrombosis. Br J Surg 64:777

Leandoer L (1968) Fibrinogen in blood and lymph after massive haemorrhage in dogs. Acta Chir Scand 134:511

Leandoer L, Bergentz S-E, Nilsson IM (1968) Effect of heparin and AMCA on coagulation and fibrinolysis in blood and lymph following massive haemorrhage in dogs. Acta Chir Scand 134:1

Lea-Thomas M, Browse NL (1972) Internal iliac vein thrombosis. Acta Radiol 12:660

Lea-Thomas M, Carty H (1975) The appearances of artefacts on lower limb phlebograms. Clin Radiol 26:527

Lee B, Trainer F, Kavner D, Madden J, Dratz H, Ejercito E (1976) Non-invasive prevention of thrombosis of deep veins of the thigh using intermittent pneumatic compression. Surg Gynecol Obstet 142:705

Lehmann J (1943) Thrombosis (treatment and prevention with methyl-bis-hydroxy-coumarin). Lancet I:611

Lehmann J (1942a) Hypoprothrombinaemia produced by methylene bis (hydroxycoumarin). Its use in thrombosis. Lancet I:318

Lehmann J (1942b) A trial of curative and prophylactic treatment of thrombosis with a peroral agent (3,3'-Methylene-di-[4-hydroxy-coumarin]) (In Swedish). Sven Läkartidn 39:73

Lehmann J (1959) Historical notes on the early development of anticoagulant therapy with dicumarol in Sweden. Circulation 19:122

Lehmann J (1976) From rotten sweet clover to AP (In Swedish). Obs Med Ferrosan, Tema AP

LeMoine R, Moser K (1980) Leg scanning with radio-isotope-labeled fibrinogen in patients undergoing hip surgery. Comparison with contrast phlebography and lung scans. JAMA 243:2035

Lennander KG (1899) Über die Möglichkeit Thrombose in den Venen der unteren Extremitäten nach Operationen zu verhüten. Zbl Chir 20:553

LeQuesne LP (1978) The prevention of deep vein thrombosis and pulmonary embolism. Am J Surg 135:421

Lerner R, Weiner J, Goldstein R (1974) Experimental venous thrombosis in agranulocytic rabbits. Thromb Res 4:165

Lerner R, Goldstein R, Nelson J (1977) Production of thromboplastin (tissue factor) and thrombi by polymorphonuclear neutrophilic leucocytes adhering to vein walls. Thromb Res 11:11

Leslie IJ, Dorgan JC, Bentley G, Galloway RW (1981) A prospective study of deep vein thrombosis of the leg in children in halofemoral traction. J Bone Joint Surg [Br] 63-B:168

Levesque G, Samama M, Kher A, Barbier P, Horellou MH, Conard J (1981) Low-dose heparin in gynecologic surgery; effect on blood coagulation tests. Haemostasis 10:97

Levy R, Laus V, Miraldi F (1975) The frequency and detection of serious postoperative thromboembolic disease. Surg Gynecol Obstet 140:903

Lewis C, Mueller C, Edwards S (1972) Venous stasis on operating table. Am J Surg 124:780

Lewis C, Antoine J, Mueller C, Talbot W, Swaroop R, Edwards S (1976) Elastic compression in the prevention of venous stasis. A critical reevaluation. Am J Surg 132:739

Lewis GP, Westwick J (1977) An in vivo model for studying arterial thrombosis. In: Mitchell JRA (ed) Thromboembolism — A new approach to therapy. Academic Press, London, p 40

Lieb L (1964) Über die "Kumarinnekrose" und ihre Beziehung zum Shwartzman-Sanarelli-Phänomen. Zentralbl Chir 89:81

Lieberman GE, Lewis GP, Peters TJ (1977) A membrane-bound enzyme in rabbit aorta capable of inhibiting adenosine-diphosphate-induced platelet aggregation. Lancet II:330

Lim RC, Bergentz S-E, Lewis DH (1969) Metabolic and tissue blood flow changes resulting from aortic cross-clamping. Surgery 65:304

Lindahl U (1966) Further characterization of the heparin-protein linkage region. Biochim Biophys Acta 130:368

Lindahl U, Höök M (1978) Glucosaminoglucans and their binding to biological macromolecules. Ann Rev Biochem 47:385

Lindahl U, Bäckström G, Höök M, Thunberg L, Fransson L-Å, Linker A (1979) Structure of the anti-thrombin-binding site in heparin. Proc Natl Acad Sci USA 76:3198

Lindblad B, Bergqvist D (to be published a) Central hemodynamic effects of dextran 70, dihydroergotamine and their combination. A study in dogs.

Lindblad B, Bergqvist D (to be published b) Tissue blood flow and blood flow distribution after administration of dextran 70, dihydroergotamine and their combination. A study in dogs using the radioactive microsphere technique.

Lindblad B, Bergqvist D, Hallböök T (1979) Prevention of thromboembolism with dextran 70, dihydroergotamine and a sulphated polysaccharide. Final report (In Swedish). Sven Läkaresällsk Förh 88:150

Linde S (1941) Postoperative Thrombose-Embolie-Komplikationen, Frequenz, Zeit des Auftretens und Dauer des Krankheitsverlaufes. Eine statistische Untersuchung. Acta Chir Scand 84:310

Linder F, Schmitz W, Encke A, Trede M, Storch HH (1967) A study of 605 fatal pulmonary embolisms and two successful embolectomies. Surg Gynecol Obstet 125:82

Lindhagen A, Bergqvist D, Hallböök T, Efsing HO (to be published a) Venous function in the leg after postoperative thrombosis diagnosed with ^{125}I-fibrinogen uptake test. Ann Surg

Lindhagen A, Bergqvist D, Hallböök T, Lindroth B (1982 b) After exercise thermography (AET) and prediction of deep vein thrombosis. Brit Med J 1:1825

Lindquist O, Rammer L, Saldeen T (1972) Pulmonary insufficiency, microembolism and fibrinolysis inhibition in a post-traumatic autopsy material. Acta Chir Scand 138:545

Lindström B (1982) On the prophylaxis of postoperative thromboembolism in general surgery. The importance of venous pooling in the calves. Thesis, University of Göteborg

Lindström B, Ahlman H, Jonsson O, Sivertsson R, Stenqvist O (1977) Blood flow in the calves during surgery. Acta Chir Scand 143:335

Lindström B, Jonsson O, Petrusson B, Korsan-Bengtsen K, Pettersson S, Wikstrand J (1979) Optimized electrical calf muscle stimulation as prophylaxis against postoperative DVT. Acta Chir Scand [Suppl] 493:42

Lindvall S (1946) Three years experience with early postoperative mobilization (In Swedish). Nord Med 29:345

Link KP (1943) The anticoagulant from spoiled sweet clover hay. Harvey Lec 39:162

Link KP (1959) The discovery of dicumarol and its sequels. Circulation 19:97

Lippmann M, Fein A (1981) Pulmonary embolism in the patients with chronic obstructive pulmonary disease. A diagnostic dilemma. Chest 79:39

Lips JPM, Sixma JJ, Schiphorst M (1980) The effect of Ticlopidine administration to humans on the binding of adenosine diphosphate to blood platelets. Thromb Res 17:19

Lister WA (1927) A statistical investigation into the causation of pulmonary embolism following operation. Lancet I:111

Litwin M (1972) Comparison of effects of dextran 70 and dextran 40 in postoperative animals. Surgery 71:295

Litwin M (1976) Blood viscosity changes after trauma. Use of dextran 40 in correction of microcirculatory insufficiency. Crit Care Med 4:67

Ljungerud S, Ljungh Å, Rausing A (1973) Frequency of thrombi in prostatic venous plexus in an autopsy series. Acta Chir Scand 139:306

Ljungnér H, Bergqvist D, Isacson S (to be published b) Plasminogen activator activity in patients undergoing transvesical and transurethral prostatectomy. Eur Urol

Ljungnér H, Bergqvist D, Isacson S, Nilsson IM (1981a) Comparison between the plasminogen activator activity in walls of superficial, muscle and deep veins. Thrombos Res 22:295

Ljungnér H, Bergqvist D, Nilsson IM (1981b) Effect of intermittent pneumatic and graded static compression on factor VIII and the fibrinolytic system. Acta Chir Scand 147:657

Ljungnér H, Bergqvist D, von Hebel I, Isacson S (to be published a) The influence of major surgery on plasminogen activator activity in superficial hand veins. Eur Surg Res

Ljungnér H, Isacson S (1979) The fibrinolytic activity in vein walls in patients undergoing prostatectomy (In Swedish). Sven Läkaresällsk Förh 88:23

Ljungqvist U, Bergentz S-E, Leandoer L, Nilsson IM (1969) Coagulation and fibrinolysis after renal transplantation. Scand J Urol Nephrol 3:23

Ljungqvist U, Appelgren L, Bergentz S-E, Leandoer L (1970) Fibrinogen turnover in healthy and uremic patients (In Swedish). Nord Med 84:964

Ljungqvist U, Bergentz S-E, Lewis DH (1971) The distribution of platelets, fibrin and erythrocytes in various organs following experimental trauma. Europ Surg Res 3:293

Ljungström KG (1975) Dextran 70 as prophylaxis against lethal postoperative pulmonary embolism (In Swedish). Sven Läkartidn 72:2284

Ljungström KG (1971) Prospective study on the value of a single infusion of dextran 70 during surgical operation in the prevention of fatal pulmonary embolism (PE). Thromb Haemost 38:197

Loeliger EA (1976) Thromboseprophylaxe mit Cumarin, Heparin in kleinen Dosen, Dextran und Blutplättchenfunktionshemmern. In: Neuhaus K, Duckert F (eds) Blutgerinnung und Antikoagulation. Schattauer, Stuttgart New York

Loeliger EA, van der Esch B, Mattern MJ, den Brabander ASA (1963) Behaviour of factors II, VII, IX and X during long-term treatment with coumarin. Thromb Diath Haemorrh 9:74

Loew D, Vinazzer H (1974) Influence of simultaneous administration of low-dose heparin and acetylsalicylic acid on blood coagulation and platelet functions. Haemostasis 3:319

Loew D, Wellmer HK, Baer U, Merguet H, Rumpf P, Petersen H, Bromig G, Persch WF, Marx FJ, von Bary SM (1974) Postoperative Thromboembolie-Prophylaxe mit Acetylsalicylsäure. Dtsch Med Wochenschr 99:565

Loew D, Brücke P, Simma W, Vinazzer H, Dienstl E, Boehme K (1977) Acetylsalicylic acid, low dose heparin, and a combination of both substances in the prevention of postoperative thromboembolism. A double blind study. Thromb Res 11:81

Lofgren E, Coates H, O'Brien P (1976) Clinically suspect pulmonary embolism after vein stripping. Mayo Clin Proc 51:77

Lopez-Majano V, Leininger B, Friedman F (1978) Incidence of pulmonary embolism in deep venous thrombosis. Respiration 36:223

Lorentzen JE, Røder OC, Buchardt-Hansen HJ (1980) Peripheral arterial embolism. A follow-up of 130 consecutive patients submitted to embolectomy. Acta Chir Scand [Suppl] 502:111

Loudon JR, McGarritz G, Vallance R, Bayliss AL, Graham J (1978) The fibrinogen uptake test after hip surgery. Br J Surg 65:616

Low J, Briggs JC (1978) Comparative plasma heparin levels after subcutaneous sodium and calcium heparin. Thromb Haemost 40:397

Lowe GDO (1978) Prevention of deep vein-thrombosis by subcutaneous ancrod. Scott Med J 23: 329

Lowe GDO, Morrice JJ, Fulton A, Forbes CD, Prentice CRM, Barbanel JC (1978) Subcutaneous ancrod after operation for fractured hip – a dose-ranging and feasability study. Thromb Haemost 40:134

Lowe GDO, Campbell AG, Meek DR, Forbes CD, Prentice CRM, Cummings SW (1979a) Subcutaneous ancrod in prevention of deep-vein thrombosis. Lancet I:51

Lowe GDO, McKillop JH, Prentice AG (1979b) Fatal retroperitoneal haemorrhage complicating anticoagulant therapy. Postgrad Med J 55:18

Lowe L (1981) Venous thrombosis and embolism. J Bone Joint Surg [Br] 63-B:155

Lüders H, Konold P, Otten GL, Koslowski L (1973) Postoperative Thromboseprophylaxe. Randomisierte, prospektive Untersuchung zum Vergleich einer Thromboemboliprophylaxe mit Antikoagulantien (Heparin-Marcumar) und Dextran 60 (Macrodex). Chirurgie 44:563

MacFarlane RG (1937) Fibrinolysis following operation. Lancet I:10

MacGowan WAL, Mooneeram R (1973) A review of 174 patients with arterial embolism. Br J Surg 60:894

MacIntyre DB, Gorden JL (1975) Duration of aspirin's effect on human platelet aggregation. J Pharm Pharmacol 27:19

Macintyre IMC, Ruckley CV (1974) Pulmonary embolism – a clinical and autopsy study. Scott Med J 19:20

Macintyre IMC, Webber RG, Crispin JR, Jones DRB, Wood JK, Allan NC, Prescott RJ, Ruckley CV (1976) Plasma fibrinolysis and postoperative deep vein thrombosis. Br J Surg 63:694

Mac Millan RL, Brown KWG (1953) Haemorrhage in anticoagulant therapy. Can Med Assoc J 69: 279

Macon W, Morton J, Adams J (1970) Significant complications of anticoagulant therapy. Surgery 68:571

Maddi VL, Wyso EM, Zinner EN (1969) Dextran anaphylaxis. Angiology 20:243

Mahadoo J, Hiebert LM, Jaques LB (1977) Vascular sequestration of heparin. Thromb Res 12:79

Mahairas GH, Weingold AB (1963) Fetal hazard with anticoagulant therapy. Am J Obstet Gynecol 85:234

Mahorner H (1969) Results of surgical operations for venous thrombosis. Surg Gynaecol Obstet 129:66

Makin GS, Mayes FB, Holroyd AM (1969) Studies on the effect of "Tubigrip" on the flow in the deep veins of the calf. Br J Surg 56:369

Malcolm I, Wigmore T, Steinbecher U (1979) Heparin-associated thrombocytopenia: Low frequency in 104 patients treated with heparin of intestinal mucosal origin. Canadian Medical Association Journal 120:108

Malmsten C, Hamberg M, Svensson J, Samuelsson B (1975) Physiological role of an endoperoxide in human platelets: Hemostatic defect due to platelet cyclo-oxygenase deficiency. Proc Natl Acad Sci USA 72:1146

Malone PC, Hamer JD, Silver IA (1979) Oxygen tension in venous valve pockets. Thromb Haemost 42:230

Mannucci PM, Åberg M, Nilsson IM, Robertson B (1975) Mechanism of plasminogen activator and factor VIII increase after vasoactive drugs. Br J Haematol 30:81

Mannucci PM, Citterio L, Panajotopoulos N (1976) Low-dose heparin and deep-vein thrombosis after total hip replacement. Thromb Haemost 36:157

Mansberger AR, Cox EF, Flotte CT, Buxton RW (1966) "Washout" acidosis following resection of aortic aneurysms. Clinical metabolic study of reactive hyperemia and effect of dextran on excess lactate and pH. Ann Surg 163:778

Mansfield A (1972) Alteration in fibrinolysis associated with surgery and venous thrombosis. Br J Surg 59:754

Margulies EH, White AM, Sherry S (1980) Sulfinpyrazone: a review of its pharmacological properties and therapeutic use. Drugs 20:179

Marin HM (1961) Coagulation of blood in isolated venous segments. Surg Gynaecol Obstet 113: 293

Markwardt F, Glusa E, Barthel W (1978) Blood level of dihydroergotoxine and inhibition of platelet aggregation. Thromb Res 12:943

Marshall R, Esnouf MP (1968) The effect of crude and purified Agkistrodon rhodostoma venom in the dog. Clin Sci 35:251

Martin DL, Hollinger RE, Suwanwela N, Fedor EJ (1971) Experimental defibrination produced by Abbott-3841 4 (Ancrod) and associated effects on some other factors of the hemostatic system. Fed Proc 30:424

Mason R, Sharp D, Chuang H, Mohammed F (1977) The endothelium. Roles in thrombosis and haemostasis. Arch Pathol Lab Med 101:61

Matheson NA, Diomi P (1970) Renal failure after the administration of dextran 40. Surg Gynecol Obstet 131:661

Matis P (1968) Postoperative anticoagulant therapy. Clin Obstet Gynecol 11:281

Matsuda T, Murakami M (1976) Relationship between fibrinogen and blood viscosity. Thromb Res [Suppl II]:25

Matt EM, Gruber UF (1977) Prophylaxe postoperativer thromboembolischer Komplikationen mit subkutan verabreichten kleinen Heparin-Dosen. Fortschr Med 95:669

Mattock P, Esnouf MP (1971) Differences in the subunit structure of human fibrin formed by the action of arvin, reptilase and thrombin. Nature 233:277

Maurer PH (1953) Dextran, an antigen in man. Proc Soc Exp Biol Med 83:879

Mavor GE, Galloway JMD (1967) The iliofemoral venous segment as a source of pulmonary emboli. Lancet I:371

Mavor GE, Galloway JMD (1969) Iliofemoral venous thrombosis. Pathological considerations and surgical management. Br J Surg 56:45

May R (1979) Varicose veins. In: May R (ed) Surgery of the veins of the leg and pelvis. Thieme, Stuttgart

May R, Thurner J (1956) Ein Gefäßsporn in der Vena iliaca com. sin. als wahrscheinliche Ursache der überwiegend linksseitigen Beckenvenenthrombosen. Z Kreislaufforsch 45:912

Mayo ME, Halil T, Browse NL (1971) The incidence of deep vein thrombosis after prostatectomy. Br J Urol 43:738

McAvoy T (1979) The biologic half-life of heparin. Clin Pharmacol Ther 25:372

McBride JA, Turpie AGG, Kraus V, Hiltz C (1975) Failure of aspirin and dipyridamole to influence the incidence of leg scan detected venous thrombosis after elective hip surgery. Thromb Diath Haemorrh 34:564

McCarthy TG, McQueen J, Johnstone FD, Weston J, Campbell S (1974) A comparison of low-dose subcutaneous heparin and intravenous dextran 70 in the prophylaxis of deep venous thrombosis after gynaecological surgery. J Obstet Gynaecol Br Commonw 81:486

McDuffe NM, Dietrich CP, Nader HB (1975) Electrofocusing of heparin-fractionation of heparin into 21 components distinguishable from other acidic mucopolysaccharides. Biopolymers 14:1473

McGovern VJ (1956) Mast cells and their relationship to endothelial surfaces. J Path Bacteriol 71:1

McKenna R, Bachmann F, Kaushal S, Galante J (1976) Thromboembolic disease in patients undergoing total knee replacement. J Bone J Surg Am Vol 58:928

McKenna R, Cole ER, Vasan US (1981) Is warfarin sodium absolutely contraindicated during lactation? Thromb Haemost 46:119

McKenna R, Galante J, Bachmann F, Wallace DL, Kaushal SP, Meredith P (1980) Prevention of venous thromboembolism after total knee replacement by high-dose aspirin or intermittent calf and thigh compression. Br Med J 1:514

McKenzie FN, Arfors K-E, Tangen O (1973) Effect of arvin on rabbit platelet activity in vitro and in vivo. Thromb Res 3:565

McKenzie FN, Arfors K-E, Matheson NA (1974) Measurement of the platelet response to laser-induced microvascular injury. Assessment of determinants of platelet aggregation in vivo. Thromb Diath Haemorrh 32:704

McLachlan MSF, Thomson JG, Taylor DW, Kelly M, Sackett DL (1979) Observer variation in the interpretation of lower limb venograms. Am J Radiol 132:227

McLachlin AD, McLachlin JA, Jory T, Rawling EG (1960) Venous stasis in the lower extremities. Ann Surg 152:678

McLean J (1916) The thromboplastic action of cephalin. Am J Physiol 41:250

McManus F (1976) The incidence of deep venous thrombosis after total hip replacement using dextran 70 prophylaxis – a venographic study. Ir J Med Sci 145:201

McNamara M, Takaki H, Yao J (1977) Venous disease. Surg Clin North Am 57:1201

McNamara M, Creasy J, Takaki H, Conn J, Yao J, Bergan J (1978) Vena caval surgery to prevent recurrent pulmonary embolism. In: Bergan J, Yao J (eds) Venous problems. Year Book Med Publishers, Chicago London

McNeil B (1976) A diagnostic strategy using ventilation-perfusion studies in patients suspect for pulmonary embolism. J Nucl Med 17:613

McNeil BJ, Holman BL, Adelstein J (1974) The scintigraphic definition of pulmonary embolism. JAMA 227:753

McNichol GP, Fletcher AP, Alkjaersig N, Sherry S (1961) The use of epsilon aminocaproic acid, a potent inhibitor of fibrinolytic activity, in the management of postoperative hematuria. J Urol 86:829

Medén-Britth G, Rådegran K (1980) Fibrinopeptide A as a measure of coagulation activity induced by surgery. An experimental study in dogs. Thromb Res 18:333

Medén-Britth G, Teien A (1979) Infusion of purified antithrombin III to patients with fracture of the neck of the femur. Eur Surg Res 11:289

Medén-Britth G, Miller-Andersson M, Olsson P (1976) Studies on plasma antithrombin isolated on heparin gel. Thromb Res 9:369

Medical Research Council (1972) Effect of aspirin on postoperative venous thrombosis. Report of the steering committee of a trial. Lancet II:441

Meier-Ruge W, Iwangoff P (1976) Biochemical effect of ergot alkaloids with special reference to the brain. Postgrad Med J [Suppl 1] 52:47

Meissner F (1961) Allergische Reaktionen nach Dextraninfusion. Allerg Asthmaforsch 4:33

Mellander S, Nordenfelt I (1970) Comparative effects of dihydroergotamine and noradrenaline on resistance, exchange and capitance functions in the peripheral circulation. Clin Sci 39:183

Menon S, McCollum JPK, Gibson AL 1971a) Blood fibrinolytic activity in deep vein thrombosis. Lancet I:292

Menon S, Gibson AL, Weightman D, Dewar HA (1971b) Comparison between blood fibrinolytic activity in the legs and arms and its possible role in phlebothrombosis. Angiologica 8:83

Merck D, Hardy J, Cannon R, Gronvall J (1964) Experimental pulmonary artery-vena cava anastomosis (Glenn Operation). Efficacy of low molecular weight dextran vs heparin in preventing thrombosis, with notes on pressure changes. J Thorac Cardiovasc Surg 47:367

Messmer K, Ljungström K-G, Gruber U, Richter W, Hedin H (1980) Prevention of dextran-induced anaphylactoid reactions by hapten inhibition. Lancet I:975

Metcalf M (1980) The lysis of artificial thrombi. Thromb Haemostas 43:34

Metcalf MJ, Arfors K-E, McKenzie FN, Smith G, Tangen O (1974) Effect of dextran on the lysis of artificial thrombi. Eur Surg Res 6:28

Meyerowitz B, Nelson R (1964) Measurement of the velocity of blood in lower limb veins with and without compression. Surgery 56:481

Michalski R, Lane DA, Kakkar VV (1977) Comparison of heparin and a semi-synthetic heparin analogue, A73025. II. Some effects on platelet function. Br J Haematol 37:247

Michelson E (1968) Anaphylactic reaction to dextrans. N Engl J Med 278:552

Mielke CH, Britten AFH (1970) Aspirin as an antithrombotic agent: template bleeding time-test of antithrombotic effect. Blood 36:855

Mielke CH, Kaneshiro MM, Maher IA, Weiner JM, Rapaport SI (1969) The standardized normal Ivy bleeding time and its prolongation by aspirin. Blood 34:204

Mielke CH, Ramos JC, Britten AFH (1973) Aspirin as an antiplatelet agent: template bleeding time as a monitor of therapy. Am J Clin Pathol 59:236

Miller R, Lies J, Carretta R, Wampold D, DeNardo G, Krans J, Amsterdam E, Mason D (1976) Prevention of lower extremity venous thrombosis by early mobilisation. Confirmation in patients with acute myocardial infarction by ^{125}I-fibrinogen uptake and venography. Ann Intern Med 84:700

Miller S, Eyster E, Saleem A, Gottleib L, Buch D, Graham W (1979) Intravascular coagulation and fibrinolysis within primate extremities during tourniquet ischemia. Ann Surg 190:227

Miller WE, DeWolfe VG (1966) Osteoporosis resulting from heparin therapy. Cleve Clin Q 33:31
Mills DC (1972) Drugs that affect platelet behaviour. In: O'Brien JR (ed) Clinics of haematology. Platelet disorders. 1:295
Mills DC, Smith JB (1971) The influence on platelet aggregation of drugs that affect the accumulation of adenosine 3':5'-cyclic monophosphate in platelets. Biochem J 121:185
Mills H, Lucia SP (1949) Familial hypochromic anemia associated with postsplenectomy erythrocytic inclusion bodies. Blood 4:891
Milne RM, Griffiths JMT, Gunn AA, Ruckley CV (1971) Postoperative deep venous thrombosis. A comparison of diagnostic techniques. Lancet II:445
Mims JA, Sarji KE, Kleinfelder J, Eurenius K (1977) Heparin-induced platelet aggregation in burn patients. Thromb Res 10:291
Minkes M, Stanford N, Chi MM-Y, Roth GJ, Needleman P, Majerus PW (1977) Cyclic AMP inhibits the availability of arachidonate to PG synthetase in human platelets. J Clin Invest 59:449
Mirkovitch V, Borgeaud J, Meyer S, Niebes P (1972) Prevention de thrombose experimentale par O-(β-hydroxyetyl)-rutosides. Helv Chir Acta 39:379
Misgeld V, Mende C (1974) Dextran-Unverträglichkeit. Med Klin 69:1452
Mitchell JRA (1979) Can we really prevent postoperative pulmonary emboli? Br Med J 1:1523
Miyamoto A, Miller L (1980) Pulmonary embolism in stroke: prevention by early heparinization of venous thrombosis detected by iodine-125 fibrinogen leg scans. Arch Phys Med Rehabil 61: 584
Mobin-Uddin K, McLean R, Bolooki H (1969) Caval interruption for prevention of pulmonary embolism. Arch Surg 99:711
Modig J, Borg T, Karlström G, Sahlstedt B, Rikner L (1981) Effects of tocainide, an oral analogue of lidocaine, on thromboembolism after total hip replacement. Upsala J Med Sci 86:269
Modig J, Malmberg P, Karlström G (1980b) Effect of epidural versus general anaesthesia on calf blood flow. Acta Anaesth Scand 24:305
Modig J, Malmberg P, Saldeen T (1980a) Comparative effects of epidural and general anaesthesia on fibrinolysis function, lower limb rheology and thromboembolism after total hip replacement. Anesthesiol 53:534
Mok CK, Hoaglund FT, Rozoff SM, Chow SP, Ma A, Yau ACMG (1979) The incidence of deep vein thrombosis in Hongkong Chinese after hip surgery for fracture of the proximal femur. Br J Surg 66:640
Mollison AW, Rennie JB (1954) Treatment of renal oedema with dextran. Br Med J 1:893
Moncada S, Korbut R (1978) Dipyridamole and other phosphodiesterase inhibitors act as antithrombotic agents by potentiating endogenous prostacyclin. Lancet I:1286
Moncada S, Vane JR (1977) The discovery of prostacyclin – a fresh insight into arachidonic acid metabolism. In: Kharasch N, Fried J (eds) Biochemical aspects of prostaglandins and thromboxanes. Academic Press, New York
Moncada S, Vane JR (1978) Instable metabolites of arachidonic acid and their role in haemostasis and thrombosis. Br Med Bull 34:129
Moncada S, Vane JR (1981) Prostacyclin and blood coagulation. Drugs 21:430
Moncada S, Gryglewski R, Bunting S, Vane JR (1976) An enzyme isolated from arteries transforms prostaglandin endoperoxides to an unstable substance that inhibits platelet aggregation. Nature 263:663
Moncada S, Korbut R, Bunting S (1978) Prostacyclin is a circulation hormone. Nature 273:767
Moore S, Pepper DS, Cash JD (1975) The isolation and characterisation of a platelet specific β-globulin (β-thromboglobulin) and the detection of antiurokinase and antiplasmin released from thrombin-aggregated washed human platelets. Biochim Biophys Acta 379:360
Morin JP, Faroul E, Lamas JP, Leoni J, Lassner J (1978) La prevention des thromboses veineuses profondes par le polysulfate de pentosane. Cah Anesthesiol 26:297
Morrell T, Dunnill MS (1968) The post-mortem incidence of pulmonary embolism in a hospital population. Br J Surg 55:347
Morrell MT, Truelove SC, Barr A (1963) Pulmonary embolism. Br Med J 5361:830
Morris GK (1980) Prevention of venous thrombocmbolism. A survey of methods used by orthopaedic and general surgeons. Lancet II:572

Morris GK, Mitchell JA (1976a) Prevention and diagnosis of venous thrombosis in patients with hip fractures. A survey of current praxis. Lancet II:867

Morris GK, Mitchell JRA (1976b) Warfarin sodium in prevention of deep venous thrombosis and pulmonary embolism in patients with fractured neck of femur. Lancet II:869

Morris GK, Mitchell JRA (1977a) Evaluation of ^{125}I-fibrinogen test for venous thrombosis in patients with hip fractures: comparison between isotope scanning and necropsy findings. Br Med J 1:264

Morris GK, Mitchell JRA (1977b) Preventing venous thromboembolism in elderly patients with hip fractures: studies of low-dose heparin, dihyridamole, aspirin, and flurbiprofen. Br Med J 1: 535

Morris GK, Mitchell JRA (1978) Can death from venous thromboembolism be prevented in elderly patients with hip fractures? Am Heart J 95:139

Morris GK, Henry APJ, Preston BJ (1974) Prevention of deep-vein thrombosis by low-dose heparin in patients undergoing total hip replacement. Lancet II:797

Morris WT, Hardy AE (1981) The effect of dihydroergotamine and heparin on the incidence of thromboembolic complications following total hip replacement; a randomized controlled clinical trial. Br J Surg 68:301

Morrison AD, Orci L, Berwick L, Perrelet A, Winegrad AI (1977) The effects of anoxia on the morphology and composite metabolism of the intact aortic intima-media preparation. J Clin Invest 59:1027

Morrison MCT (1963) Is pulmonary embolectomy obsolete? Br J Dis Chest 57:187

Morrison ND, Stephenson CBS, Maclean D, Stanhope JM (1976) Deep vein thrombosis after femoropopliteal bypass grafting with observations on the incidence of complications following the use of dextran 70. N Z Med J 84:233

Moseley P, Kerstein M (1980) Pregnancy and thrombophlebitis. Surg Gynecol Obstet 150:593

Moser G, Froidevaux A (1976) Prophylaxie des thromboses veineuses profondes postoperatoires par des petites doses d'heparin sous-cutanées, associées ou non au port de pas compressifs: étude comparative et resultats. Schweiz Rundschau Med 65:1015

Moser G, Krähenbühl B, Barroussel R, Bene J-J, Rohner A (1981a) Mechanical versus pharmacologic prevention of deep venous thrombosis. Surg Gynecol Obstet 152:448

Moser K, Le Moine JR, Nachtney F, Spragg R (1981b) Deep venous thrombosis and pulmonary embolism. Frequency in a respiratory care unit. JAMA 246:1422

Moser K, Spragg R, Bender F, Konopka R, Hartman M, Fedullo P (1980) Study of factors that may condition scintigraphic detection of venous thrombi and pulmonary emboli with Indium-111-labelled platelets. J Nucl Med 21:1051

Moses RG, Warren MB (1973) Coumarin necrosis. Med J Aust 2:76

Moskovitz PA, Ellenberg SS, Feffer HL, Kenmore PI, Neviaser RJ, Rubin BE, Varma VM (1978) Low-dose heparin for prevention of venous thromboembolism in total hip arthroplasty and surgical repair of hip fractures. J Bone Joint Surg Am Vol 60:1065

Mosley JG (1978) Low-dose heparin in breast-cancer surgery. Lancet I:161

Mostbeck A, Partsch H (1978) Umverteilung regionaler Blutvolumina durch Dihydroergotamin und Beinkompression. Med Klin 73:801

Mozes MH, Bogokowsky E, Antebein N, Tzur S, Penchas S (1966) Inferior vena cava ligation for pulmonary embolism: Review of 118 cases. Surgery 60:1250

Mudge M, Hughes LE (1978) The long term sequelae of deep vein thrombosis. Br J Surg 65:692

Mühe E (1977) Physikalische Möglichkeiten der Thromboseprophylaxe. Langenbecks Arch Chir 345:Kongreßbericht

Mühe E, Burghardt K-H, Kolb W, Strobel G (1975) Eine neue Methode zur Prophylaxe postoperativer Venenthrombosen. Klinikarzt 4:88

Müller-Schweinitzer E (1974) Studies on the peripheral mode of action of dihydroergotamine in human and canine veins. Eur J Clin Pharmacol 27:231

Müller-Schweinitzer E, Brundell J (1975a) Enhanced prostaglandin synthesis contributes to the venoconstrictor activity of ergotamine. Blood Vessels 12:193

Müller-Schweinitzer E, Brundell J (1975b) Modification of canine vascular smooth muscle responses to dihydroergotamine by endogenous prostaglandin synthesis. Eur J Clin Pharmacol 34:197

Mulcare RJ, Royster TS, Phillips LL (1976) Intravascular coagulation in surgical procedures on the abdominal aorta. Surg Gynaecol Obstet 143:730

A multi-unit controlled trial (1974) Heparin versus dextran in the prevention of deep-vein thrombosis. Lancet II:118

Murata K, Nakazawa K, Hamai A (1975) Distribution of acidic glycosaminoglycans in the intima, media and adventitia of bovine aorta and their anticoagulant properties. Artherosclerosis 21: 93

Murphy M, Dalrymple G, Rivarola C (1972) Silent pulmonary embolism in the elderly surgical patient. Geriatrics 27:87

Murray G (1947) Anticoagulants in venous thrombosis and the prevention of pulmonary embolism. Surg Gynaecol Obstet 84:665

Mustard JF, Packham MA (1970) Factors influencing platelet function: adhesion, release and aggregation. Pharmacol Rev 22:97

Mustard JF, Rowsell HC, Smythe HA, Senyi A, Murphy EA (1967) The effect of sulfinpyrazone on platelet economy and thrombus formation in rabbits. Blood 29:859

Muzaffar TZ, Young GG, Bryce WAJ, Dhall DP (1972a) Studies on fibrin formation and effects of dextran. Thromb Diath Haemorrh 28:244

Muzaffar TZ, Stalker AL, Bryce WAJ, Dhall DP (1972b) Structural alterations in fibrin clots with dextran. Thromb Diath Haemorrh 28:257

Myhre H, Holen A (1969) Thrombosis prophylaxis. Dextran or sodium warfarin? A controlled clinical study (In Norwegian). Nord Med 82:1534

Myhre H, Støren E, Auensen C (1973) Pre- or postoperative start of anticoagulation prophylaxis in patients with fractured hips? J Oslo City Hosp 23:15

Myhre HO, Støren EJ, Ongre A (1974) The incidence of deep venous thrombosis in patients with leg oedema after arterial reconstruction. Scand J Thor Cardiovasc Surg 8:73

Myrvold HF, Persson J-E, Svensson B, Wallensten S, Vikterlöf KJ (1973) Prevention of thromboembolism with dextran 70 and heparin in patients with femoral neck fractures. Acta Chir Scand 139:609

Nader HF, McDuffe NM, Dietrich CP (1974) Heparin fractionation by electrofocusing: presence of 21 components of different molecular weights. Biochem Biophys Res Commun 57:488

Naeye RL (1962) Thrombotic state after hemorrhagic diathesis, possible complication of therapy with epsilon aminocaproic acid. Blood 19:694

Nalbandian R, Mader I, Barrett J, Pearce J, Rupp E (1965) Petechiae, echymoses, and necrosis of the skin induced by coumarin congeners. JAMA 192:603

Nalbandian R, Beller F, Kamp A, Henry R, Wolf P (1971) Coumarin necrosis of skin treated successfully with heparin. Obstet Gynecol 38:395

Naleczynska A, Gregor A, Kostrzewka E (1970) The effect of Fluidex polfa (dextran 40) on the plasma coagulation factors. In: Ditzel J, Lewis DH (eds) Proc 6th Eur Conf Microcirc. Aalborg

Nandi P, Wong KP, Wei WI, Ngan H, Ong GB (1980) Incidence of postoperative deep vein thrombosis in Hong Kong Chinese. Br J Surg 67:251

Natelson EA, Lynch EC, Alfrey CP (1969) Heparin-induced thrombocytopenia: an unexpected response to treatment of consumption coagulopathy. Ann Intern Med 71:1121

Needleman P (1979) Prostacyclin in blood vessel-platelet interaction: perspectives and questions. Nature 279:14

Needleman P, Moncada S, Bunting S, Vane JR (1976) Identification of an enzyme in platelet microsomes which generates thromboxane A_2 from prostaglandin endoperoxides. Nature 261:558

Neglén P (1980) Aortic clamping. Skeletal muscle metabolism and central circulation during abdominal reconstructive vascular surgery for arteriosclerotic disease. Bull 23 Dep Surg. Univ Lund

Negus D (1978) Diagnosis of deep vein thrombosis: results of a survey. J R Soc Med 71:796

Negus D, Pinto DJ, Le Quesne LP, Brown N, Chapman M (1968) ^{125}I-labelled fibrinogen in the diagnosis of deep-vein thrombosis and its correlation with phlebography. Br J Surg 55:835

Negus D, Pinto DJ, Brown N (1969) Platelet adhesiveness in postoperative deep-vein thrombosis. Lancet I:220

Negus D, Pinto DJ, Slack WW (1971) Effect of small doses of heparin on platelet adhesiveness and lipoprotein-lipase activity before and after surgery. Lancet I:1202

Negus D, Friedgood A, Cox SJ, Peel ALG, Wells BW (1980) Ultra-low dose intravenous heparin in the prevention of postoperative deep-vein thrombosis. Lancet I:891

Nelsestuen GL, Suttie JW (1972) The purification and properties of an abnormal prothrombin produced by dicumarol-treated cows. A comparison to normal prothrombin. J Biol Chem 247: 8176

Nelsestuen GL, Zytkovicz T, Howard JB (1974) The mode of action of vitamin K. Identification of gamma-carboxyglutamic acid as a component of prothrombin. J Biol Chem 249:6347

Nelson JC, Lerner RG, Goldstein R (1978) Heparin-induced immune thrombocytopenia. Arch Intern Med 138:548

Nelson PG (1970) Effect of heparin on serum free-fatty acids, plasma catecholamines and the incidence of arrhytmias following acute myocardial infarction. Br Med J 3:735

Nenci G, Agnelli G, Berrettini M (1981) Biphasic sulphinpyrazone-warfarin interaction. Br Med J 282:1361

Nettelblad Å (1931) Studien an den Krankengeschichten des Thrombosenmaterials der Gebäranstalt Stockholm-Süd aus den Jahren 1912–1927. Acta Obstet Gynecol Scand 11:165

Neu LT, Waterfield JR, Ash CJ (1965) Prophylactic anticoagulant therapy in the orthopaedic patient. Ann Intern Med 62:463

Neumann R, Sostman D, Gottschalk A (1980) Current status of ventilation-perfusion imaging. Semin Nucl Med 10:198

Nicolaides AN (1973) Prevention of deep vein thrombosis. Geriatrics 28:69

Nicolaides AN (1975) Venous stasis in the lower limb. In: Nicolaides AN (ed) Thromboembolism. Aetiology, advances in prevention and management. MTP, Lancaster

Nicolaides AN (1978a) The current status of small-dose subcutaneous heparin in the prevention of venous thromboembolism. In: Bergan J, Yao J (eds) Venous problems. Year Book Medical Publishers, Chicago London

Nicolaides AN (1978b) Invited commentary. World J Surg 2:13

Nicolaides AN, Gordon-Smith I (1975) A rational approach to prevention. In: Nicolaides AN (ed) Thromboembolism. Aetiology, advances in prevention and management. MTP, Lancaster

Nicolaides AN, Irving D (1975) Clinical factors and the risk of deep venous thrombosis. In: Nicolaides AN (ed) Thromboembolism. Aetiology, advances in prevention and management. MTP, Lancaster

Nicolaides AN, Kakkar VV, Renney JTG, Kidner PH, Hutchinson DCS, Clarke MB (1971) Myocardial infarction and deep-vein thrombosis. Br Med J 1:432

Nicolaides AN, Clark CT, Thomas RD, Lewis JD (1972a) Soleal veins and local fibrinolytic activity. Br J Surg 59:914

Nicolaides AN, Desai S, Douglas JN, Fourides G, Dupont PA, Lewis JD, Dodsworth H, Luck RJ, Jamieson CW (1972b) Small doses of subcutaneous sodium heparin in preventing deep venous thrombosis after major surgery. Lancet II:890

Nicolaides AN, Field ES, Kakkar VV, Yates-Bell AJ, Taylor S, Clarke MB (1972c) Prostatectomy and deep-vein thrombosis. Br J Surg 59:487

Nicolaides AN, Kakkar VV, Field ES, Fish P (1972d) Soleal veins, stasis and prevention of deep vein thrombosis. In: Kakkar VV, Jouhar AJ (eds) Thromboembolism: diagnosis and treatment. Churchill Livingstone, Edinburgh London

Nicolaides AN, Kakkar VV, Field ES, Fish P (1972e) Venous stasis and deep-vein thrombosis. Br J Surg 59:713

Nicolaides AN, Kakkar VV, Field ES, Spindler J (1972f) Antibiotics, postoperative infection, and deep-vein thrombosis. Br J Surg 59:303

Nicolaides AN, Fernandes F, Pollock AV (1980) Intermittent sequential pneumatic compression of the legs in the prevention of venous stasis and postoperative deep venous thrombosis. Surgery 87:69

Nicolaon KG, Barnette WE, Gasic GP (1977) 6,9-thiaprostacyclin. A stable and biologically potent analogue of prostacyclin (PGI$_2$). J Am Chem Soc 99:7736

Nielsen A (1942) Prophylactic postoperative heparin treatment (In Danish). Nord Med 16:2873

Nillius A (1978) On thromboembolism after total hip replacement. Thesis. Malmö

Nillius A, Nylander G (1979) Deep vein thrombosis after total hip replacement: a clinical and phlebographic study. Br J Surg 66:324

Nillius SA, Ahlberg Å, Arborelius M, Hellgren T, Nylander G (1979a) Antiembolism stockings as thromboembolism prophylaxis in patients undergoing total hip replacement (In Swedish). Sven Läkaresällsk 87:47

Nillius SA, Ahlberg Å, Arborelius Jr M, Rosberg B (1979b) Preoperative normovolemic haemodilution with dextran 70 as a thromboembolic prophylaxis in total hip replacement. Int Orthop 3:197

Nilsen D, Jeremic M, Weisert O (1980) An attempt at predicting postoperative deep vein thrombosis by preoperative coagulation studies in patients undergoing total hip replacement. Thromb Haemost 43:194

Nilsson B, Nilsson IM, Hedner U (1981) Δ 4-ethylestrenol in recurrent deep venous thrombosis. Acta Med Scand 209:45

Nilsson IM (1977) Coagulation, fibrinolysis, and venous thrombosis. Triangle 16:19

Nilsson IM (1979) Biochemical and clinical aspects of factor VIII. In: Saldeen T (ed) The microembolism syndrome. Almqvist & Wiksell, Stockholm

Nilsson IM, Eiken O (1964) Further studies on the effect of dextran of various molecular weight on the coagulation mechanism. Thromb Diath Haemorrh 11:38

Nilsson IM, Pandolfi M (1970) Fibrinolytic response of the vascular wall. Thromb Diath Haemorrh [Suppl] 40:231

Nilsson IM, Robertson B (1968) Effects of venous occlusion on coagulation and fibrinolytic components in normal subjects. Thromb Diath Haemorrh 20:397

Nilsson IM, Krook H, Sternby NH, Söderberg E, Söderström N (1961) Severe thrombotic disease in a young man with bone marrow and skeletal changes and with a high content of an inhibitor in the fibrinolytic system. Acta Med Scand 169:323

Nilsson IM, Hedner U, Isacson S (1975) Phenformin and ethyloestrenol in recurrent venous thrombosis. Acta Med Scand 198:107

Nilsson IM, Holmberg L, Åberg M, Vilhardt H (1980a) The release of plasminogen activator and factor VIII after injection of DDAVP in healthy volunteers and in patients with von Willebrand's disease. Scand J Haematol 24:351

Nilsson IM, Vilhardt H, Åberg M (1980b) Association between VIIIR: Ag and plasminogen activator. Sixth Int Congr on Thrombosis of the Mediterranean League against Thromboembolic diseases. Monte Carlo 1980. Abstract book, No. 31

Nishizawa EE, Nynalda DJ, Suydum DE, Molony GA (1973) Flurbiprofen, a new potent inhibitor of platelet aggregation. Thromb Res 3:577

Nittis G, Ladapoulos C, Schwimmer M (1953) Effect of dextran infusion on bleeding time. Bull NY Univ Med Coll 16:86

Norgren L (1979) Does low-dose heparin prevent thrombosis after surgery? (In Swedish). Läkartidningen 76:3981

Nossel HL, Yudelman I, Canfield RE, Butler VP, Spanondis K, Wilner GD, Qureshi GD (1974) Measurement of fibrinopeptide A in human blood. J Clin Invest 54:43

Nudelman H, Kempson R (1966) Necrosis of the breast. A rare complication of anticoagulant therapy. Am J Surg 111:728

Nunn B, Lindsay R (1980) Effect of Ticlopidine on human platelet responsiveness ex vivo: comparison with aspirin. Thromb Res 18:807

Nylander G, Olivecrona H (1976) The phlebographic pattern of acute leg thrombosis within a defined urban population. Acta Chir Scand 142:505

Nylander G, Semb H (1972) Veins of the lower part of the leg after tibial fractures. Surg Gynaecol Obstet 134:974

Nylander G, Olivecrona H, Hedner U (1977) Earlier and concurrent morbidity of patients with acute lower leg thrombosis. Acta Chir Scand 143:425

Nyman D, Eriksson AW, Lehmann W, Blombäck M (1979) Inherited defective platelet aggregation with arachidonate as the main expression of a defective metabolism of arachidonic acid. Thromb Res 14:739

O'Brien JR (1968) Effects of salicylates on human platelets. Lancet I:779

O'Brien JR (1977) Lignocaine and deep-vein thrombosis. Lancet II:928

O'Brien JR, Etherington MD, Shuttleworth RD (1978) Ticlopedine — an antiplatelet drug; effects in human volunteers. Thromb Res 13:245

O'Brien JR, Tulevski V, Etherington M (1971) Two in-vivo studies comparing high and low aspirin dosage. Lancet I:399

O'Brien JR, Jamieson S, Etherington M, Klaber MR (1972) Platelet function in venous thrombosis and low-dosage heparin. Lancet I:1302

O'Brien TE, Woodford M, Irving MH (1979) The effect of intermittent compression of the calf on the fibrinolytic responses in the blood during a surgical operation. Surg Gynaecol Obstet 149: 380

Ochsner A, DeBakey ME (1940) Therapy phlebothrombosis and thrombo-phlebitis. Arch Surg 40: 208

Ockelford PA, Carter CJ, Hirsh J (1981) The lack of relationship between anti-Xa activity and antithrombotic activity of molecular weight heparin. Thromb Haemost 46:116

O'Donnell T, Browse N, Burnaud K, Lea Thomas M (1977) The socioeconomic effects of an iliofemoral venous thrombosis. J Surg Res 22:483

O'Grady J, Moncada S (1978) Aspirin: a paradoxical effect on bleeding time. Lancet II:780

Oh TH, Naidoo SS, Jaques LG (1973) The uptake and disposition of ^{35}S-heparin by macrophages in vitro. J Reticuloendothel Soc 13:134

Olbert F, Ender HG, Gaudernak T, Kuderna H, Pelinka H, Renner K, Russe O, Schlag G (1977) Häufigkeit der Beinvenenthrombosen nach Unterschenkelfrakturen unter Berücksichtigung der Besonderheiten der Technik und der Deutung der Phlebographie. In: Ehringer H (ed) Akute tiefe Becken- und Beinvenenthrombosen. Huber, Bern Stuttgart Vienna

Oliver MF, Kurien VA, Greenwood TW (1968) Relation between serum free fatty acids and arrhytmias and death after acute myocardial infarction. Lancet I:710

Olow B (1963) Effect of streptokinase on post-operative changes in some coagulation factors and the fibrinolytic system. Acta Chir Scand 126:197

Olsen EGJ, Pitney WR (1969) The effect of arvin on experimental pulmonary embolism in the rabbit. Br J Haematol 17:425

Olsson P (1963) Variations in antithrombin activity in plasma after major surgery. Acta Chir Scand 126:24

Olsson P, Lagergren H, Ek S (1963) The elimination from plasma of intravenous heparin. An experimental study on dogs and humans. Acta Med Scand 173:169

Olsson R, Korsan-Bengtsen P-M, Korsan-Bengtsen K, Lennartsson J, Waldenström J (1978) Serum aminotransferases after low-dose heparin treatment. Short communication. Acta Med Scand 204:229

Olsson S (1974) Platelets and fibrin in the early development of arterial and venous thrombi. Experimental and methodological studies. Thesis. University of Malmö

Olver I, Jenning G, Bobik A, Esler M (1980) Low bioavailability as a cause of apparent failure of dihydroergotamine in orthostatic hypotension. Br Med J 281:275

Orme M, Lewis PJ, de Swiet M, Serlin MJ, Sibeon R, Baty JD, Breckenridge AM (1977) May mothers given warfarin breast-feed their infants? Br Med J 2:1564

Orning OM, Syse PR, Hjort PF (1967) Side effects of phenylindandione (In Norwegian). Tisdkr Nor Laegeforen 87:1273

Osime U (1978) Incidence of postoperative deep vein thrombosis in Nigerians using ^{125}I-labelled fibrinogen. Br Med J 2:1607

Østerud B, Miller-Andersson M, Abildgaard U, Prydz H (1976) The effect of antithrombin III on the activity of the coagulation factors VII, IX and I. Thromb Haemost 35:295

O'Sullivan EF, Renney JTG (1972) Anti-platelet drugs in the prevention of postoperative deep vein thrombosis. III Congr Int Soc Thromb Haemostas. Abstracts p 438, Washington DC

O'Toole RD (1973) Heparin: adverse reaction. Letter. Ann Intern Med 79:759

Pachter L, Riles T (1977) Low dose heparin: bleeding and wound complications in the surgical patient. A prospective randomized study. Ann Surg 186:669

Packham MA, Warrior ES, Glynn MF, Senyi AS, Mustard JF (1967) Alteration of the response of platelets to surface stimuli by pyrazole compounds. J Exp Med 126:171

Packham MA, Nishizawa EE, Mustard JF (1968) Response of platelets to tissue injury. Biochem Pharmacol [Suppl] 171

Palacios-Macedo X, Diaz-Devis C, Escudero J (1969) Fetal risk with the use of coumarin anticoagulant agents in pregnant patients with intracardiac ball valve prosthesis. Am J Cardiol 24:853

Paleirac G, Meynadier J, Guilhou JJ, Castaigne JP (1979) Comparison des proprietes inhibitrices plaquettaires de la Ticlopidine et du dipyridamole. Etude comparative croisée et aveugle. Mediterr Med 2:182

Palmberg S, Hirsjärvi E (1977) Deep vein thrombosis and pulmonary embolism in aged surgical patients. Gerontology 21:46

Pandolfi M (1970) Persistence of fibrinolytic activity in fragments of human veins cultured in vitro. Thromb Diath Haemorrh 24:43

Pandolfi M, Isacson S, Nilsson IM (1969) Low fibrinolytic activity in the walls of veins of patients with thrombosis. Acta Med Scand 186:1

Pandolfi M, Hedner U, Nilsson IM (1970) Bilateral occlusion of the retinal veins in a patient with inhibition of fibrinolysis. Ann Ophthalmol 2:481

Papadimitriou J, Tsiftsis D, Peros C, Kelekis D, Papadimitriou K, Tountas C (1977) Incidence of silent phlebothrombosis in bed-ridden patients. In: Louros NC, Le Vay D (eds) Proceedings of the XX biennal world congress of the International College of Surgeons. Excerpt Med, Amsterdam New York

Pareti FI, Mannucci PM, D'Angelo A, Smith JB, Sautebin L, Galli G (1980) Congenital deficiency of thromboxane and prostacyclin. Lancet I:898

Pasternack R, Baughman K, Fallon J, Block P (1981) Scanning electron microscopy after coronary transluminal angioplasty of normal canine coronary arteries. Am J Cardiol 45:591

Paterson JC (1969) The pathology of venous thrombi. In: Sherry S, Brinkhous KM, Genton E, Stengle JM (eds) Thrombosis. Natl Acad Sci. Washington

Paterson JC, McLachlin J (1954) Precipitating factors in venous thrombosis. Surg Gynaecol Obstet 98:36

Paterson N, Dhall DP (1971) The release of adenosine diphosphate (ADP) from human platelets by dextran. 6th Eur Conf Microcirc. Aalborg 1970, p 324, Karger, Basel

Patrano C, Ciabattoni G, Pinca E, Pugliese F, Castrucci G, De Salvo A, Satta A, Peskar B (1980) Low dose aspirin and inhibition of thromboxane B_2 production in healthy subjects. Thromb Res 17:317

Paul C, Medén-Britth G (1975) Coagulation alterations after routine surgery (In Swedish). Sven Läkartidn 72:4385

Pay G, Wallis R, Zelaschi D (1981) The effect of sulphinpyrazone and its metabolites on platelet function in vitro and in vivo. Haemost 10:165

Payling Wright H (1942) Changes in the adhesiveness of blood platelets following parturition and surgical operations. J Path Bact 54:461

Pedegana L, Burgess E, Moore J, Carpenter M (1977) Prevention of thromboembolic disease by external pneumatic compression in patients undergoing total hip arthroplasty. Clin Orthop Rel Res 128:190

Pedersen K, Jakobsen P (1979) Two new metabolites of sulfinpyrazone in the rabbit: a possible cause of the prolonged in vivo effect. Thromb Res 16:871

Petrén G (1930) On the causes of postoperative deaths. Ann Surg 92:1

Pettersson G (1941) Drei Fälle von Lungenembolie auf dem Operationstisch. Acta Chir Scand 84:321

Pettifor JM, Benson R (1975) Congenital malformations associated with the administration of oral anticoagulants during pregnancy. J Pediatr 86:459

Phillips RS (1963) Prognosis in deep venous thrombosis. Arch Surg 87:732

Pinto DJ (1970) Controlled trial of an anticoagulant (warfarin-sodium) in the prevention of venous thrombosis following hip surgery. Br J Surg 57:349

Pitney WR, Bell WR, Bolton G (1969a) Blood fibrinolytic activity during arvin therapy. Br J Haematol 16:165

Pitney WR, Holt PJL, Bray C, Bolton G (1969b) Acquired resistance to treatment with arvin. Lancet I:79

Pitt A, Andersson S, Habersberger P, Rosengarten D (1980) Low dose heparin in the prevention of deep-vein thrombosis in patients with acute myocardial infarction. Am Heart J 99:574

Pizzo S, Schwartz M, Hill R, McKee P (1972) Mechanism of ancrod anticoagulation. A direct proteolytic effect of fibrin. J Clin Invest 51:2841

Plante J, Boneu B, Vaysse C, Barret A, Gouzi M, Bierme R (1979) Dipyridamol-aspirin versus low doses of heparin in the prophylaxis of deep venous thrombosis in abdominal surgery. Thromb Res 14:399

Plate G, Einarsson E, Eklöf B, Ohlin P (1981) Incidence of pulmonary embolism in acute iliofemoral vein thrombosis. Acta Chir Scand [Suppl] 506:35

Pletscher MC, Gruber UF (1977) Hämatokrit und Häufigkeit postoperativer tiefer Venenthrombosen. Prakt Anästh 12:307

Pollock AV (1977) Calf-muscle stimulation as a prophylactic method against deep vein thrombosis. Triangle 16:41

Pollock AV, Evans M (1978) Cigarette smoking and postoperative deep-vein thrombosis. Br Med J 2:637

Pollock AV, Rosenberg IL, Evans M (1976) Prevention of postoperative leg vein thrombosis: a comparison of low-dose heparin and electrical calf muscle stimulation. In: Kakkar VV, Thomas DP (eds) Heparin. Chemistry and clinical usage. Academic Press, London

Polterauer P, Zekert F, Gottlob R (1975) Azetylsalizylsäure und Dipyridamol: Aggregationshemmung im Experiment am Kaninchen. Vasa 4:397

Ponder E, Ponder RV (1961) Age and molecular weight of dextrans, their coating effects, and their interaction with serum albumin. Nature 190:277

Popov-Cenić S, Müller N, Kladetsky RG, Hack G, Lang U, Safer A, Rahlfs VW (1977) Durch Prämedikation, Narkose und Operation bedingte Änderungen des Gerinnungs- und Fibrinolysesystems und der Thrombozyten. Einfluß von Dextran und Hydroxyäthylstärke während und nach Operation. Anaesthesist 26:77

Porter J, Lindell T, Lakin P (1972) Leg edema following femoropopliteal autogenous vein bypass. Arch Surg 105:883

Poulose K, Kapcar A, Reba R (1976) False positive ^{125}I-fibrinogen test. Angiology 27:258

Powers P, Cuthbert D, Hirsh J (1979) Thrombocytopenia found uncommonly during heparin therapy. JAMA 241:2396

Powley JM, Doran FSA (1973) Galvanic stimulation to prevent deep-vein thrombosis. Lancet I:406

Prentice C, Hassanein AA, Turpie AGG, McNicol GP, Douglas AS (1969) Changes in platelet behaviour during arvin therapy. Lancet I:644

Prentice C, Lowe G, Forbes C (1979) Preventing postoperative thromboembolism. Br Med J 2:127

Prerovsky I, Roztocil K, Hlavova A, Koleilat Z, Razgova L, Oliva I (1972) The effect of hydroxyethylrutosides after acute and chronic oral administration in patients with venous diseases. A double-blind study. Angiologia 9:408

Prescott RJ, Jones DB, Vasilescu C, Henderson JT, Ruckley CV (1978) Smoking and risk factors in deep vein thrombosis. Thromb Haemost 40:128

Prescott S, Richards K, Tikoff G, Armstrong J, Shigeoka J (1981) Venous thromboembolism in decompensated chronic obstructive pulmonary disease. A prospective study. Am Rev Respir Dis 123:32

Preston E, Whipps S, Jackson CA, French AJ, Wyld PJ, Stoddard CJ (1981) Inhibition of prostacyclin and platelet thromboxane A_2 after low-dose aspirin. N Engl J Med 304:76

Preter B, Pescia R, Spieler U, Brunner U (1972) Über das Ausmaß und den Verlauf von traumatischen Schäden am tiefen Venensystem bei Unterschenkelfrakturen. Radiologe 12:305

Prexl HJ, Suppan G, Kronberger D, Fueger GF (1976) Prospektive Untersuchung der Häufigkeit postoperativer Beinvenenthrombosen und ihre medikamentöse Beeinflussung durch Aescin. Wiener Klin Wochenschr 88:326

Protoulis C, Bouvier C, Vaucher J, Krähenbühl B (1976) Incidence et prévention de la thrombose veineuse profonde dans la chirurgie de la hanche. Schweiz Rundschau Med 65:1298

Pulaski EJ (1951) Present status of plasma volume expanders in the treatment of shock. Arch Surg 63:745

Pyörälä T, Lampinen V (1970) Preoperative anticoagulant treatment in gynaecological surgery. Acta Obstet Gynecol Scand 49:215

Quenneville G, Barton B, McDevitt E (1959) The use of anticoagulants for thrombophlebitis during pregnancy. Am J Obstet Gynecol 77:1135

Quick AJ (1966) Salicylates and bleeding. The aspirin tolerance test. Am J Med Sci 252:265

Quinn J (1971) Perfusion scanning in chronic obstructive lung disease. Sem Nucl Med 1:185

Raberger G, Schwarz M, Benke T, Kraupp O (1981) Die Wirkung von Dihydroergotamin auf den großen und kleinen Kreislauf. In: Tscherne H, Deutsch E (eds) Postoperative Thromboembolie-Prophylaxe aus aktueller Sicht. Thieme, Stuttgart New York

Raich P, Hahn P, Korst D (1974) Heparin therapy. Am Fam Physician 10:163

Rajah SM, Penny A, Kester R (1978) Aspirin and bleeding time. Lancet II:1104

Rakoczi I, Chamone D, Collen D, Verstraete M (1978) Prediction of postoperative leg-vein thrombosis in gynaecological patients. Lancet I:509

Rakoczi I, Chamone D, Verstraete M, Collen D (1980) The relevance of clinical and hemostasis parameters for the prediction of postoperative thrombosis of the deep veins of the lower extremity in gynecologic patients. Surg Gynaecol Obstet 151:225

Rampling MW (1974) The solubility of fibrinogen in solutions containing dextran of various molecular weights. Biochem J 143:767

Rampling MW (1976) Interactions between dextran, fibrinogen and plasma membranes. Biochem Pharm 25:751

Rao G, Zikria E, Miller W, Samadani S, Ford W (1975) Incidence and prevention of pulmonary embolism after coronary artery surgery. Vasc Surg 9:37

Rawles JM, Warlow C, Ogston D (1975) Fibrinolytic capacity of arm and leg veins after femoral shaft fracture and acute myocardial infarction. Br Med J 2:61

Redman CWG (1979) Coagulation problems in human pregnancy. Postgrad Med J 55:367

Regoeczi E, Gergely J, McFarlane AS (1966) In vivo effects of Agkistrodon rhodostoma venom: studies with fibrinogen-^{131}I. J Clin Invest 45:1202

Rehnqvist N (1978) Intrahepatic jaundice due to warfarin therapy. Acta Med Scand 204:335

Reichelt W, Piepenbrock S, Schleussner E, Stegmann T (1980) Die Wirkungen von Dihydroergotamin auf Volumengehalt und Compliance der extrathorakalen Kapazitätsgefässe des Menschen unter Narkosebedingungen während extrakorporaler Zirkulation in Hypothermie. Z Kardiol 69:67

Reid HA, Chan KE, Thean PC (1963a) Prolonged coagulation defect (defibrination syndrome) in Malayan viper bite. Lancet I:621

Reid HA, Thean PC, Chan KE, Baharom AR (1963b) Clinical effects of bites of Malayan pit viper (Agkistrodon rhodostoma). Lancet I:617

Reilly DT, Burden AC, Fossard DP (1980) Fibrinolysis and the prediction of postoperative deep vein thrombosis. Br J Surg 67:66

Relihan M, Litwin M (1973) Morbidity and mortality associated with flail chest injury: a review of 85 cases. J Trauma 13:663

Rem J, Duckert F, Fridrich R, Gruber UF (1975) Subkutane kleine Heparindosen zur Thromboseprophylaxe in der allgemeinen Chirurgie und Urologie. Schweiz Med Wochenschr 105:827

Rem J, Feddersen C, Brandz MR, Kehlet H (1981) Postoperative changes coagulation and fibrinolysis independent of neurogenic stimuli and adrenal hormones. Br J Surg 68:229

Renney JTG, Kakkar VV, Nicolaides AN (1970) The prevention of postoperative deep vein thrombosis, comparing dextran-70 and intensive physiotherapy. Br J Surg 57:388

Renney JTG, O'Sullivan EF, Burke PF (1976) Prevention of postoperative deep vein thrombosis with dipyridamole and aspirin. Br Med J 1:992

Renschler HE, Schmidt FW, Mammen EF (1963) Untersuchungen über die Auswirkungen langdauernder Antikoagulantientherapie auf die Leber. Dtsch Arch Klin Med 208:524

Revenäs B (1979) Anaphylactic shock in the monkey: Early circulatory and respiratory response in aggregate anaphylaxis. Acta Univ Ups Abstr Ups Diss Fac Med 320

Revenäs B, Smedegård G, Hedin H, Richter W, Saldeen T (1980) Immune complex mediated anaphylactic shock in humans? 7th World Congr Anaesthesiologists. Hamburg Sept 1980

Rhodes GR, Dixon RH, Silver D (1973) Heparin induced thrombocytopenia with thrombotic and hemorrhagic manifestations. Surg Gynecol Obstet 136:409

Rhodes GR, Dixon RH, Silver D (1977) Heparin induced thrombocytopenia. Eight cases with thrombotic-hemorrhagic complications. Ann Surg 186:752

Ribaudo M, Hoellrich R, McKinnon W, Schuler S (1975) Evaluation of mini-dose heparin administration as a prophylaxis against postoperative pulmonary embolism: a prospective double-blind study. Am Surg 41:289

Rich N, Spencer F (1978) Vascular trauma. Saunders, Philadelphia London Toronto

Richardson MH (1904) On certain unavoidable calamities following surgical operations. Boston Med Surg J 151:583

Richter W (1966) Normalizing effect of low molecular weight dextran fractions on the reduced suspension stability of human erythrocytes in vitro. Acta Chir Scand 131:1

Richter W (1971) Hapten inhibition of passive antidextran anaphylaxis in guinea pigs. Role of molecular size in anaphylactogenicity and precipitability of dextran fraction. Int Arch Allergy Appl Immunol 41:826

Richter W (1973a) Built-in hapten inhibition of anaphylaxis by the low molecular weight subfractions of a B512 dextran fraction of M_W 3400. Int Arch Allergy Appl Immunol 45:930

Richter W (1973b) Immunological in vivo and in vitro studies of the dextran antidextran system. Diss, Uppsala Alltryck Östervåla

Richter W, Seeman D, Hedin H, Ring J, Messmer K (1980) Dextranunverträglichkeit. Immunologische, tierexperimentelle und klinische Studien. Med Welt 31:365

Ricketts CR (1952) Interaction of dextran and fibrinogen. Nature 169:970

Ricketts CR, Cope E, Thomlinson J (1966) Dextran and the placental barrier. Br Med J 1:1050

Ricketts CR, Lorentz L, Maycock WA (1950) Molecular composition of dextran solutions for intravenous use. Nature 165:770

Ricotta J, Collins G, Rich N (1979) Effects of aspirin and dextran on patency of bovine heterografts in the venous system. Ann Surg 189:116

Rieckert H (1971) Primäre Therapieziele bei der hypotonen Fehlregulation. Fortschr Med 89:173

Ries E (1899) Some radical changes in the aftertreatment of cheiliotomy cases. JAMA 33:454

Ring J (1978) Anaphylaktoide Reaktionen nach Infusion natürlicher und künstlicher Kolloide. Springer, Berlin Heidelberg New York

Ring J, Messmer K (1976) Anaphylaktoide Reaktionen nach Infusion kolloidaler Volumenersatzmittel. Internist Prax 16:579

Ring J, Messmer K (1977) Incidence and severity of anaphylactoid reactions to colloid volume substitutes. Lancet I:466

Risberg B (1977) Fibrinolysis and tourniquet. Lancet II:360

Rish L, Rodriquez JC (1972) Effect of O-(beta-hydroxyethyl)-rutosides on oedema in chronic venous insufficiency of the lower limb. A double blind trial. Angiologica 9:62

Rø JS, Kluge TH, Taksdal S, Skrede S (1974) Haemostatic parameters and erythrocyte sedimentation rate in dextran-warfarin treated vascular surgical patients. Scand J Thor Cardiovasc Surg 8:206

Roberts B, Rosato FE, Rosato EF (1964) Heparin – a cause of arterial emboli? Surgery 55:803

Roberts JVC (1975) Fibrinogen uptake scanning for diagnosis of deep vein thrombosis – a plea for standardization. Br Med J 3:455

Roberts MH, Johnston FR (1975) Hepatic rupture from anticoagulant therapy. Arch Surg 110:1152

Roberts VC, Cotton LT (1974) Prevention of postoperative deep vein thrombosis in patients with malignant disease. Br Med J 1:358

Roberts VC, Cotton LT (1975) Failure of low-dose heparin to improve efficacy of peroperative intermittent calf compression in preventing postoperative deep vein thrombosis. Br Med J 3:458

Roberts VC, Sabri S, Pietroni MC, Gurewich V, Cotton LT (1971) Passive flexion and femoral vein flow: a study using a motorized foot mover. Br Med J 3:78

Roberts VC, Sabri S, Beeley AH, Cotton LT (1972) The effect of intermittently applied external pressure on the haemodynamics of the lower limb in man. J Surg 59:223

Robertson B, Pandolfi M, Nilsson IM (1972a) "Fibrinolytic capacity" in healthy volunteers as estimated from effect of venous occlusion of arms. Acta Chir Scand 138:429

Robertson B, Pandolfi M, Nilsson IM (1972b) "Fibrinolytic capacity" in healthy volunteers at different ages as studied by standardized venous occlusion of arms and legs. Acta Med Scand 191:199

Robertson B, Pandolfi M, Nilsson IM (1972c) Response of local fibrinolytic activity to venous occlusion of arms and legs in healthy volunteers. Acta Chir Scand 138:437

Robin E (1977) Overdiagnosis and overtreatment of pulmonary embolism: The emperor may have no clothes. Ann Int Med 87:775

Roderick L (1929) The pathology of sweet clover disease in cattle. J Am Vet Med Ass 74:314

Rogers P, Walsh P, Marder V, Bosak GC, Lachman J, Ritchie W, Oppenheimer L, Sherry S (1978) Controlled trial of low-dose heparin and sulfinpyrazone to prevent venous thromboembolism after operation on the hip. J Bone Joint Surg [Am] 60:758

Romanus M, Risberg B (1978) Fibrinolysis in ischemic hamster cheek pouch. Thromb Res 12:42

Rose SS (1970) A report on the use of an hydroxyethylrutoside in symptoms due to venous back pressure and allied conditions in the lower limbs. Br J Clin Pract 24:161

Rosenberg IL, Evans M, Pollock AV (1975) Prophylaxis of postoperative leg vein thrombosis by low dose subcutaneous heparin or preoperative calf muscle stimulation: a controlled clinical trial. Br Med J 1:649

Rosenberg JS, McKenna P, Rosenberg RD (1975) Inhibition of antithrombin-heparin cofactor. J Biol Chem 250:8883

Rosenberg R (1976) The function of heparin. In: Kakkar VV, Thomas DP (eds) Heparin. Chemistry and clinical usage. Academic Press, London New York San Francisco

Rosenberg RD (1977) Chemistry of the hemostatic mechanism and its relationship to the action of heparin. Fed Proc 36:10

Rosenberg RD, Lam L (1979) Correlation between structure and function of heparin. Proc Natl Acad Sci USA 76:1218

Rosenberg RD, Damus PS (1973) Purification and mechanism of action of human antithrombin-heparin cofactor. J Biol Chem 248:6490

Rosenberg RD, Dosta GM, Jordan RE, Gardner WT (1980) The interaction of heparin with thrombin and antithrombin. Biochem Biophys Res Comm 96:1200

Rosenfeld EL, Lukomskaja IS (1957) The splitting of dextran and isomaltase by animal tissues. Clin Chim Acta 2:105

Rosengarten D, Laird J (1971) The effect of leg elevation on the incidence of deep-vein thrombosis after operation. Br J Surg 58:182

Rosengarten D, Laird J, Jeyasingh K, Martin P (1970) The failure of compression stockings (Tubigrip) to prevent deep venous thrombosis after operation. Br J Surg 57:296

Rosenthal D, Cossman D, Matsumoto G, Callow A (1979) Prophylactic interruption of the inferior vena cava. A retrospective evaluation. Am J Surg:389

Rosenthal N (1925) Clinical and hematological studies on Banti's disease. 1. The blood platelet factor with reference to splenectomy. JAMA 84:1887

Rosner SW (1965) Heparin administration as an aerosol. Vasc Dis 2:131

Ross S, Ebert R (1959) Microelectrophoresis of blood platelets and the effect of dextran. J Clin Invest 38:155

Rossi E, Green D, Rosen J, Spies S, Jao J (1980) Sequential changes in factor VIII and platelets preceeding deep vein thrombosis in patients with spinal cord injury. Br J Haematol 45:143

Rössle R (1937) Über die Bedeutung und Entstehung der Wadenvenenthrombosen. Virch Arch 300:180

Roth GJ, Siok CJ (1978) Acetylation of the NH_2-terminal serine of prostaglandin synthetase by aspirin. J Biol Chem 253:3782

Roth GJ, Stanford N, Majerus PW (1975) Acetylation of prostaglandin synthetase by aspirin. Proc Natl Acad Sci USA 72:3073

Roth GJ, Ozols J, Siok CJ (1978) Modification by aspirin of the amino terminal serine of prostaglandin synthetase. Clin Res 26:356

Rothman S, Adelson E, Schwebel A, Langdell RD (1957) Adsorption of carbon-14-dextran to human blood platelets and red blood cells in vitro. Vox Sang 2:104

Roztocil K, Prerovsky I, Oliva I (1977) The effect of hydroxyethylrutosides on capillary filtration rate in the lower limb of man. Eur J Clin Pharmacol 11:435

Ruckley CV (1975) ^{125}I-fibrinogen test in diagnosis of deep venous thrombosis. Br Med J 2:498

Ruckley CV (1976) A multi-unit controlled trial of heparin and dextran in the prevention of venous thromboembolic disease. In: Kakkar VV, Thomas DP (eds) Heparin. Chemistry and clinical usage. Academic Press, London

Ruckley CV (1981) Pulmonary embolism; trends in Edinburgh surgical units over twenty years. Thromb Haemost 46:18

Russo JV, Friesinger GC, Margolis S, Ross RS (1970) Heparin and ventricular arrhytmias after myocardial infarction. Lancet II:1271

Rustad H (1970) Prophylactic treatment with anticoagulants against venous thrombosis and pulmonary embolism in surgical patients. Norwegian Monographs on Medical Science. Universitetsforlaget, Oslo

Ryde M, Eriksson H, Tangen O (1981) Studies on the different mechanisms by which heparin and polysulphated xylan (PZ68) inhibit blood coagulation in man. Thromb Res 23:435

Saameli K (1978) Effects on the uterus. In: Berde B, Schild HO (eds) Ergot alkaloids and related compounds. Springer, Berlin Heidelberg New York, p 233

Saba H, Saba S, Blackburn C, Hartmann R, Mason R (1979) Heparin neutralization of PGI_2: Effects upon platelets. Science 205:499

Saba T, Antikatzides T (1979) Heparin induced alterations in clearance and distribution of blood-borne microparticles following operative trauma. Ann Surg 189:426

Sabri S, Roberts VC, Cotton LT (1971a) Effects of externally applied pressure on the haemodynamics of the lower limb. Br Med J 3:503

Sabri S, Roberts VC, Cotton LT (1971b) Prevention of early postoperative deep vein thrombosis by intermittent compression of the leg during surgery. Br Med J 4:394

Sabri S, Roberts VC, Cotton LT (1971c) Prevention of early postoperative deep vein thrombosis by passive exercise of leg during surgery. Br Med J 3:82

Sabri S, Roberts VC, Cotton LT (1972) The effects of intermittently applied external pressure on the haemodynamics of the hind-limb in greyhound dogs. Br J Surg 59:219

Sachs JJ, Labate JS (1949) Dicumarol in the treatment of antenatal thromboembolic disease. Report of a case with hemorrhagic manifestations in the fetus. Am J Obstet Gynecol 57:965

Sagar S (1974) Heparin prophylaxis against fatal postoperative pulmonary embolism. Br Med J 2: 153

Sagar S, Massey J, Sanderson JM (1975) Low-dose heparin prophylaxis against fatal pulmonary embolism. Br Med J 4:257

Sagar S, Stamatakis JD, Higgins AF, Nairn D, Maffei FH, Thomas DP, Kakkar VV (1976a) Efficacy of low-dose heparin in prevention of extensive deep-vein thrombosis in patients undergoing total-hip replacement. Lancet I:151

Sagar S, Stamatakis JD, Thomas DP, Kakkar VV (1976b) Oral contraceptives, antithrombin III activity and postoperative deep-vein thrombosis. Lancet I:509

Sahud MA, Cohen RJ (1971) Aspirin-induced prolongation of the Ivy bleeding time: its diagnostic usefulness. Calif Med 115:10

Sakamoto S, Sakamoto M, Goldhaber P, Glimcher MJ (1975) Studies on the interaction between heparin and mouse bone collagenase. Biochim Biophys Acta 395:41

Saldeen T (1977) The microembolism syndrome and dextran. In: Lewis D (ed) Dextran – 30 years. Acta Univ Upsal Symp Univ Ups Ann 500 Celebrantis 3. Uppsala 1977

Saldeen T, Hedin H, Revenäs P, Smedegård G (1979) Morphologic alterations in human aggregate anaphylaxy (In Swedish). Sven Läkaresällsk Förh 88:4

Saldeen T, Hjelmstedt Å, Modig J, Sahlstedt B (1981) Effect of epidural block on deep venous thrombosis and fibrinolysis after total hip replacement. In: Davidson J, Nilsson IM, Åstedt B (eds) Progress in fibrinolysis, vol V. Churchill Livingstone, Edinburgh London Melbourne New York

Salzman A, Axilrod H (1971) The value of preoperative lung scanning in the assessment of postoperative perfusion abnormalities. J Urol 106:581

Salzman E (1963) Measurement of platelet adhesiveness. A simple in vitro technique demonstrating an abnormality in von Willebrand's disease. J Lab Clin Med 62:724

Salzman E (1979) The surgeon's comments. In: Verstraete M, Vermylen J, Roberts H (eds) The challenge of clinical trials in thrombosis. Schattauer, Stuttgart New York

Salzman E, Davies G (1980) Prophylaxis of venous thromboembolism. Analysis of cost effectiveness. Ann Surg 191:207

Salzman E, Harris WH, DeSanctis RW (1966) Anticoagulation for prevention of thromboembolism following fractures of the hip. N Engl J Med 75:122

Salzman E, Harris W, DeSanctis R (1971) Reduction of venous thromboembolism by agents affecting platelet function. New Engl J Med 284:1287

Salzman E, Ploetz J, Bettmann M, Skillman J, Klein L (1980a) Intraoperative external pneumatic calf compression to afford longterm prophylaxis against deep vein thrombosis in urological patients. Surgery 87:239

Salzman E, Rosenberg R, Smith M, Linden J, Favreau L (1980b) Effect of heparin and heparin fractions on platelet aggregation. J Clin Invest 65:64

Salzman R, Bucher T (1978) Actions of ergot alkaloids at adrenoreceptors. In: Berde B, Schild HO (eds) Ergot alkaloids and related compounds. Springer, Berlin Heidelberg New York

Sandritter W, Felix H (1967) Geographical pathology of fatal lung embolism. Pathol Microbiol 30: 742

Sas G, Blasko G, Bankegyi D, Jako J, Palos A (1974) Abnormal antithrombin III (antithrombin III "Budapest") as a cause of a familial thrombophilia. Thromb Diath Haemorrh 32:105

Satiani B, Kuhns M, Evans W (1980) Deep venous thrombosis following operations upon the abdominal aorta. Surg Gynaecol Obstet 151:241

Sautter R, Lavson D, Bhattacharyya S, Chen H-M, Treuhalf P, Milbauer J, Mazza J, Emanuel D, Kock E, Lolley D, Myers W, Ray J, Plotka E, Nycz G, Wenzel F (1979) The limited utility of fibrinogen I 125 leg scanning. Arch Intern Med 139:148

Sawyer PN, Srinivasan S (1973) The role of surface phenomena in intravascular thrombosis. Bibl Anat 12:106

Sawyer PN, Stanczewski B, Pomerance A, Lucas T, Stoner G, Srinivasan S (1973) Utility of anticoagulant drugs in vascular thrombosis: Electron microscopic and biophysical study. Surgery 74:263

Schaub N, Duckert F, Fridrich R, Gruber UF (1975) Häufigkeit postoperativer tiefer Venenthrombosen bei Patienten der allgemeinen Chirurgie und Urologie. Langenbecks Arch Chir 340:23

Schaul W, Emery H, Hall J (1975) Chondrodysplasia punctata and maternal warfarin use during pregnancy. Am J Dis Child 129:360

Schipper HG (1980) Antithrombin III and human antithrombin III concentrates. Clinical and experimental studies. Thesis. Rodopi, Amsterdam

Schipper HG, Roos J, van der Menlen F, ten Cate JW (1981) Antithrombin III deficiency in surgical intensive care patients. Thromb Res 21:73

Schlag G, Grünwald M, Redl H (1981) Experimenteller Beitrag zur Thromboseproblematik. In: Tscherne H, Deutsch E (eds) Postoperative Thromboembolie-Prophylaxe aus aktueller Sicht. Thieme, Stuttgart New York

Schlosser V (1977) Klinik, Prophylaxe und Therapie der Lungenembolie aus chirurgischer Sicht. Med Klin 72:1947

Schmid-Schönbein H, Volger E, Weiss J, Brandhuber M (1975) Effect of O-(beta-hydroxyethyl)-rutosides on the microrheology of human blood under defined flow conditions. Vasa 4:263

Schmitt HE (1977) Phlebography in the diagnosis of deep venous thrombosis. In: Kappert A (ed) New trends in venous diseases. Huber, Bern Stuttgart Vienna

Schneider J, Bierbaum D, Mross I, Capp-Schwoerer H (1967) Medikamentöse Thrombose- und Embolieprophylaxe mit SP-54 bei der Therapie gynäkologischer Karzinome mit Radium und Telekobaltbestrahlung. Med Welt 23:1446

Schofield F (1924) Damaged sweet clover; the cause of a new disease in cattle stimulating hemorrhagic septicemia and blackleg. J Am Vet Med Ass 64:553

Scholkens BA, Bartman W, Beck G (1979) Vasodilation and inhibition of platelet aggregation by prostacyclins with modified omega side chain. Prostaglandins 3:7

Schönbauer L (1928) Über postoperative Thrombose und Embolie. Arch Klin Chir 149:1

Schöndorf T (1978) Thromboembolieprophylaxe mit Heparin bei elektiven Hüftgelenksoperationen. Deutsch Med Wochenschr 103:1877

Schöndorf T, Hey D (1976) Combined administration of low dose heparin and aspirin as prophylaxis of deep vein thrombosis after hip joint surgery. Haemostasis 5:250

Schöndorf T, Weber U (1979) Heparin prophylaxis combined with DHE or dextran in hip operations. Thromb Diath Haemorrh 42:249

Schöndorf T, Weber U (1980) Prevention of deep vein thrombosis in orthopedic surgery with the combination of low dose heparin plus either dihydroergotamine or dextran. Scand J Haematol [Suppl] 36:126

Schöning B, Koch H (1975) Pathergiequote verschiedener Plasmasubstitute an Haut und Respirationstractus orthopädischer Patienten. Anaesthetist 24:507

Schoolman HM, Becktel JM, Best WR (1968) Statistics in medical research: principles versus practices. J Lab Clin Med 71:357

Schuster J, Meier-Ruge W, Elgi F (1969) Zur Pathologie der Osteopathie nach Heparinbehandlung. Dtsch Med Wochenschr 94:2334

Schütze U, Berenskötter H, Clausen C, Meybier H (1979) Die Wirkung von Dihydroergotamin auf die Darmmotilität bei funktionellen Passagestörungen. Therapiewoche 29:5887

Schütze U, Wiedemann K, Hanf K, Bauer PK (1980) Der Einfluß von Dihydroergotamin auf die Darmmobilität. Eine tierexperimentelle Untersuchung. Therapiewoche 30:1355

Schwartz N, Feigl W, Neuwirth E, Holzner JH (1976) Venöse Thrombosen und Lungenembolien in Obduktionsgut. Wien Klin Wochenschr 88:423

Schwartz S, Shay H, Beebe H, Rob C (1964) Effect of low molecular weight dextran on venous flow. Surgery 55:106

Schwartzkopff W (1965) Determination of permeability of the abdominal capillary membranes with low and high molecular substances. Bibl Anat 7:156

Scott Blair GW, Matchett RH (1972) On the interpretation of thromboelastograms. Haemostasis 1:93

Scurr JH, Ibrahim SZ, Faber RG, LeQuesne LP (1977) The efficacy of graduated compression stockings in the prevention of deep vein thrombosis. Br J Surg 64:371

Scurr JH, Robbe I, Ellis H (1979) Thromboembolism — prophylaxis using a mechanical device to dorsiflex the foot. Thromb Haemost 42:250

Scurr J, Robbe I, Ellis H, Goldsmith H (1981) Simple mechanical method for decreasing the incidence of thromboembolism. Am J Surg 141:582

Scurr JH, Bucknall TE, Ellis H, Wastell C (1981) Sequential pneumatic compression — an effective method of preventing deep venous thrombosis. Thromboembolism 46:191

Sebeseri O, Kummer H, Zingg E (1975) Controlled prevention of post-operative thrombosis in urological diseases with depot heparin. Eur Urol 1:229

Sechas M, Papachristodoulou A, Mandalaki T, Gogas S, Skalkeas G (1977) Prophylaxis of postoperative venous thrombosis of the lower extremities. In: Louros NC, Le Vay D (eds) Proceedings of the biennial world congress of the International College of Surgeons. Excerpt Med, Amsterdam Oxford

Sechas M, Mandalaki T, Fouridis G, Loizou C, Dimitriadou C, Bekopoulos T, Kranidis A (1978) Results of the action of dihydroergotamine on the prevention of postoperative venous thrombosis. Fifth Int Congr on Thromboembolism, p 64

Seeman P (1972) The membrane actions of anesthetics and tranquilizers. Pharmacol Rev 24:583

Seemann C, Hedin H, Richter W, Ring J, Dtippig S, Messmer K (1978) Hapten-Hemmung der Dextran-induzierten anaphylaktoiden Reaktion. Allergol Immunopathol 1:185

Segal S, Sadovsky E, Weinstein D, Polishuk WZ (1975) Prevention of postpartum venous thrombosis with low doses of heparin. Eur J Obstet Gynecol Reprod Biol 5/5:273

Segesser D, Gruber UF (1977) Vergleich der Wirksamkeit von Natriumheparinat und Calciumheparinat zur Verhütung thromboembolischer Komplikationen. Arzneim Forsch 27:2157

Seglias J, Gruber UF (1979) Dosage in low-dose heparin prophylaxis. Haemostasis 8:361

Seigel DG (1972) Pregnancy, the puerperium and the steroid contraceptive. In: Foster D (ed) The epidemiology of venous thrombosis. Milbank Memorial Fund Q 50:15

Seltzer MH, Quarantillo EP (1973) Spontaneous splenic rupture in an anticoagulant patient. J Med Soc N J 70:397

Semple R (1954) The effect of single large infusions of various dextran solutions on hypovolemic dogs. Can J Biochem Physiol 32:670

Senftleben W (1879) Über den Verschluß der Blutgefässe nach Unterbindung. Arch Path Anat Physiol 77:421

Sevitt S (1962) Venous thrombosis and pulmonary embolism. Their prevention by oral anticoagulants. Am J Med 33:703

Sevitt S (1974) The structure and growth of valve-pocket thrombi in femoral veins. J Clin Path 27:517

Sevitt S (1978) Pathology and pathogenesis of deep vein thrombi. In: Bergan J, Yao J (eds) Venous problems. Year Book Medical Publishers, Chicago London

Sevitt S, Gallagher NG (1959) Prevention of venous thrombosis and pulmonary embolism in injured patients. Lancet II:981

Sevitt S, Gallagher NG (1961) Venous thrombosis and pulmonary embolism. A clinico-pathological study in injured and burned patients. Br J Surg 48:475

Seyfer A, Seaber A, Dombrose F, Urbaniak J (1981) Coagulation changes in elective surgery and trauma. Ann Surg 193:210

Shah GA, Dhall TZ, Ferguson IA, Dhall DP (1980) Detection of deep vein thrombosis by ^{125}I-labelled fibrinogen scanning technique – a methodological study. Thromb Res 18:101

Shaper AG, Marsh NA, Patel I, Kater F (1975) Response of fibrinolytic activity to venous occlusion. Br Med J 3:561

Sharnoff JG (1963) An evaluation of the Dale and Laidlow coagulometer in the heparin control of thromboembolism. Proc NY State Assoc Publ Health Lab 43:10

Sharnoff JG (1966) Results in the prophylaxis of postoperative thromboembolism. Surg Gynecol Obstet 123:303

Sharnoff JG (1975) Small dose subcutaneous heparin. A safe regimen. In: Nicolaides AN (ed) Thromboembolism. Aetiology, advances in prevention and management. MTP, Lancaster

Sharnoff JG, DeBlazio G (1970) Prevention of fatal postoperative thromboembolism by heparin prophylaxis. Lancet II:1006

Sharnoff JG, Bagg JF, Breen SR, Rogliano AG, Walsh AG, Scardino V (1960) The possible indication of postoperative thromboembolism by platelet counts and blood coagulation studies in the patient undergoing extensive surgery. Surg Gynecol Obstet 111:469

Sharnoff JG, Kass HH, Mistica BA (1962) A plan of heparinization of the surgical patient to prevent postoperative thromboembolism. Surg Gynecol Obstet 115:75

Sharp AA, Wasser BA, Paxton AM, Allington MJ (1968) Anticoagulant therapy with a purified fraction of Malayan pit viper venom. Lancet I:493

Shaw LW, Cornfield J, Cole C (1974) Statistical problems in the design of clinical trials and interpretation of results. Thromb Diath Haemorrh [Suppl] 59

Shead GV, Narayanan R (1980) Incidence of postoperative venous thromboembolism in South India. Br J Surg 67:813

Sherman S, Hall BD (1976) Warfarin and fetal abnormality. Lancet I:692

Sherry S (1975) Low-dose heparin prophylaxis for postoperative venous thromboembolism. N Engl J Med 293:300

Sherry S (1976) Low-dose heparin for the prophylaxis of pulmonary embolism. Am Rev Resp Dis 114:661

Sherry S (1979) The Anturane reinfarction trial. In: Verstraete M, Vermylen J, Roberts H (eds) The challenge of clinical trials in thrombosis. Schattauer, Stuttgart New York

Shnider M, D'Souza CR (1976) Cutaneous gangrene: a rare complication of coumarin therapy. Can J Surg 19:64

Shoemaker WC, Brunius U, Gelin L-E (1965) Hemodynamic and microcirculatory effects of high and low viscosity dextrans. Surgery 58:518

Shull K, Nicolaides A, Fernandes F, Miles C, Horner J, Neddham T, Cooke E, Eastcott F (1979) Significance of popliteal reflux in relation to ambulatory venous pressure and ulceration. Arch Surg 114:1304

Siegerstetter J, Neiss A (1977) Estimating the risk of postoperative thrombosis. The statistician's contribution. In: Pabst HW, Maurer G (eds) Postoperative Thromboembolie-Prophylaxe. Schattauer, Stuttgart New York

Sigel B, Edelstein A, Felix R, Memhardt C (1973) Compression of the deep venous system of the lower leg during inactive recumbency. Arch Surg 106:38

Sigel B, Edelstein A, Savitch L, Hasty J, Felix R (1975) Type of compression for reducing venous stasis. A study of lower extremities during inactive recumbency. Arch Surg 110:171

Sigel B, Justin J, Gibson R, Felix R, Popky G, Parker J, Ipsen J (1979) Risk assessment of pulmonary embolism by multivariate analysis. Arch Surg 114:188

Sigg K (1977) Treatment of varicose veins by injection-sclerotherapy: a method practised in Switzerland. In: Hobbs J (ed) The treatment of venous disorders. A comprehensive review of current practice in the management of varicose veins and the postthrombotic syndrome. MTP, Lancaster

Sikorsky JM, Hampson WG, Staddon GE (1981) The natural history and aetiology of deep vein thrombosis after total hip replacement. J Bone Joint Surg [Br] 63-B:171

Silberman S, Bernik M, Potter E, Kwaan H (1973) Effects of ancrod (arvin) in mice: studies on plasma fibrinogen and fibrinolytic activity. Br J Haematol 24:101

Silver MJ, Smith JB, Ingerman C, Kocsis JJ (1973) Arachidonic acid-induced human platelet aggregation and prostaglandin formation. Prostaglandins 4:863

Silvergleid R, Bernstein R, Burton DS, Tanner JB, Silverman JF, Schrier SL (1977) Aspirin-persantin prophylaxis in elective total hip replacement. Thromb Haemost 38:166

Silverstein A (1979) Neurological complications of anticoagulation therapy. A neurologist's review. Arch Intern Med 139:217

Simmons AV, Sheppard MA, Cox AF (1973) Deep venous thrombosis after myocardial infarction. Predisposing factors. Br Heart J 35:623

Simmons R, Uranga V, La Plante S, Buselmeier T, Kjellstrand C, Najarian J (1972) Pulmonary complications in transplant recipients. Arch Surg 105:260

Simon T, Stengle J (1974) Antithrombin practice in orthopaedic surgery. Results of a survey. Clin Orthopaed Rel Res 102:181

Sinclair J, Forbes CD, Prentice CRM, Scott R (1976) The incidence of deep vein thrombosis in prostatectomised patients following the administration of the fibrinolytic inhibitor, aminocaproic acid (EACA). Urol Res 4:129

Sinzinger H, Silberbauer K, Winter M (1978) Prostacyclin – Hemmwirkung auf die Thrombozytenanlagerung an die Gefäßwand in vivo? Vasa 7:350

Sixma JJ (1978) Techniques for diagnosing prethrombotic states. A review. Thromb Haemost 40:252

Sjöberg HE, Blombäck M, Granberg PO (1976) Thromboembolic complications, heparin treatment and increase in coagulation factors in Cushing's syndrome. Acta Med Scand 199:95

Skillman J, Collins R, Coe N, Goldstein B, Shapiro R, Zervas N, Bettman M, Salzman E (1978) Prevention of deep vein thrombosis in neurosurgical patients: A controlled, randomized trial of external pneumatic compression boots. Surgery 83:354

Slade L, Taylor L, Wechsler A, McKee P (1973) Postsurgical haemorrhage in dogs anticoagulated with ancrod (arvin). Ann Surg 178:721

Slade L, Andes A, Mason A (1976) Platelet aggregation following defibrination with ancrod. Thromb Haemost 36:424

Smedegård G (1980) Anaphylactic shock. Pathophysiology of aggregate and cytotropic anaphylaxis in the monkey. Acta Univ Ups Abstr Upps Diss Fac Sci 548, Uppsala

Smith GW (1968) Iliofemoral venous thrombectomy indications, technique and results in forty-five cases. Circulation 37:847

Smith JB, Willis AL (1971) Aspirin selectively inhibits prostaglandin production in human platelets. Nature 231:235

Smith JB, Ingerman C, Kocsis JJ, Silver MJ (1973) Formation of prostaglandins during the aggregation of human blood platelets. J Clin Invest 52:965

Smith JB, Ingerman C, Kocsis JJ, Silver MJ (1974) Formation of an intermediate in prostaglandin biosynthesis and its association with the platelet release reaction. J Clin Invest 53:1468

Smith JB, Ingerman C, Silver MJ (1976a) Malondialdehyde formation as an indicator of prostaglandin production by human platelets. J Lab Clin Med 88:167

Smith JB, Ingerman C, Silver MJ (1976b) Persistence of thromboxane A2-like material and platelet release-inducing activity in plasma. J Clin Invest 58:1119

Smith R, Blick E, Coalson J, Stein P (1972) Thrombus production by turbulence. J Appl Physiol 32:261

Smith RC, Duncancson J, Ruckley CV, Webber RG, Allan NC, Dawes J, Bolton AE, Hunter WM, Pepper DS, Cash JD (1978a) β-thromboglobulin and deep vein thrombosis. Thromb Haemost 39:338

Smith RC, Elton RA, Orr JD, Hart AJL, Graham DF, Fuller GAG, Rundle JSH, Macpherson AIS, Ruckley CV (1978b) Dextran and intermittent pneumatic compression in prevention of postoperative deep vein thrombosis. Multiunit trial. Br Med J 1:952

Smyrnis SA, Kolios AS (1973) Deep vein thrombosis in surgical patients. A phlebographic study. Surgery 73:692

Smyrnis SA, Kolios AS, Agnantis JK (1973) Deep-vein thrombosis in patients with fracture of the upper part of the femur. A phlebography study. Br J Surg 60:447

Smythe HA, Ogryzlo MA, Murphy EA, Mustard JF (1965) The effect of sulfinpyrazone (anturan) on platelet economy and blood coagulation in man. Can Med Assoc J 92:818

Solonen K (1963) Prophylactic anticoagulant therapy in the treatment of lower limb fractures. Acta Orthop Scand 33:329

Soreff J, Johansson H, Diener L, Göransson L (1975) Acetylsalicylic acid in a trial to diminish thromboembolic complications after elective hip surgery. Acta Orthop Scand 46:246

Soria C, Soria J, Caen J (1978) Action du polysufate de pentosane sur la coagulation. Cah d'Anesthesiol 26:1

Spebar M, Collins G, Rich N, Kang I, Clagett P, Salander J (1981) Perioperative heparin prophylaxis of deep venous thrombosis in patients with peripheral vascular disease. Am J Surg 142:649

Special report (1977) Prevention of venous thromboembolism in surgical patients by low-dose heparin. Prepared by the Council on thrombosis by The American Heart Association. Circulation 55:423

Spieler U, Preter B, Brunner U (1972) Traumatische Thrombosen im tiefen Venensystem bei frischen Unterschenkelfrakturen. Schweiz Med Wochenschr 102:1535

Spiro M, Roberts VC, Richards JB (1970) Effect of externally applied pressure on femoral vein blood flow. Br Med J 1:719

Spittle CR (1973) Vitamin C and deep vein thrombosis. Lancet II:199

Sripad S, Antcliff AC, Martin P (1971) Deep-vein thrombosis in two district hospitals in Essex. Br J Surg 58:563

Stadil F (1970) Prevention of postoperative vein thrombosis with dextran 70 (In Danish). Ugeskr Laeg 132:1817

Stalker AL (1964) Intravascular erythrocyte aggregation. Bibl Anat 4:108

Stamatakis JD, Kakkar VV, Lawrence D, Ward V (1977a) Synergistic effect of heparin and dihydroergotamine in the prophylaxis of postoperative deep vein thrombosis. In: Pabst HW, Maurer G (eds) Postoperative Thromboembolie-Prophylaxe. Schattauer, Stuttgart New York

Stamatakis JD, Kakkar VV, Sagar S, Lawrence D, Nairn D, Bentley PG (1977b) Femoral vein thrombosis and total hip replacement. Br Med J 2:223

Stamatakis JD, Lawrence D, Kakkar VV (1977c) Surgery, venous thrombosis and anti-Xa. Br J Surg 64:709

Stamatakis JD, Sagar S, Lawrence D, Kakkar VV (1977d) Dihydroergotamine in the prevention of postoperative deep venous thrombosis. Br J Surg 64:294

Stamatakis JD, Kakkar VV, Lawrence D, Bentley PG, Nairn D, Ward V (1978) Failure of aspirin to prevent postoperative deep vein thrombosis in patients undergoing total hip replacement. Br Med J 1:1031

Stanton J, Freis E, Wilkins R (1949) The acceleration of linear flow in the deep veins of the lower extremity of man by local compression. J Clin Invest 28:553

Stanton-Hicks M (1981) Low-dose heparin therapy and spinal anaesthesia. JAMA 246:886

Starksen N, Day A, Gazzaniga A (1978) Does splenectomy result in a higher incidence of limb deep venous thrombosis? Am J Surg 135:202

Stathatkis N, Papayannis AG, Gardikas CD (1973) Postoperative antithrombin-III concentration. Lancet I:430

Stead N, Kaplan AP, Rosenberg RD (1976) Inhibition of activated factor XII by antithrombin-heparin cofactor. J Biol Chem 251:6481

Steele M, Lim R (1975) Advances in management of splenic injuries. Am J Surg 130:159

Steele P (1980) Trial of dipyridamole-aspirin in recurring venous thrombosis. Lancet II:1328

Stein P, Sabbah H (1974) Measured turbulence and its effect on thrombus formation. Circ Res 35:608

Stein P, Willis P, De Mets D (1981) History and physical examination in acute pulmonary embolism in patients without preexisting cardiac or pulmonary disease. Am J Cardiol 47:218

Steinmann E, Duckert F, Gruber UF (1975) Wert von Dextran 70 zur Thromboembolieprophylaxe in der allgemeinen Chirurgie, Orthopädie, Urologie und Gynäkologie. Eine Literaturübersicht. Schweiz Med Wochenschr 105:1637

Stella L, Donati MB, de Gaetano G (1975) Bleeding time in laboratory animals. I. Aspirin does not prolong bleeding time in rats. Thromb Res 7:709

Stenflo J (1975) Structural comparison of normal and dicoumarol-induced prothrombin. In: Hemker HC, Veltkamp JJ (eds) Prothrombin and related coagulation factors. Leiden University Press. Leiden

Stenflo J, Ganrot PO (1973) Binding of Ca^{2+} to normal and dicoumarol-induced prothrombin. Biochem Biophys Res Comm 50:98

Stenflo J, Suttie JW (1977) Vitamin K-dependent formation of γ-carboxyglutamic acid. Ann Rev Biochem 46:157

Stenflo J, Fernlund P, Egan W (1974) Vitamin K dependent modification of glutamic acid residues in prothrombin. Proc Natl Acad Sci USA 71:2730

Stephenson CBS, Wallace JG, Vaughan JV (1973) Dextran 70 in the prevention of postoperative deep-vein thrombosis with observations on pulmonary embolism. Report on a pilot study. N Z Med J 77:302

Stevens J, Fardin R, Freeark R (1968) Lower extremity thrombophlebitis in patients with femoral neck fractures. A venographic investigation and a review of the early and late significance of the findings. J Trauma 8:527

Stevenson M, Rohr P, Davidson A, Byars E, Hopkins G, Tarney T (1977) Changes in euglobulin lysis following intermittent pneumatic calf compression. Thromb Haemost 38:263

Stevenson R, Burton M, Ferlauto G, Taylor H (1980) Hazards of oral anticoagulants during pregnancy. JAMA 243:1549

Stewart G (1975) The role of the vessel wall in deep venous thrombosis. In: Nicolaides AN (ed) Thromboembolism. Aetiology, advances in prevention and management. MTP, Lancaster

Stewart G, Ritchie WG, Lynch PR (1973) A scanning and transmission electron microscopic study of canine jugular veins. Proc Workshop on Scanning Electron Microscopy in Pathology. IIT Res Inst, Chicago

Stewart G, Ritchie WG, Lynch PR (1974) Venous endothelial damage produced by massive sticking and emigration of leukocytes. Am J Pathol 74:507

Stewart G, Stern HR, Schaub RG (1978) Endothelial alterations, deposition of blood elements and increased accumulation of ^{131}I-albumin in canine jugular veins following abdominal surgery. Thromb Res 12:555

Stinchfield FE, Sankaran B, Samilson R (1956) The effect of anticoagulant therapy on bone repair. J Bone Joint Surg [Am] 38-A:270

Stone H, Fabian T (1979) Management of duodenal wounds. J Trauma 19:334

Størsen E, Auensen C (1971) The clinical and roentgenological course of deep-vein thrombosis. J Oslo City Hosp 21:141

Storm O (1958) Anticoagulant protection in surgery. Thromb Diath Haemorrh 2:484

Stovner J, Lund I (1970) The muscle relaxants and their antagonists. A ten-year survey. Br J Anaesth 42:235

Strand L, Bank-Mikkelsen OK, Lindewald H (1975) Small heparin doses as prophylaxis against deep-vein thrombosis in the major surgery. Acta Chir Scand 141:624

String T, Barcia P (1975) Complications of small dose prophylactic heparinization. Am J Surg 130:570

Strömbeck JP (1942) Some viewpoints on etiology and prophylaxis of thrombosis (In Swedish) Nord Med 13:522

Strömbeck JP (1948) An attempt to evaluate the different modern methods for the prevention and treatment of thromboembolism. Acta Chir Scand 97:113

Stuart RK, Thomas DP (1967) Comparative effects of ADP and thrombin in producing stasis thrombosis. Thromb Diath Haemorrh 18:537

Stubbs R (1979) Preventing thromboembolic complications in high-risk surgical patients. Br Med J 1:1707

Sturm V, Gruber UF (1974) Wert der Kumarinderivate zur Thromboembolieprophylaxe in der Chirurgie, Orthopädie und Gynäkologie. Schweiz Med Wochenschr 104:1507

Stürmer E (1976) Pharmacological basis of the treatment of orthostatic disorders with ergot alkaloids. Cardiology 61 [Suppl 1]:290

Stutz P, Gruber UF (1978) Einfluß verschiedener medikamentöser Prophylaxeformen auf die Lokalisation von tiefen Venenthrombosen. Schweiz Rundschau Med 67:1355

Sullivan JM, Harker DH, Gorlin R (1968) Pharmacologic control of thromboembolic complications of cardiac-valve replacement. A preliminary report. N Engl J Med 279:576

Sun FF, McGuire JC, Taylor BM (1978) Metabolism of prostacyclin (PGI_2). Prostaglandins 15:724

Sundqvist S-B, Hedner U, Kullenberg HKE, Bergentz S-E (1981) Deep venous thrombosis of the arm: a study of coagulation and fibrinolysis. Br Med J 2:265

Suomalainen O (1980) Thromboembolism in elective hip surgery. A clinical study, with special re-reference to the incidence, reliability of diagnostic methods, and risk factors of postoperative thromboembolism. Thesis. University of Kuopio

Sutherland WA, Klein RL (1973) Heparin absorption during heparin-saline lung lavage in a patient with pulmonary alveolar proteinosis. Chest 63:1033

Suttie J (1979) How coumarin anticoagulants work. Drug Ther 9:63

Suttie JW, Grant GA, Esmon CT, Shah DV (1974) Postribosomal function of vitamin K in prothrombin synthesis. Mayo Clin Proc 49:933

Svanberg L, Bernstein K, Kullander S, Åstedt B (1980) Effect of dihydroergotamine on coagulation factors and components of the fibrinolytic system. Acta Obstet Gynaecol Scand 59:251

Svend–Hansen H, Bremerskov V, Gøtrik J, Ostri P (1981) Low-dose heparin in proximal femoral fractures. Failure to prevent deep vein thrombosis. Acta Orthop Scand 52:77

Svensjö E (1977) Is a further trial comparing low dose heparin and dextran needed? In: Lewis D (ed) Dextran – 30 years. Acta Univ Ups Symp Univ Ups Ann 500 Celebrantis 3

Svensjö E (1978) Characterization of leakage of macromolecules in postcapillary venules. An intravital and electron microscopy study in the hamster cheek pouch. Acta Univ Ups Diss Fac Pharm, No. 34

Swank RL (1958) Suspension stability of the blood after injections of dextran. J Appl Physiol 12:125

Szczepanski KP (1979) Results of surgical treatment of arterial embolism. Scand J Thor Cariovasc Surg 13:71

Taberner DA, Poller L, Burslem RW, Jones JB (1978) Oral anticoagulants controlled by the British comparative thromboplastin versus low-dose heparin in prophylaxis of deep vein thrombosis. Br Med J 1:272

Taberner DA, Poller L, Burslem RW (1979) Antiplasmin concentrations after surgery: failure of alpha$_2$-antiplasmin to rise in patients with venous thrombosis. Br Med J 1:1122

Takkunen O (1975) The effect of different modes of artificial ventilation and of some prophylactic means on the incidence of postoperative deep vein thrombosis. Ann Chir Gynaecol Fenn [Suppl] 191

Talbot S, Griffiths PD (1974) The diagnosis of pulmonary embolism. Postgrad Med J 50:675

Talbot S, Wakley EJ, Langman MJS (1972) A_1, A_2, B and O Blood-groups, Lewis blood-groups, and serum triglyceride and cholesterol concentrations in patients with venous thromboembolic disease. Lancet I:1152

Tammisto T, Palmu A, Elfving G, Silvonen E, Tiitinen P (1970) Postoperative thromboembolism after different modes of artificial respiration. Acta Chir Scand 136:39

Tangen O, Wik KO, Almqvist IAM, Arfors K-E, Hint HC (1972) Effects of dextran on the structure and plasmin induced lysis of human fibrin. Thromb Res 1:487

Tanner W, Delaney P, Hennessy T (1980) The influence of heparin on intravenous infusions: a prospective study. Br J Surg 67:311

Tansik RL, Namm DH, White HL (1978) Synthesis of prostaglandin 6-keto-$F_{1\alpha}$ by cultured aortic smooth muscle cells and stimulation of its formation in a system with platelet lysates. Prostaglandins 15:399

Tarnay T, Rohr P, Davidson A, Stevenson M, Byars E, Hopkins G (1980) Pneumatic calf compression, fibrinolysis, and the prevention of deep venous thrombosis. Surgery 88:489

Tateson JE, Moncada S, Vane JR (1977) Effect of prostacyclin (PGX) on cyclic AMP concentration in human platelets. Prostaglandins 13:389

Taylor TV, Raftery ABT, Elder JB, Loveday C, Dymock IW, Gibbs ACC, Jeacock J, Lucas SB, Pell MA (1979) Leucocyte ascorbate levels and postoperative deep venous thrombosis. Br J Surg 66:583

Teger-Nilsson A-C, Gyzander E, Hedner U, Myrvold H, Hoppa H, Olsson R, Wallmo L (1978) Antiplasmin and other natural inhibitors of fibrinolysis in clinical material. In: Davidson JF, Rowan RM, Samama MM, Desnoyers PC (eds) Progress in clinical fibrinolysis and thrombolysis. Vol 3. Raven, New York

Teien A, Bjørnson J (1976) Heparin elimination in uraemic patients on haemo-dialysis. Scand J Haematol 17:29

Teien A, Abildgaard U, Höök M (1976a) The anticoagulant effect of heparan sulfate and dermatan sulfate. Thromb Res 8:859

Teien A, Lie M, Abildgaard U (1976b) Assay of heparin in plasma using a chromogenic substrate for activated factor X. Thromb Res 8:413

Terry R, Yuile CL, Golodetz A, Philips C, White RR (1953) Metabolism of dextran – a plasma volume expander. Studies of radioactive carbonlabeled dextran in dogs. J Lab Clin Med 42:6

Thebault JJ, Blatrix CE, Blanchard JF, Panak EA (1975) Effects of Ticlopidine, a new platelet aggregation inhibitor in man. Clin Pharmacol Ther 18:485

Thomas DP (1978a) Biological standardization of sulphated mucopolysaccharides. Fifth Int Congr on Thromboembolism, Bologna:92

Thomas DP (1978b) Heparin in the prophylaxis and treatment of venous thromboembolism. Semin Hematol 15:1

Thomas DP, Barrowcliffe TW, Lindahl U, Thunberg L, Merton LE, Hiller KF, Eggleton CA (1981) A comparative study of heparin and heparin fractions in preventing experimental venous thrombosis. Thromb Haemost 46:185

Thomas DP, Sagar S, Stamatakis JD, Maffei FHA, Erdi A, Kakkar VV (1976) Plasma heparin levels after administration of calcium and sodium salts of heparin. Thromb Res 9:241

Thomas DP, Lane DA, Michalski R, Johnson EA, Kakkar VV (1977) A heparin analogue with specific action on antithrombin III. Lancet I:120

Thomas DP, Merton RE, Barrowcliffe TW, Mulloy B, Johnson EA (1979) Anti-factor Xa activity of heparin sulphate. Thromb Res 14:501

Thomas DP, Barrowcliffe TW, Merton RE, Stocks J, Dawes J, Pepper DS (1980a) In vivo release of anti-Xa clotting activity by a heparin analogue. Thromb Res 17:831

Thomas DP, Barrowcliffe TW, Johnson EA (1980b) The influence of tissue source, salt and molecular weight on heparin activity. Scand J Haematol [Suppl] 36:40

Thomas ML, Browse NL (1972) Internal iliac vein thrombosis. Acta Radiol 12:660

Thorburn J, Loudon JR, Vallance R (1980) Spinal and general anaesthesia in total hip replacement: frequency of deep vein thrombosis. Br J Anaesth 52:1117

Thorén L (1978) Dextran as a plasma volume substitute. In: Blood substitutes and plasma expanders. Liss, New York

Thorsén G (1947) Dextran as substitute for plasma. North Surg Assoc 23:126

Thorsén G, Hint H (1950) Aggregation, sedimentation and intravascular sludging of erythrocytes. An experimental study. Acta Chir Scand [Suppl] 154

Thulesius O, Gjöres J-E (1972) Studies on blood viscosity in chronic venous insufficiency with regard to treatment with flavonoids. Angiologica 9:390

Tibbutt DA, Williams EW, Walker MW, Chesterman CN, Holt JM, Sharp AA (1974) Controlled trial of ancrod and streptokinase in the treatment of deep vein thrombosis of lower limb. Br J Haematol 27:407

Tietze C, Lewit S (1972) Joint program for the study of abortion (JPSA): Early medical complications of legal abortion. Stud Fam Plann 3:97

Tillberg B (1974) Prophylaxis of postoperative venous thrombosis by combined leg bandaging and oxyphenbutaxone. Clinical and experimental investigations. Acta Orthop Scand [Suppl] 158

Tilsner V, Müller U, Reuter H, Raedler A (1980) Results of low-dose heparin prophylaxis of venous thrombosis considering plasma heparin and anti-thrombin III concentration. Thromb Res 17:519

Törngren S (1979a) Optimal regimen of low-dose heparin prophylaxis in gastrointestinal surgery. Acta Chir Scand 145:87

Törngren S (1979b) Prophylaxis of postoperative deep venous thrombosis. Studies on low-dose heparin, blood coagulation, infection as a risk factor and the half-life of fibrinogen in patients after gastrointestinal surgery. Acta Chir Scand [Suppl] 495

Törngren S (1980) Low dose heparin and compression stockings in the prevention of postoperative deep venous thrombosis. Br J Surg 67:482

Törngren S, Forsberg K (1978) Concentrated or diluted heparin prophylaxis of postoperative deep venous thrombosis. Acta Chir Scand 144:283

Törngren S, Norén I, Savidge G (1979) The effect of low-dose heparin on fibrinopeptide A, platelets, fibrinogen degradation products and other haemostatic parameters measured in connection with intestinal surgery. Thromb Res 14:871

Törngren S, Hägglund G, Molin K, Rieger Å (1980a) Postoperative deep venous thrombosis and infectious complications. A clinical study of patients undergoing colo-rectal surgery. Scand J Infect Dis 12:123

Törngren S, Forsberg K, Rieger Å (1980b) Fibrinogen catabolism in patients with postoperative infectious complications. Scand J Infest 12:55

Tomikawa M, Ashida S, Kakihata K, Abiko Y (1978) Antithrombotic action of Ticlopidine, a new platelet aggregation inhibitor. Thromb Res 12:1157

Trowbridge AA, Caraveo J, Green JB, Amaral B, Stone MJ (1978) Heparin related immune thrombocytopenia. Am J Med 65:277

Tsapogas MK, Goussos H, Peabody RA, Karmody AM, Eckert C (1971) Postoperative venous thrombosis and the effectiveness of prophylactic measures. Arch Surg 103:561

Tscherne H, Westermann K, Trentz O, Pretscher P, Mellmann J (1978) Thromboembolische Komplikationen und ihre Prophylaxe beim Hüftgelenkersatz. Unfallheilkunde 81:178

Tso SC, Wong V, Chan V, Chan TK, Ma HK, Todd D (1979) The effect of oral contraceptives on venous thrombosis and coagulation parameters after gynaecological operation in Chinese. Thromb Haemost 42:26

Tso SC, Wong V, Chang V, Chang TK, Ma HK, Todd D (1980) Deep vein thrombosis and changes in coagulation and fibrinolysis after gynaecological operations in chinese: the effect of oral contraceptives and malignant disease. Br J Haematol 46:603

Turitto VT, Weiss HJ (1980) Red blood cells: Their dual role in thrombus formation. Science 207:541

Turpie A (1976) Nonpharmacologic prophylaxis against venous thrombosis: prevention of venous thrombosis in neurosurgical patients with intermittent calf compression. In: Madden J, Hume M (eds) Venous thromboembolism. Prevention and treatment. Appleton-Century-Crafts, New York

Turpie A, Hirsh J (1979) Prophylaxis and therapy of venous thromboembolism. CRC Crit Rev Clin Lab Sci 10:247

Turpie A, Prentice CRM, McNicol GP, Douglas AS (1971) In-vitro studies with ancrod (arvin). Br J Haematol 20:217

Turpie A, Gallus A, Beattie W, Hirsh J (1977) Prevention of venous thrombosis in patients with intracranial disease by intermittent pneumatic compression of the calf. Neurology 27:435

Turpie A, Hirsh J, Genton E, Ilan P, Gent M (1978) Comparative effects of sodium and calcium heparin on plasma heparin concentration, partial thromboplastin time, platelet count and bleeding. Circ 57 [58 Suppl II] 206

Turpie A, Delmore T, Hirsh J, Hull R, Genton E, Hiscoe C, Gent M (1979) Prevention of venous thrombosis by intermittent sequential calf compression in patients with intracranial disease. Thromb Res 15:611

Tyler H, Saxton C, Parry J (1981) Administration to man of UK-37, 248-01, a selective inhibitor of thromboxane synthetase. Lancet I:629

Udén A (1979) Thromboembolic complications following scoliosis surgery in Scandinavia. Acta Orthop Scand 50.175

Ulrich J, Jessen B, Siggaard-Andersen J (1973) Comparative effects of dihydroergotamine and hydergin on the blood flow, capillary filtration rate and the capacitance vessels in the human calf studied by plethysmography. Angiologia 24:657

Vagher JP, Caprini J, Zuckerman L (1979) Multi system analysis of intravenous calcium and sodium heparin. Thromb Res 14:881

Valladares JB, Hankinson J (1980) Incidence of lower extremity deep vein thrombosis in neurosurgical patients. Neurosurgery 6:138

van den Berg E, Walterbusch G, Gotzen L, Rumpf K-D, Otten B, Fröhlich H (1982a) Ergotism leading to threatened limb amputation or to death in two patients given heparin-dihydroergotamine prophylaxis. Lancet I:955

van den Berg E, Rumpf K-D, Fröhlich H, Walterbusch G, Müller-Vahl H, Reilmann H, Graen J (1982b) Vascular spasm during thromboembolism prophylaxis with heparin-dihydroergotamine. Lancet I:268

van der Linde DL (1975) Postoperative deep vein thrombosis (In Dutch). Thesis. University of Nijmegen

van der Meer J, Hemker HC, Loeliger EA (1968) Pharmacological aspects of vitamin K_1. Clinical and experimental study in man. Thromb Diath Haemorrh [Suppl] 29

van Dulken H, Thomeer R (1977) Mini-dose heparin. J Neurosurg 47:974

Vance BM (1934) Thrombosis of the veins of the lower extremity and pulmonary embolism as a complication of trauma. Am J Surg 26:19

van Geloven F, Wittebol P, Sixma JJ (1977) Comparison of postoperative coumarin, dextran 40 and subcutaneous heparin in the prevention of postoperative deep vein thrombosis. Acta Med Scand 202:367

van Haeringen NJ, Glasius E, ten Cate JW, Gerritsen J, van Geet J (1973) Effect of O-(beta-hydroxyethyl)-rutoside on red cell and platelet functions in man. Bibl Anat 12:459

van Vroonhoven TJMV, van Zijl J, Muller H (1974) Low-dose subcutaneous heparin versus oral anticoagulation in the prevention of postoperative deep-venous thrombosis. A controlled clinical trial. Lancet I:375

Varenhorst E (1980) Metabolic changes during endocrine treatment in carcinoma of the prostate. A prospective study in man with special reference to cardiovascular complications during treatment with oestrogens or cyproterone acetate or after orchidectomy. Linköping Univ Med Diss No. 103, Linköping

Vasalli P, Simon G, Rouiller C (1963) Production of ultrastructural glomerular lesions resembling those of toxemia of pregnancy by using thromboplastin infusion in rabbits. Nature 199:1105

Veltkamp JJ, Muis H, Muller AD (1971) Additional evidence for the existence of a precursor molecule of the prothrombin complex in oral anticoagulation. Thromb Diath Haemorrh 25:312

Vennerød AM, Laake K (1975) Inhibition of purified plasma kallikrein by antithrombin III and heparin. Thromb Res 7:223

Venous Thrombosis Clinical Study Group (1975) Small doses of subcutaneous sodium heparin in the prevention of deep vein thrombosis after elective hip operations. Br J Surg 62:348

Vere MF, Sellers SM, Joyce DN, Staddon GE (1979) Use of ethamsylate in vaginal surgery and deep-vein thrombosis. Br Med J 2:528

Vermylen J, Chamone DAP, Verstraete M (1979) Stimulation of prostacyclin release from vessel wall by Bay G 6575, an antithrombotic compound. Lancet I:518

Verstraete M (1976a) Oral anticoagulants, dextran or low-dose subcutaneous heparin: which is it to be in the prophylaxis of deep vein thrombosis of operated patients. Acta Clin Belg 31:106

Verstraete M (1976b) The prevention of postoperative deep vein thrombosis and pulmonary embolism with low dose subcutaneous heparin and dextran. Surg Gynecol Obstet 143:981

Vessey MP (1979) Comments of an epidemiologist. In: Verstraete M, Vermylen J, Roberts H (eds) The challenge of clinical trials in thrombosis. Schattauer, Stuttgart New York

Vessey MP, Doll R (1968) Investigation of relation between use of oral contraceptives and thromboembolic disease. Br Med J 2:199

Vessey MP, Mann JI (1978) Female sex hormones and thrombosis. Epidemiological aspects. Br Med Bull 34:157

Vinazzer H, Bergmann H (1968) Steigerung der Streptokinasewirkung durch niedermolekulares Dextran. Wien Med Wochenschr 118:337

Vinazzer H, Bergmann H (1975) Zur Beeinflussung postoperativer Änderungen der Blutgerinnung durch Hydroxyäthylstärke. Anaesthesist 24:517

Vinazzer H, Pütter J, Loew D (1975) Influence of intravenously administered acetylsalicylic acid on platelet functions. A pharmacodynamic and pharmacokinetic study. Haemostasis 4:12

Vinnicombe J, Shuttleworth KED (1966) Aminocaproic acid in the control of haemorrhage after prostatectomy. Safety of aminocaproic acid — a controlled trial. Lancet I:232

Virchow R (1856) Gesammelte Abhandlungen zur wissenschaftlichen Medizin. Von Meidinger Sohn, Frankfurt a M

Vogel G, Marek ML, Oertner R (1970) Untersuchungen zum Mechanismus der therapeutischen und toxischen Wirkung des Roßkastanien-Saponins Aescin. Arzneim Forsch 20:699

Vogel G, Ströcker H (1966) Die Wirkung von Pharmaka — insbesondere von Flavonoiden und Aescin — auf den Lymphfluß und die Permeabilität der intakten Plasma-Lymph-Schranke von Ratten für Flüssigkeit und definierte Makromoleküle. Arzneim Forsch 16:1630

Vollmar J (1968) Plastische Eingriffe an den tiefen Venen. In: Kappert A, May R (eds) Das postthrombotische Zustandsbild der Extremitäten. Huber, Bern

Vollmar J, Rüdiger KD (1972) Statistische Untersuchungen zur Häufigkeit von Lungenembolien und hämorrhagischen Infarkten im Obduktionsgut. Zbl Allg Path 115:138

von Hugo R, Hafter R, Graeff H (1981) A comparative study of heparin and a heparin analogue in the prevention of thrombosis in patients with gynaecological cancer under radiotherapy. Thromb Haemost 46:191

von Hospenthal J, Frey C, Rutishauser G, Gruber UF (1977) Thromboseprophylaxe bei transurethraler Prostataresektion. Urologe [A] 16:88

von Kreiter H, Fink U (1967) Ein Fall von Leberschädigung nach Cumarin-Medikation. Med Klin 62:12

von Strauch M (1894) Über Venenthrombose der unteren Extremitäten nach Koliotomien bei Beckenhochlagerung und Aethernarkose. Zentralbl Gynekol 18:304

von Sydow G (1947) Hypoprothrombinemia and brain damage in the child of a dicumarol-treated mother (In Swedish). Nord Med 34:1172

Wahl TO, Lipschitz DA, Stechschulte DJ (1978) Thrombocytopenia associated with antiheparin antibody. JAMA 240:2560

Walker SH, Duncan DB (1967) Estimation of the probability of an event as a function of several independent variables. Biometrika 54:167

Wallenbeck I, Tangen O (1975) On the lysis of fibrin formed in the presence of dextran and other macromolecules. Thromb Res 6:75

Wallenbeck I, Bergqvist D, Hallböök T, Yin ET (1979) XaI (antithrombin III) activity in relation to postoperative deep vein thrombosis (DVT). Thromb Haemost 42:375

Wallenius G (1950) The relief of nephrotic edema by dextran infusions. Scand J Clin Lab Invest 2: 228

Wallenius G (1954) Renal clearance of dextran as a measure of glomerular permeability. Acta Soc Med Ups [Suppl] 4

Walser A, Moser G, Krähenbühl B (1980) Per- und postoperative Stase als Thrombosefaktor? Vasa 9:306

Walsh JJ, Bonnar J, Wright FM (1974) A study of pulmonary embolism after deep leg vein thrombosis after major gynaecological surgery using labelled fibrinogen, phlebography and lung-scanning. J Obstet Gynaecol Br Commonw 81:311

Warlow C, Ogston D (1973) The ^{125}I-fibrinogen technique in the diagnosis of venous thrombosis. Clin Haematol 2:199

Warlow C, Ogston D, Douglas AS (1976) Deep venous thrombosis of the legs after strokes. Part I. Incidence and predisposing factors. Br Med J 1:1178

Warlow C, Terry G, Kenmure ACF, Bealtie AG, Ogston D, Douglas AS (1973) A double-blind trial of low doses of subcutaneous heparin in the prevention of deep-vein thrombosis after myocardial infarction. Lancet II:934

Warren R, Lauridsen J, Belko J (1953) Alterations in numbers of circulating platelets following surgical operation and administration of adrenocorticotropic hormone. Circulation 7:481

Wasteson Å, Glimelius B, Busch C, Westermark B, Heldin C-H, Norling B (1977) Effect of a platelet endoglycosidase on cell surface associated heparan sulphate of human cultured endothelial and glial cells. Thromb Res 11:309

Watson W, Chang T (1975) Platelet-surface interaction: effects of dextran 70 on platelet retention in extracorporeal surfaces. Biomater Med Devices Art Organs 3:489

Wautier JL, Caen JP (1979) Pharmacology of platelet-suppressive agents. Semin Thromb Haemost 5:293

Weber W, Wolff V, Bromig G (1971) Postoperative Thrombo-Embolie-Prophylaxe mit Colfarit. Ther Berichte 43:229

Weiss HJ (1967) The effect of clinical dextran on platelet aggregation, adhesion and ADP-release in man: In vivo and in vitro studies. J Lab Clin Med 69:37

Weiss HJ, Aledort LM (1967) Impaired platelet/connective tissue reaction in man after aspirin ingestion. Lancet II:495

Weiss HJ, Lages BA (1977) Possible congenital defect in platelet thromboxane synthetase. Lancet I:760

Weiss HJ, Aledort LM, Kochwa S (1968) The effect of salicylates on the hemostatic properties of platelets in man. J Clin Invest 47:2169

Weiss V, Jekiel M, Ritschard J, Bouvier CA (1977) Prévention de la maladie thromboembolique post-operatoire par les anti-agrégants en chirurgie gynécologique. Méd Hyg 35:943

Weissmann RE, Tobin RW (1958) Arterial embolism occurring during systemic heparin therapy. Arch Surg 76:219

Wells RE (1969) Rheological aspects of stasis in thrombus formation. In: Sherry S (ed) Thrombosis. Natl Acad Sci. Washington

Weseley AC, Neustadter MI, Levine W (1957) Massive intraperitoneal hemorrhage of overian follicular origin during anticoagulant therapy. Am J Obstet Gynaecol 73:683

Wessler S (1952) Studies in intravascular coagulation. I. Coagulation changes in isolated venous segments. J Clin Invest 31:1011

Wessler S (1962) Thrombosis in the presence of vascular stasis. Am J Med 33:648

Wessler S (1975a) Factors in the initiation of deep venous thrombosis. In: Nicolaides AN (ed) Thromboembolism. Aetiology, advances in prevention and management. MTP, Lancaster

Wessler S (1975b) Mini-dose heparin. Thromb Diath Haemorrh 34:718

Wessler S (1976) Heparin as an antithrombotic agent. Low-dose prophylaxis. JAMA 236:389

Wessler S, Gitel S (1979) Heparin: New concepts relevant to clinical use. Blood 53:525

Wessler S, Yin ET (1968) Experimental hypercoagulable state induced by factor X: comparison of the nonactivated and activated forms. J Lab Clin Med 72:256

Wessler S, Yin ET (1969) On the mechanism of thrombosis. Progr Haematol 6:201

Westerborn A (1946) Thrombi and emboli at early ambulation and mobilization (In Swedish). Nord Med 29:347

Westerholm B (1966) Dextran-induced release of 5-hydroxytryptamine from rabbit platelets. Acta Physiol Scand 67:236

Wetterdal P (1941) The use of heparin as a prophylactic agent against thrombosis following gynecologic operations. Acta Med Scand 107:123

Wheeler CG, Thompson JE, Austin DJ, Patman DR, Stockton RL (1966) Interruption of the inferior vena cava for thromboembolism. Ann Surg 163:199

White P, Sadd J, Nensel R (1979) Thrombotic complications of heparin therapy. Including six cases of heparin-induced skin necrosis. Ann Surg 190:595

Whitehead MI, McCarthy TG (1976) A comparative trial of subcutaneous sodium and calcium heparin as assessed by local haematoma formation and pain. In: Kakkar VV, Thomas DP (eds) Heparin. Chemistry and clinical usage. Academic Press, London New York San Francisco

Widmer LK (ed) (1978) Peripheral venous disorders. Prevalence and socio-medical importance. Observations in 4529 apparently healthy persons. Basle study III. Huber, Bern Stuttgart Vienna

Wiedeman MP (1980) Microscopic observation of small blood vessels in sulfinpyrazone-treated animals. In: McGregor D, Mustard JF, Sherry S (eds) Cardiovascular actions of sulfinpyrazone: basic and clinical research. Symposium Specialists Inc, Miami 1980, p 99

Wijnja I (1976) Single dose ampoules, undertreatment and low-dose heparin prophylaxis. N Engl J Med 294:116

Wilhelm K, Brader JJ, Beer H-P, Lauterjung KL, Messmer K (1978) Thromboseprophylaxe mit niedrig dosiertem Dextran 60. Münch Med Wochenschr 120:223

Willén J, Bergqvist D, Hallböök T (1982) Venous insufficiency as late complication after tibial fracture. Acta Orthop Scand 53:149

Williams HT (1971) Prevention of postoperative deep-vein thrombosis with perioperative subcutaneous heparin. Lancet II:950

Williams J, Britt L, Eades T, Sherman R (1975) Pulmonary embolism after amputation of the lower extremity. Surg Gynecol Obstet 140:246

Williams J, Eikman E, Greenberg S, Hewitt C, Lopes-Cuanca E, Jones P, Madden J (1978) Failure of low dose heparin to prevent pulmonary embolism after hip surgery or above the knee amputation. Ann Surg 188:468

Williams O, McCaffrey JF, Lau OJ (1973) Deep vein thrombosis in a Queensland hospital. Br Med J 1:517

Williams O, Lyall J, Vernon M, Croft DN (1974) Ventilation-perfusion lung scanning for pulmonary embolism. Br Med J 1:600

Williams WJ (1973) Venography (editorial). Circulation 47:220

Willis AL (1974) An enzymatic mechanism for the antithrombotic and antihemostatic actions of aspirin. Science 183:325

Willis AL, Kuhn DC (1973) A new potential mediator of arterial thrombosis whose biosynthesis is inhibited by aspirin. Prostaglandins 4:127

Windsor E, Freeman L (1964) An investigation of routes of administration of heparin other than injection. Am J Med 37:408

Wolfe JHN, Morland M, Browse NL (1979) The fibrinolytic activity of varicose veins. Br J Surg 66:185

Wood E, Prentice C, McGrouther A, Sinclair J, McNicol G (1973) Trial of aspirin and RA 233 in prevention of postoperative deep vein thrombosis. Thromb Diath Haemorrh 30:18

Worowski K, Puzynski S, Szmitkowski M, Lipinski B (1970) On the mechanism of fibrinolysis activation in electroshock. Coagulation 3:23

Wray R, Maurer B, Shillingford J (1973) Prophylactic anticoagulant therapy in the prevention of calf-vein thrombosis after myocardial infarction. N Engl J Med 288:815

Wright C, Mahadoo J (1980) Long-term toxicity study of intrapulmonary heparin. In: Chemistry and biology of heparin. The Center for Thrombosis and Haemostasis. Chapel Hill

Wright C, Mahadoo J, Jaques LB (1979) Anticoagulant activity and operative blood loss after intrapulmonary heparin. Br J Surg 66:844

Wright HP, Osborn SB (1952) Effect of posture on venous velocity, measured with ^{24}NaCl. Br Heart J 14:325

Wu AVO, Mansfield A (1980) The relationship between the blood and vein wall fibrinolytic activities in response to surgical trauma. Acta Haematol 63:191

Wu T, Tsapogas M, Jordan R (1977) Prophylaxis of deep venous thrombosis by hydroxychloroquine sulfate and heparin. Surg Gynecol Obstet 145:714

Xabregas A, Gray L, Ham JM (1978) Heparin prophylaxis of deep vein thrombosis in patients with a fractured neck of the femur. Med J Austr 1:620

Yamazaki H, Motomiya T, Sonoda M, Miyagawa N (1979) Changes in platelet aggregability after ovariectomy. Thromb Haemost 42:1332

Yett H, Skillman J, Salzman E (1978) The hazards of aspirin plus heparin. N Engl J Med 298:1092

Ygge J (1970) Studies on blood coagulation and fibrinolysis in conditions associated with an increased incidence of thrombosis. Methodological and clinical investigations. Scand J Haematol [Suppl] 11

Yin ET, Tangen O (1976) Heparin, heparinoids and blood coagulation. In: Kakkar VV, Thomas DP (eds) Heparin. Chemistry and clinical usage. Academic Press, London

Yin ET, Wessler S (1970) Heparin accelerated inhibition of activated factor X by a natural plasma inhibitor. Biochim Biophys Acta 201:387

Yin ET, Bergqvist D, Arfors KE, Wallenbeck I, Tangen O (1980) Rationale for the use of heparin and heparin-like substances in the prevention of thromboembolism. In: Coccheri S (ed) Proceedings of the Vth International Congress on Thromboembolism, Bologna 1978. Quaderni della Coagulazione, p 296. Periodici Baldacci di Informazione Medica

Yin ET, Wessler S, Stoll PJ (1971a) Identity of plasma activated factor X inhibitor with antithrombin III and heparin co-factor. J Biol Chem 246:712

Yin ET, Wessler S, Stoll PJ (1971b) Rabbit plasma inhibitor of the activated species of blood coagulation factor X: Purification and some properties. J Biol Chem 246:3694

Yin ET, Wessler S, Butler JV (1973) Plasma heparin. A unique submicrogram sensitive assay. J Lab Clin Med 81:298

Youngchaiyud P, Kettel LJ, Cugell DW (1969) The effect of heparin aerosols on airway conductance in patients with chronic obstructive pulmonary disease. Am Rev Resp Dis 99:449

Zahavi J, Jones NAG, Lekton J, Dubiel M, Kakkar VV (1980a) Enhanced in vivo platelet "release reaction" in old healthy individuals. Thromb Res 17:329

Zahavi J, Westwick J, Al-Hasani SFA, Dubiel M, Price AJ, Scully MF, Honey AC, Kakkar VV (1980b) Enhanced in-vivo platelet release reaction, increased thromboxane synthesis, and decreased prostacyclin release after tourniquet ischaemia. Lancet II:663

Zahn W (1872) Untersuchungen über Thrombose. Zentralbl Med Wissenschaften 10:129

Zederfeldt B (1957) Studies on wound healing and trauma. Acta Chir Scand [Suppl] 224

Zekert F, Kohn P, Vormittag E, Poigenfürst J, Thien M (1974) Thromboembolieprophylaxe mit Acetylsalicylsäure bei Operationen wegen hüftgelenksnaher Frakturen. Münch Unfallheilkd 77:97

Zelikovski A, Zucker G, Eliashiv A, Reiss R, Shalit M (1981) A new sequential pneumatic device for the prevention of deep vein thrombosis. J Neurosurg 54:652

Zilliacus H (1946) On the specific treatment of thrombosis and pulmonary embolism with anticoagulants, with particular reference to the post-thrombotic sequelae. The results of five years treatment of thrombosis and pulmonary embolism at a series of Swedish hospitals during the years 1940–1945. Helsingfors Acta Med Scand [Suppl]

Zimpfer M, Schwarz M, Stanek B, Raberger G (1981) Cardiovascular effects of dihydroergotamine during epidural anaesthesia in dogs. Pharmacology 23:305

Zingg W, Lindsay R (1964) Rheology of blood-dextran mixtures. Surg Forum 15:228

Zozoya J (1932) Immunological reactions between dextran polysaccharides and some bacterial antisera. J Exp Med 55:353

Zucker MB, Borelli J (1955) Viscous metamorphosis of blood platelets produced by thrombine. Fed Proc 14:168

Zucker MB, Peterson J (1968) Inhibition of adenosine diphosphate-induced secondary aggregation and other platelet functions by acetylsalicylic acid ingestion. Proc Soc Exp Biol Med 127:547

Zweifler AJ (1962) Relation of prothrombin concentration to bleeding during oral anticoagulant therapy. N Engl J Med 267:283

Books and Reviews
Dealing with Thromboprophylactic Problems

Bergan J, Yao J (eds) (1978) Venous problems. Year Book Med Publishers, Chicago London

Bergentz S-E (1978) Dextran in the prophylaxis of pulmonary embolism. World J Surg 2:19

Bergqvist D (1979) Prophylaxis of postoperative thromboembolic complications with low-dose heparin. An analysis of different administration intervals. Acta Chir Scand 145:7

Bloom A, Thomas D (eds) (1981) Haemostasis and thrombosis. Churchill Livingstone, Edinburgh London Melbourne New York

Clagett P, Salzman E (1975) Prevention of venous thromboembolism. Prog Cardiovasc Dis 17:345

Gallus AS, Hirsh J (1976) Antithrombotic drugs I–III. Med Prog 10, 11, 12

Genton E, Turpie A (1980) Venous thromboembolism associated with gynecologic surgery. Clin Obstet Gynecol 23:209

Gruber UF (1975) Dextran and the prevention of postoperative thromboembolic complications. Surg Clin N Am 55:679

Gruber UF, Sturm V, Rem J, Schaub N, Rittermann WW (1975) The present state of prevention of postoperative thromboembolic complications. Bibl Haematol 41:98

Jaques LB (1980) Heparins – anionic polyelectrolyte drugs. Pharmacol Rev 31:99

Jobin F (1978) Acetylsalicylic acid, hemostasis and human thromboembolism. Semin Thromb Haemostas 4:3

Kakkar VV (1978) The current status of low-dose heparin in the prophylaxis of thrombophlebitis and pulmonary embolism. World J Surg 2:3

Nicolaides AN (ed) (1975) Thromboembolism. Aetiology. Advances in prevention and management. MTP Press, Lancaster

Salzman E, Harris W (1976) Prevention of venous thromboembolism in orthopaedic patients. J Bone Joint Surg 58-A:903

Sturm V, Gruber UF (1975) Wert der Kumarinderivate zur Thromboembolieprophylaxe in der Chirurgie, Orthopädie und Gynäkologie. Schweiz Med Wochenschr 43:1507

Thomas D (ed) (1978) Thrombosis. Br Med Bull 34

Thomas D (1978) Heparin in the prophylaxis and treatment of venous thromboembolism. Semin Hematol 15:1

Turpie A, Hirsh J (1979) Prophylaxis and therapy of venous thromboembolism. CRC Crit Rev Clin Lab Sci, p 247

Verstraete M, Vermylen J, Roberts H (eds) (1979) The challenge of clinical trials in thrombosis. Schattauer, Stuttgart New York

von Aarburg R, Gruber UF (1978) Prophylaxe postoperativer thromboembolischer Komplikationen bei hüftgelenksnahen Frakturen. Unfallheilkunde 81:475

Wessler S, Gitel S (1979) Heparin: new concepts relevant to clinical use. Blood 53:525

Subject Index

Comprehensive Manuals of Surgical Specialties

Edited by
Richard H. Egdahl

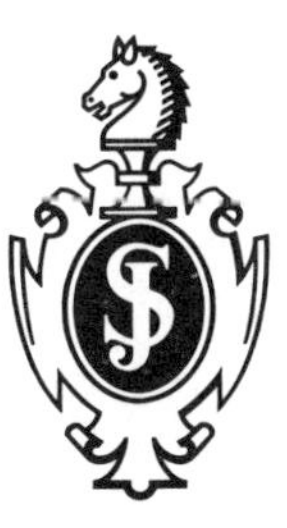

Springer-Verlag
Berlin
Heidelberg
New York

E.W. Humphrey, D.L. McKeown
Manual of Pulmonary Surgery
1982. 215 figures (190 figures in full color).
XI, 259 pages
ISBN 3-540-90732-7

Manual of Ambulatory Surgery
Editors: K.J. Kassity, J.E. McKittrick, F.W. Preston
Illustrated by J. Koelling
1982. 270 figures (172 figures in full color)
XVIII, 266 pages
ISBN 3-540-90700-9

W.P. Longmire, R.K. Tompkins
Manual of Liver Surgery
Illustrated by T. Bloodhart
1981. 230 figures (142 in full color). XVII, 267 pages
ISBN 3-540-90212-0

B.J. Harlan, A. Starr, F.M. Harwin
Manual of Cardiac Surgery
Volume 1
1980. 193 figures (183 in full color), 8 tables.
XV, 204 pages
ISBN 3-540-90393-3

Volume 2
1981. 130 figures in full color. XV, 143 pages
ISBN 3-540-90563-4

E.J. Wylie, R.J. Stoney, W.K. Ehrenfeld
Manual of Vascular Surgery
Volume 1
1980. 557 figures (471 in full color). XII, 264 pages
ISBN 3-540-90408-5

Volume 2
1983. ISBN 3-540-90409-3
In preparation

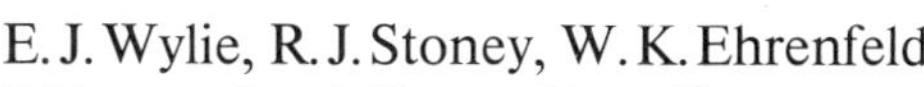

C.E.Welch, L.W.Ottinger, J.P.Welch
**Manual of Lower
Gastrointestinal Surgery**
1980. 215 figures (138 figures in color), 7 tables.
XVI, 276 pages. ISBN 3-540-90205-8

A.T.K.Cockett, K.Koshiba
Manual of Urologic Surgery
Illustrated by I.Takamoto
1979. 532 color illustrations. XVIII, 284 pages
ISBN 3-540-90423-9

B.J.Masterson
Manual of Gynecologic Surgery
With contributions by K.E.Krantz, W.J.Cameron,
J.W.Daly, J.A.Fayez, E.W.Franklin
Illustrator: D.McKeown
1979. 204 figures (192 in color), 12 tables.
XV, 256 pages. ISBN 3-540-90372-0

R.E.Hermann
**Manual of Surgery of the Gallbladder,
Bile Ducts, and Exocrine Pancreas**
With contributions by A.M.Cooperman,
C.B.Esselstyn Jr., E.Steiger, R.T.Holzbach
1979. 197 color figures (123 figures in black and
white), 16 tables. XIV, 306 pages. ISBN 3-540-90351-8

W.S.McDougal, C.L.Slade, B.A.Pruitt, Jr.
Manual of Burns
Medical Illustrators: M.Williams, C.H.Boyter,
D.P.Russel
1978. 214 color figures, 4 tables. X, 165 pages
ISBN 3-540-90319-4

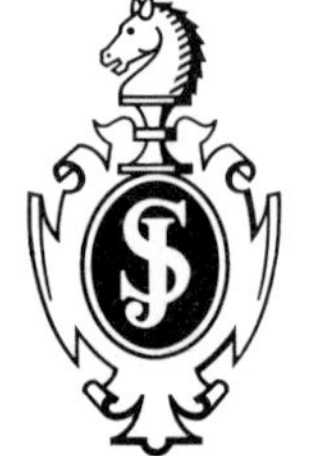

Springer-Verlag
Berlin
Heidelberg
New York

A.J.Edis, L.A.Ayala, R.H.Egdahl
Manual of Endocrine Surgery
1975. 266 figures, mostly in color. 242 color plates.
XIII, 274 pages. ISBN 3-540-07064-8